Black Jack

Volume 4

Osamu Tezuka

 VERTICAL.

Translation—Camellia Nieh
Production—Glen Isip
Akane Ishida

Published by Vertical, Inc., New York.

Originally published in Japanese as *Burakku Jakku 4*
by Akita Shoten, Tokyo, 1987.
Burakku Jakku first serialized in *Shukan Shonen Champion*,
Akita Shoten, 1973-83.

ISBN: 978-1-934287-43-9

Manufactured in the United States of America

First Edition

Vertical, Inc.
1185 Avenue of the Americas 32nd Floor
New York, NY 10036
www.vertical-inc.com

CONTENTS

FALSE IMAGE

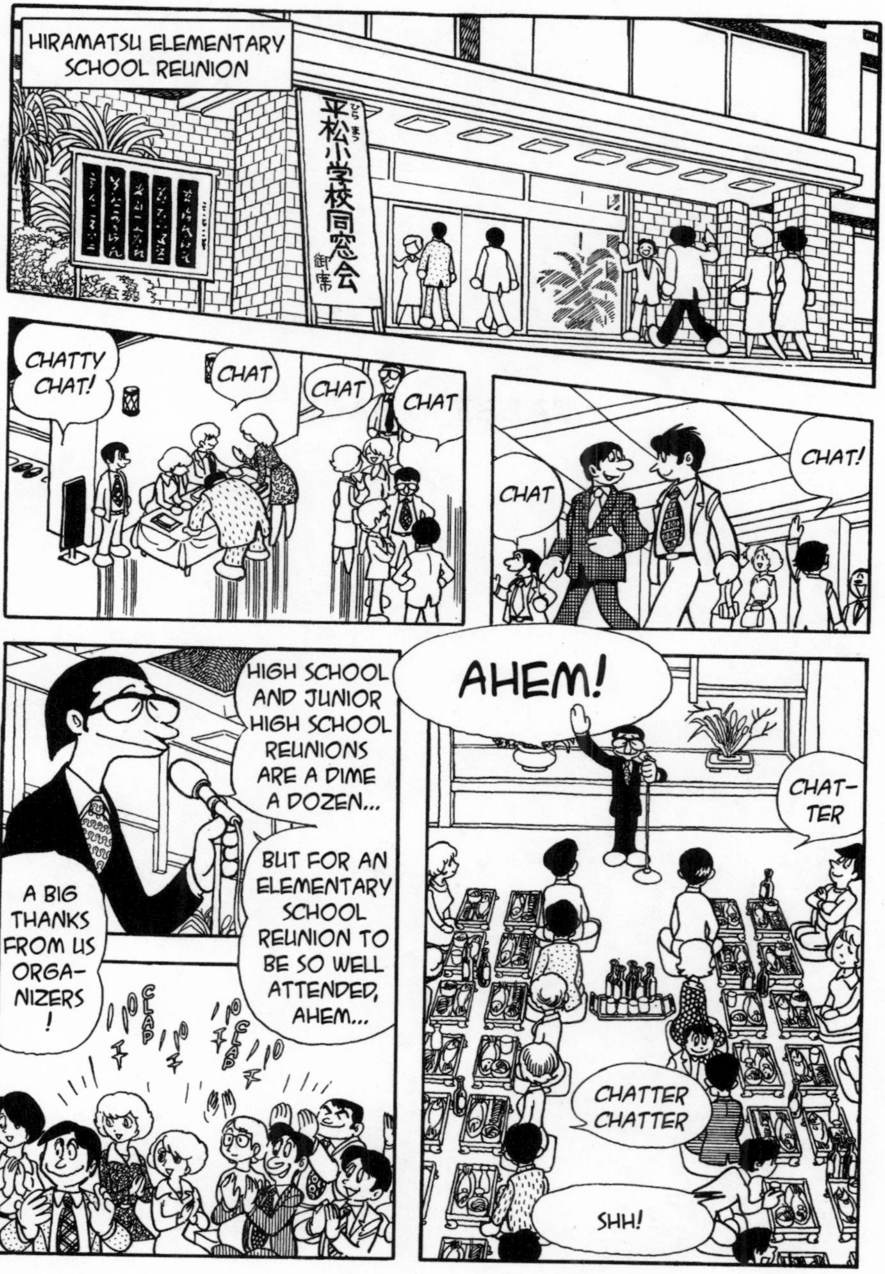
HIRAMATSU ELEMENTARY SCHOOL REUNION
平松小学校同窓会
御席
CHAT!
CHAT
CHAT
CHAT
CHAT
CHATTY CHAT!
AHEM!
CHAT-TER
CHATTER CHATTER
SHH!
HIGH SCHOOL AND JUNIOR HIGH SCHOOL REUNIONS ARE A DIME A DOZEN...
BUT FOR AN ELEMENTARY SCHOOL REUNION TO BE SO WELL ATTENDED, AHEM...
A BIG THANKS FROM US ORGA-NIZERS!
CLAP
CLAP

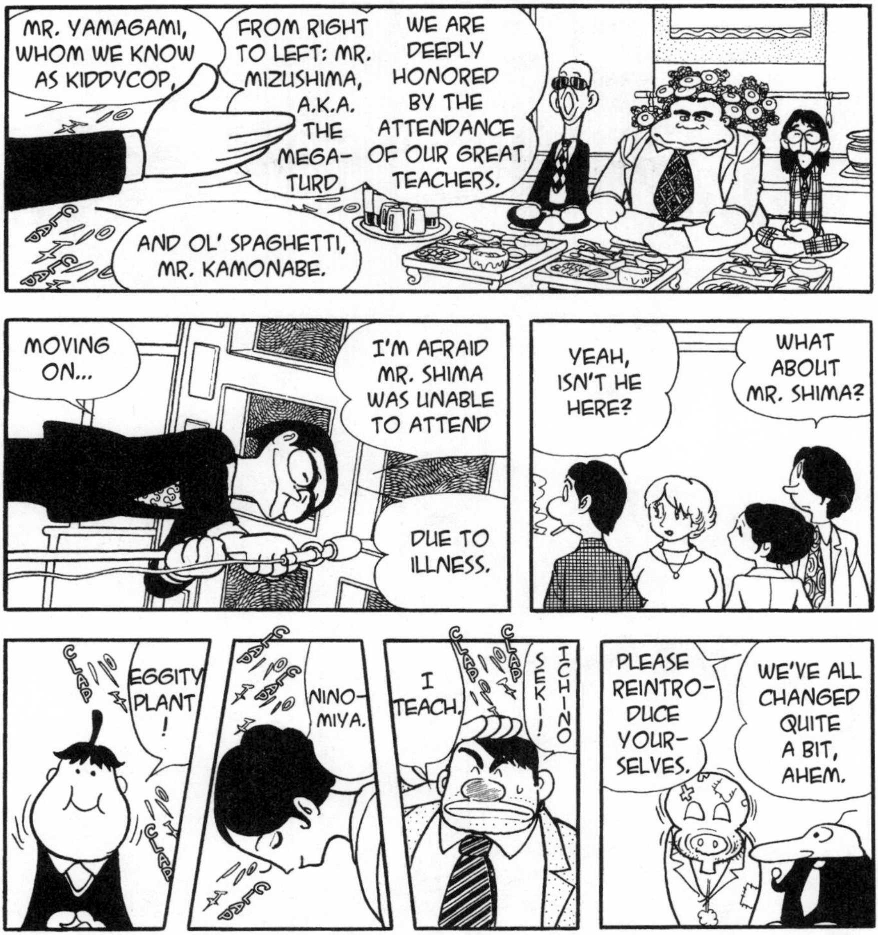
WE ARE DEEPLY HONORED BY THE ATTENDANCE OF OUR GREAT TEACHERS.
FROM RIGHT TO LEFT: MR. MIZUSHIMA, A.K.A. THE MEGA-TURD,
MR. YAMAGAMI, WHOM WE KNOW AS KIDDYCOP,
AND OL' SPAGHETTI, MR. KAMONABE.
CLAP CLAP
WHAT ABOUT MR. SHIMA?
YEAH, ISN'T HE HERE?
I'M AFRAID MR. SHIMA WAS UNABLE TO ATTEND
DUE TO ILLNESS.
MOVING ON...
WE'VE ALL CHANGED QUITE A BIT, AHEM.
PLEASE REINTRODUCE YOURSELVES.
CLAP CLAP
ICHINOSEKI!
I TEACH.
CLAP CLAP
NINOMIYA.
CLAP
EGGITY PLANT!
CLAP
CLAP CLAP CLAP
NEXT PLEASE!
UHM...
NEXT?

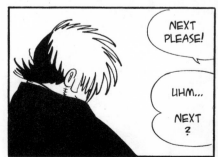

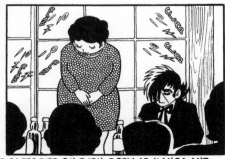

NOTE: THE TEACHERS' NAMES, NICKNAMES, AND FACES RIFF ON THEN-POPULAR MANGA AND THEIR AUTHORS.

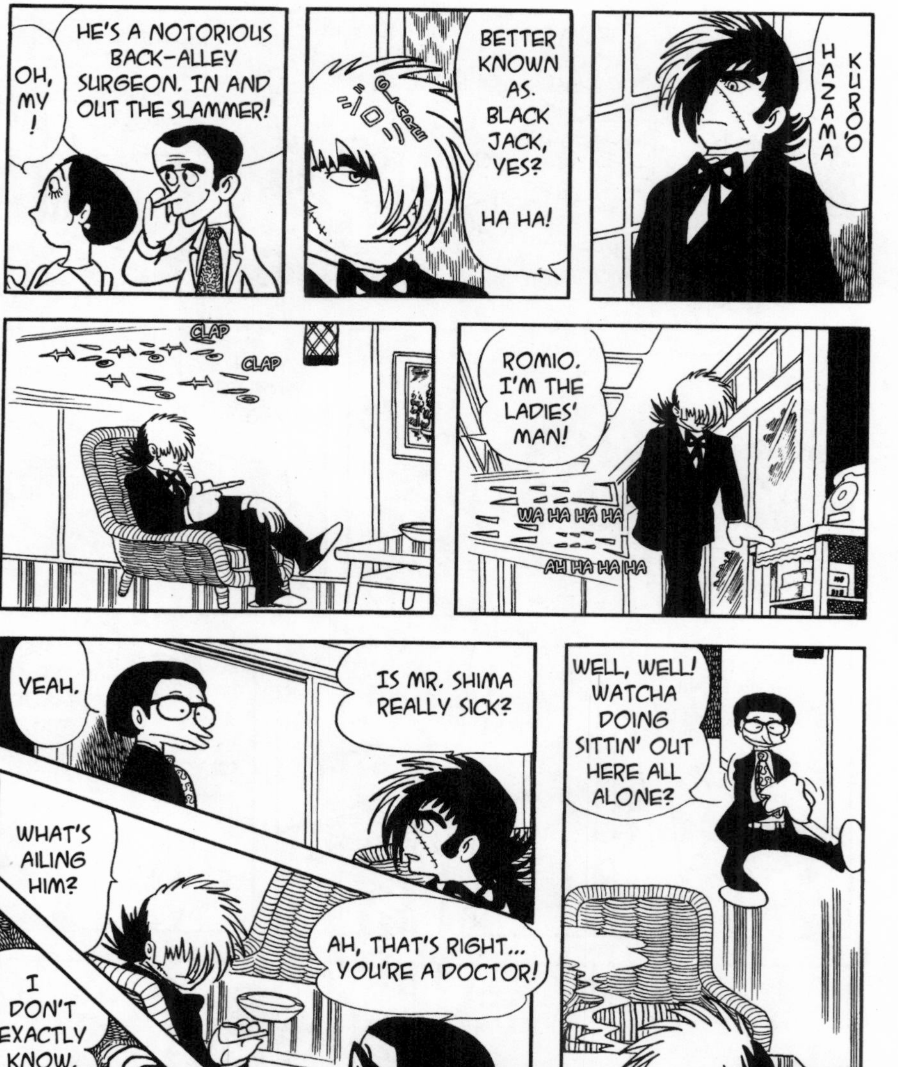
KURO'O HAZAMA
BETTER KNOWN AS. BLACK JACK, YES?
HA HA!
HE'S A NOTORIOUS BACK-ALLEY SURGEON. IN AND OUT THE SLAMMER!
OH, MY!
ROMIO. I'M THE LADIES' MAN!
WA HA HA HA
AH HA HA HA
CLAP
CLAP
WELL, WELL! WATCHA DOING SITTIN' OUT HERE ALL ALONE?
HAVING A SMOKE.
IS MR. SHIMA REALLY SICK?
YEAH.
WHAT'S AILING HIM?
AH, THAT'S RIGHT... YOU'RE A DOCTOR!
I DON'T EXACTLY KNOW.
HE'S HARD TO TRACK DOWN...

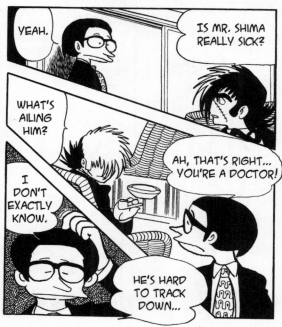

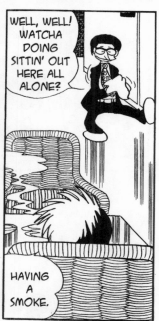

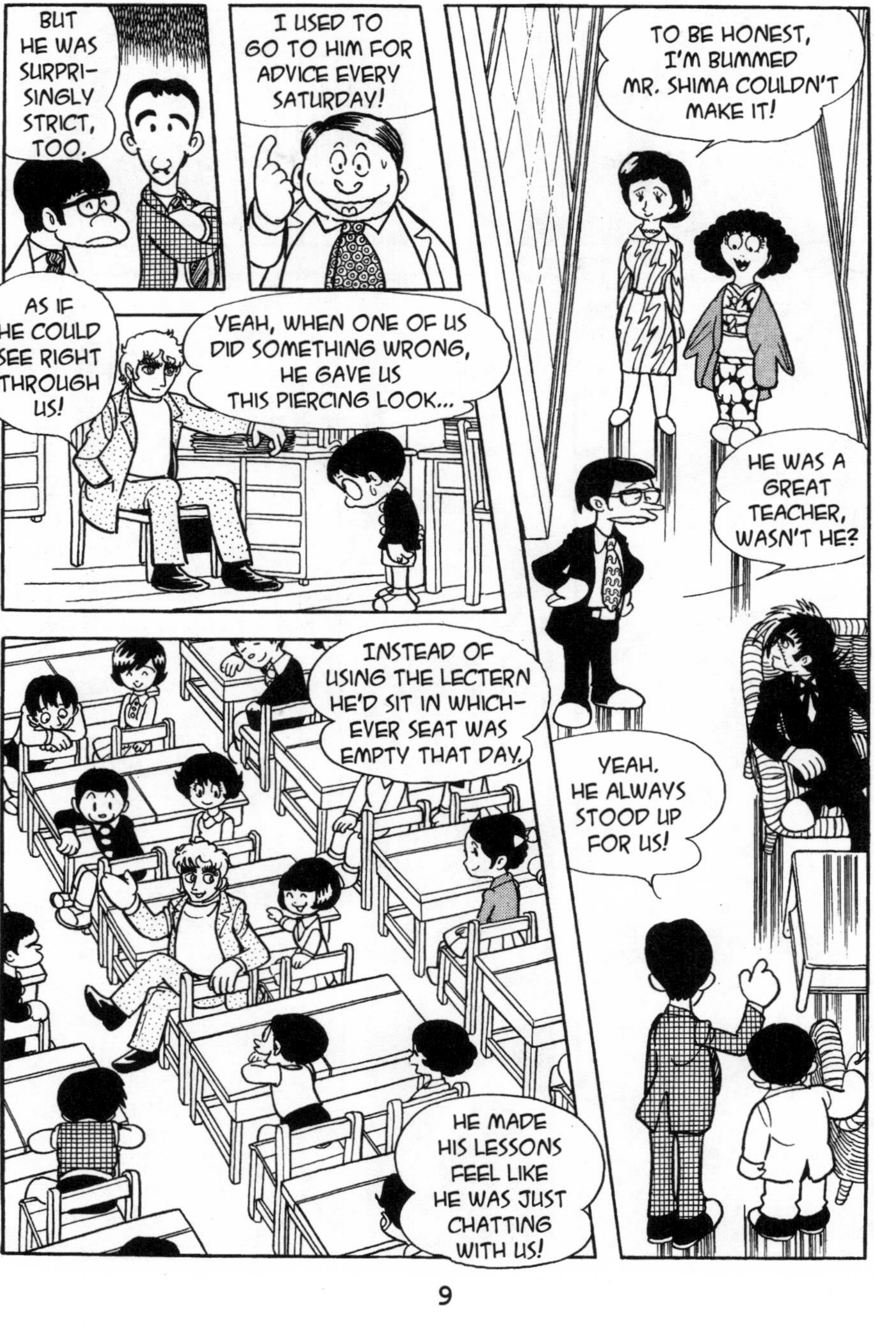
TO BE HONEST, I'M BUMMED MR. SHIMA COULDN'T MAKE IT!
HE WAS A GREAT TEACHER, WASN'T HE?
YEAH. HE ALWAYS STOOD UP FOR US!
I USED TO GO TO HIM FOR ADVICE EVERY SATURDAY!
BUT HE WAS SURPRI-SINGLY STRICT, TOO.
YEAH, WHEN ONE OF US DID SOMETHING WRONG, HE GAVE US THIS PIERCING LOOK...
AS IF HE COULD SEE RIGHT THROUGH US!
INSTEAD OF USING THE LECTERN HE'D SIT IN WHICH-EVER SEAT WAS EMPTY THAT DAY.
HE MADE HIS LESSONS FEEL LIKE HE WAS JUST CHATTING WITH US!

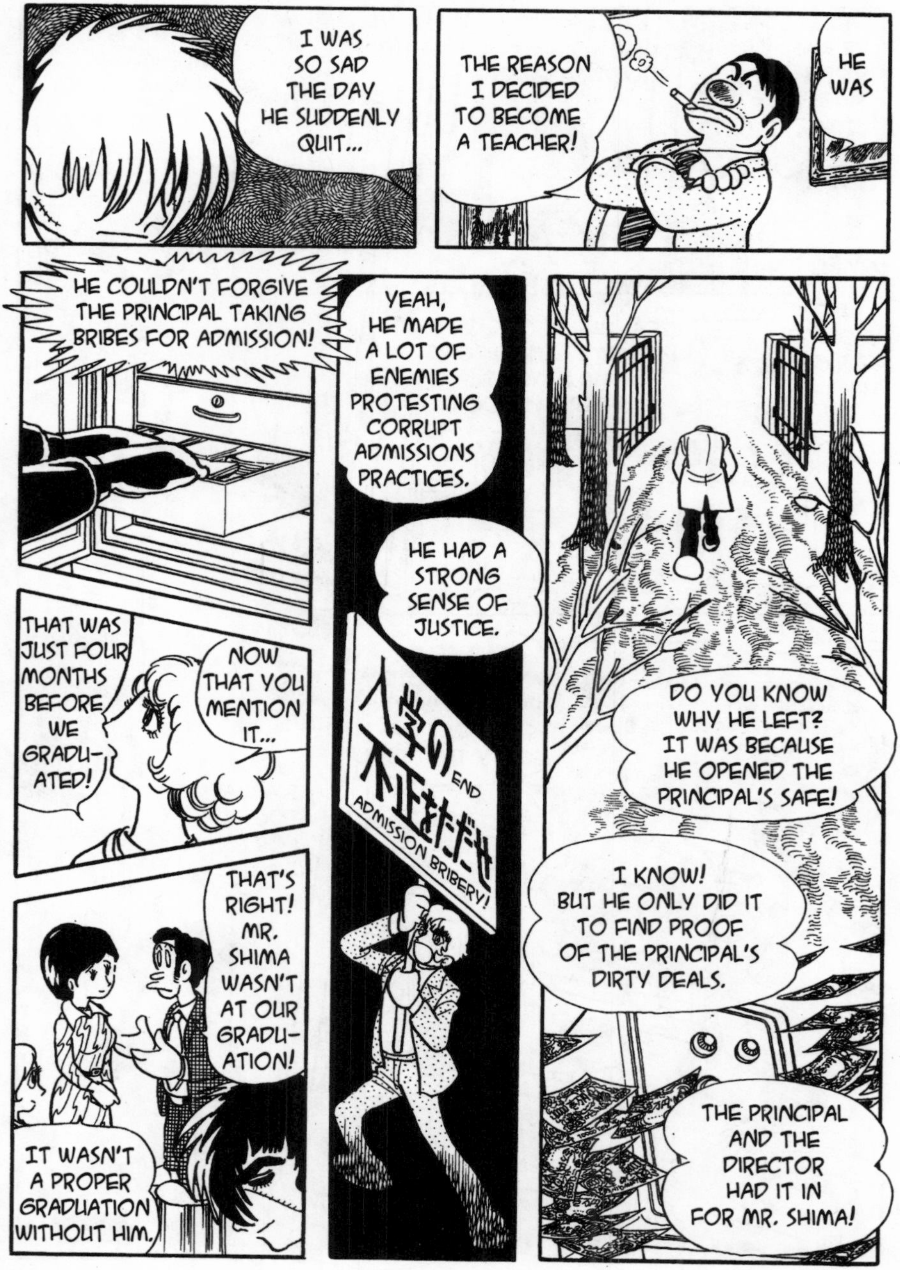
HE WAS
THE REASON I DECIDED TO BECOME A TEACHER!
I WAS SO SAD THE DAY HE SUDDENLY QUIT...
DO YOU KNOW WHY HE LEFT? IT WAS BECAUSE HE OPENED THE PRINCIPAL'S SAFE!
I KNOW! BUT HE ONLY DID IT TO FIND PROOF OF THE PRINCIPAL'S DIRTY DEALS.
THE PRINCIPAL AND THE DIRECTOR HAD IT IN FOR MR. SHIMA!
YEAH, HE MADE A LOT OF ENEMIES PROTESTING CORRUPT ADMISSIONS PRACTICES.
HE HAD A STRONG SENSE OF JUSTICE.
入学の不正をただせ
END ADMISSION BRIBERY!
HE COULDN'T FORGIVE THE PRINCIPAL TAKING BRIBES FOR ADMISSION!
NOW THAT YOU MENTION IT...
THAT WAS JUST FOUR MONTHS BEFORE WE GRADU-ATED!
THAT'S RIGHT! MR. SHIMA WASN'T AT OUR GRADU-ATION!
IT WASN'T A PROPER GRADUATION WITHOUT HIM.

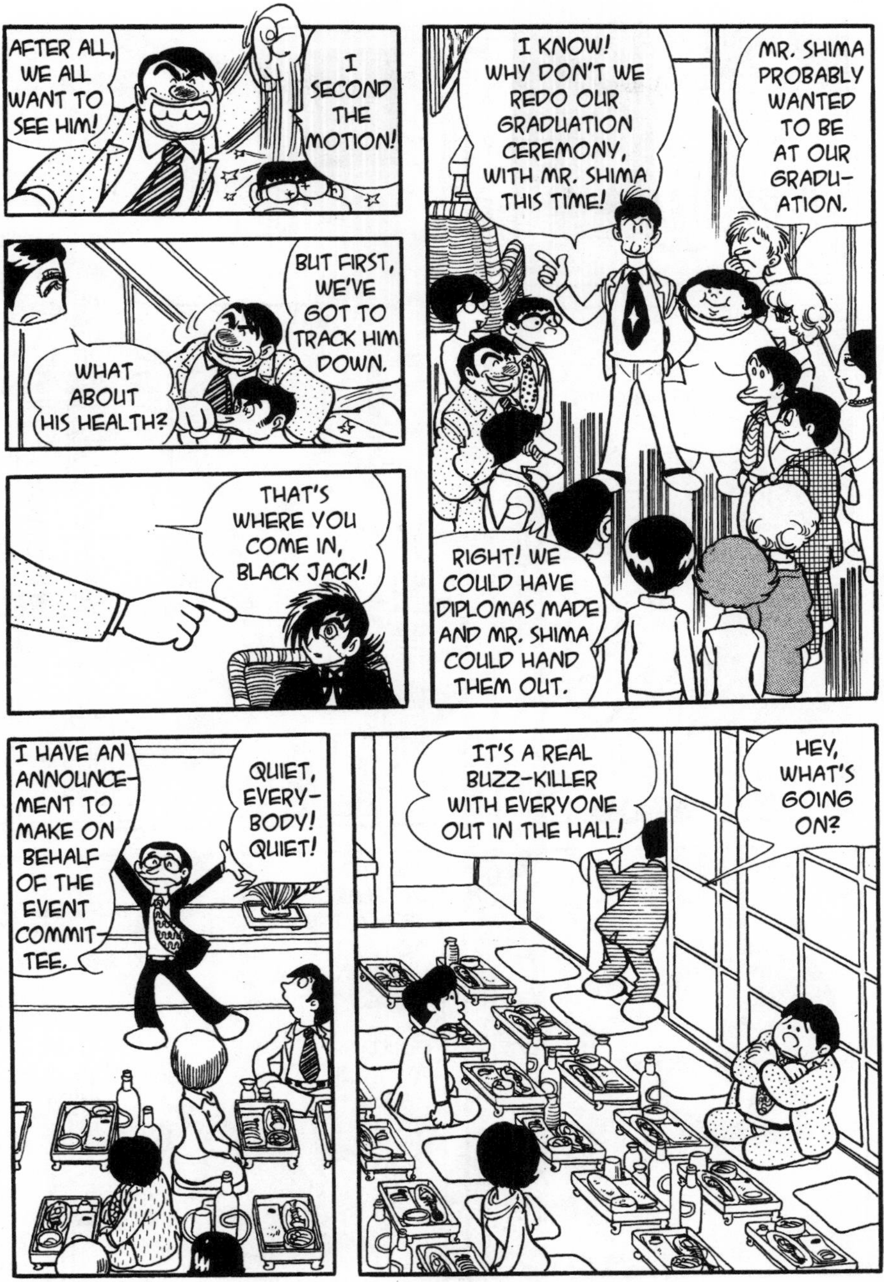
MR. SHIMA PROBABLY WANTED TO BE AT OUR GRADUATION.
I KNOW! WHY DON'T WE REDO OUR GRADUATION CEREMONY, WITH MR. SHIMA THIS TIME!
RIGHT! WE COULD HAVE DIPLOMAS MADE AND MR. SHIMA COULD HAND THEM OUT.
I SECOND THE MOTION!
AFTER ALL, WE ALL WANT TO SEE HIM!
BUT FIRST, WE'VE GOT TO TRACK HIM DOWN.
WHAT ABOUT HIS HEALTH?
THAT'S WHERE YOU COME IN, BLACK JACK!
HEY, WHAT'S GOING ON?
IT'S A REAL BUZZ-KILLER WITH EVERYONE OUT IN THE HALL!
QUIET, EVERYBODY! QUIET!
I HAVE AN ANNOUNCEMENT TO MAKE ON BEHALF OF THE EVENT COMMITTEE.

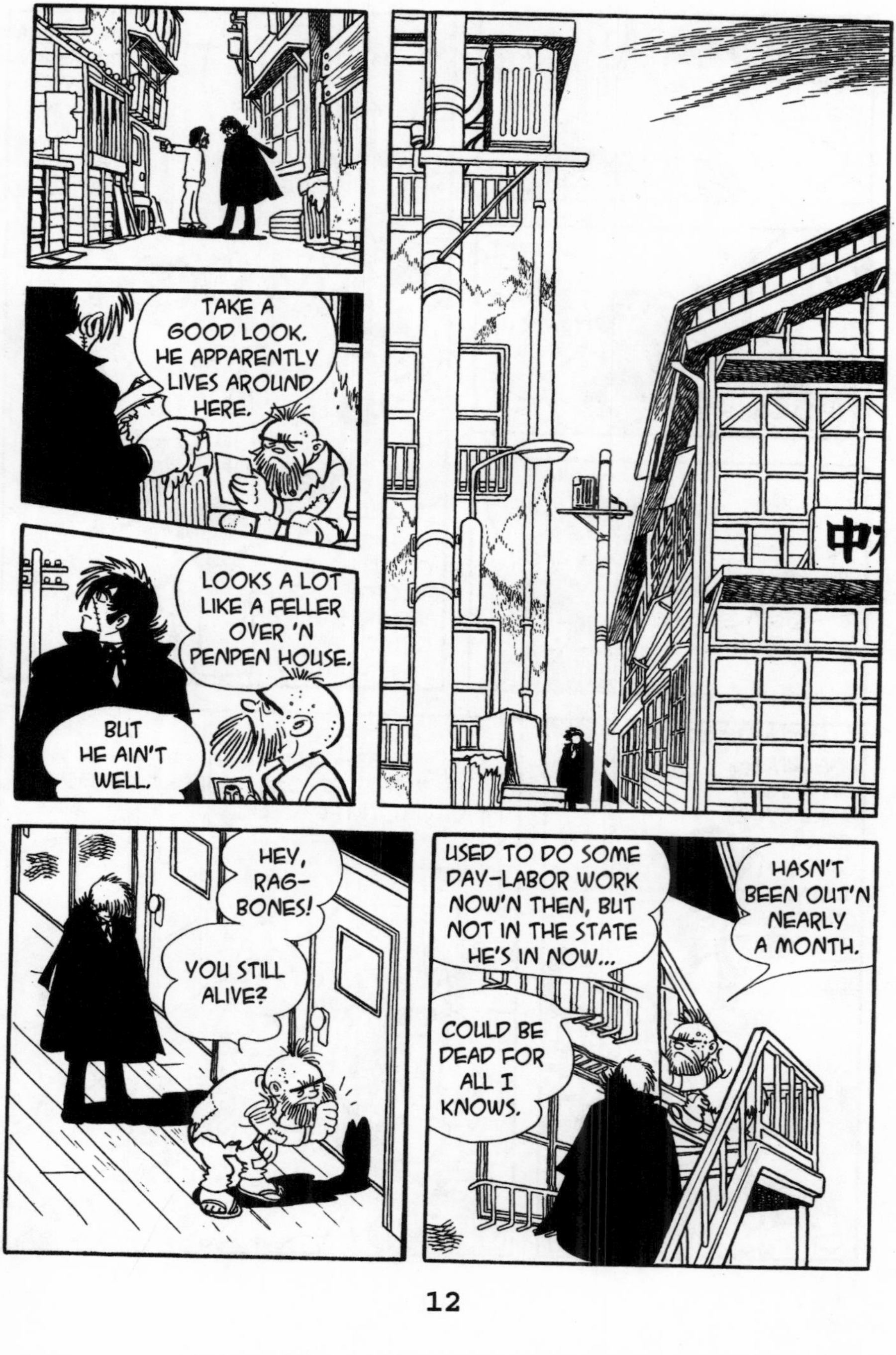
TAKE A GOOD LOOK. HE APPARENTLY LIVES AROUND HERE.
LOOKS A LOT LIKE A FELLER OVER 'N PENPEN HOUSE.
BUT HE AIN'T WELL.
HASN'T BEEN OUT'N NEARLY A MONTH.
USED TO DO SOME DAY-LABOR WORK NOW'N THEN, BUT NOT IN THE STATE HE'S IN NOW...
COULD BE DEAD FOR ALL I KNOWS.
HEY, RAG-BONES!
YOU STILL ALIVE?

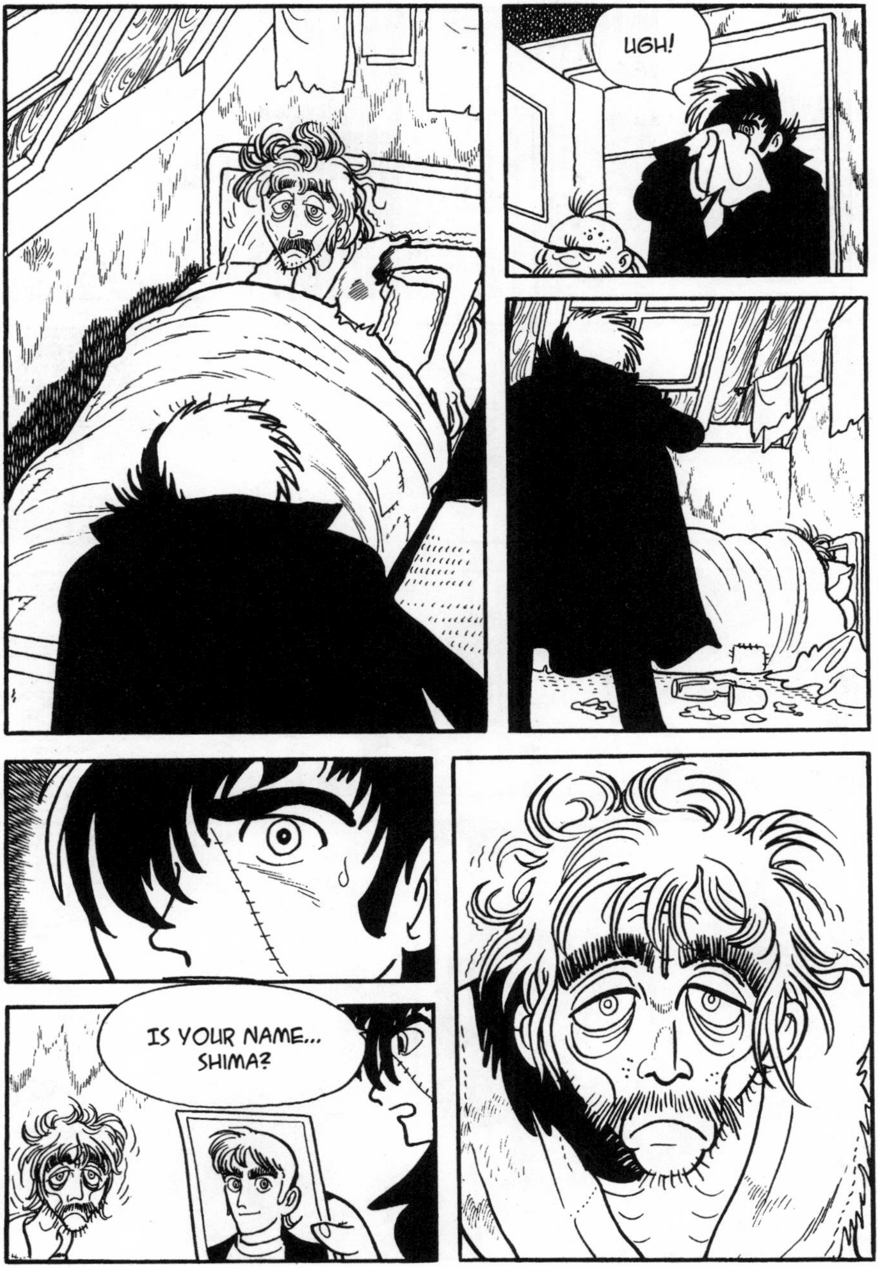
UGH!
IS YOUR NAME... SHIMA?

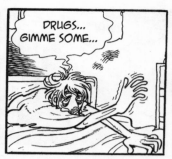

...
ARE YOU MR. SHIMA?
DRUGS... GIMME SOME...
HE'S AN ADDICT?!
PLEASE... DRUGS...
DOES THIS PICTURE MEAN ANY-THING TO YOU?
KLONK
ガクリ
FINAL STAGE ...
NEARLY AN EMPTY SHELL!
WELL, NOW! YER A DOCTOR?!
THERE MUST BE... A WAY TO DETERMINE HIS IDENTITY.
EUREKA! HIS BLOOD DONATION RECORD ...
BUT... WHAT A TRANS-FORMATION.
YOHEI SHIMA, AGE 43. IT'S HIM, ALL RIGHT!

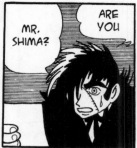

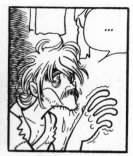

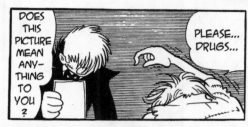

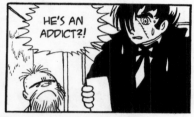

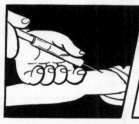

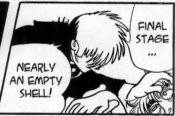

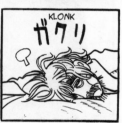

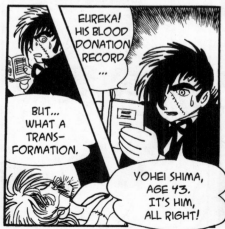

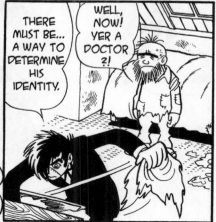

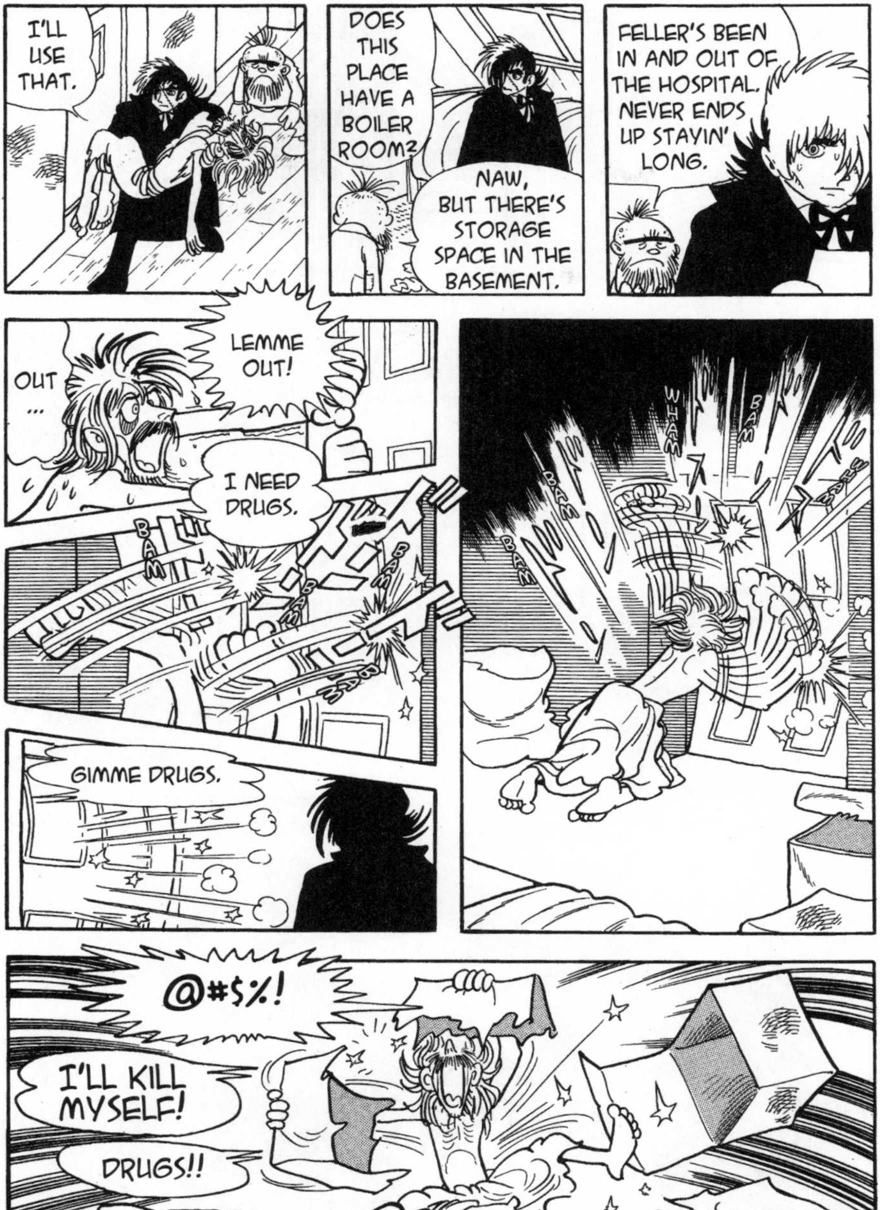
FELLER'S BEEN IN AND OUT OF THE HOSPITAL. NEVER ENDS UP STAYIN' LONG.
DOES THIS PLACE HAVE A BOILER ROOM?
NAW, BUT THERE'S STORAGE SPACE IN THE BASEMENT.
I'LL USE THAT.
BAM
WHAM
BAM
BAM
LEMME OUT!
OUT ...
I NEED DRUGS.
BAM
BAM
BAM
BAM
GIMME DRUGS.
@#$%!
I'LL KILL MYSELF!
DRUGS!!

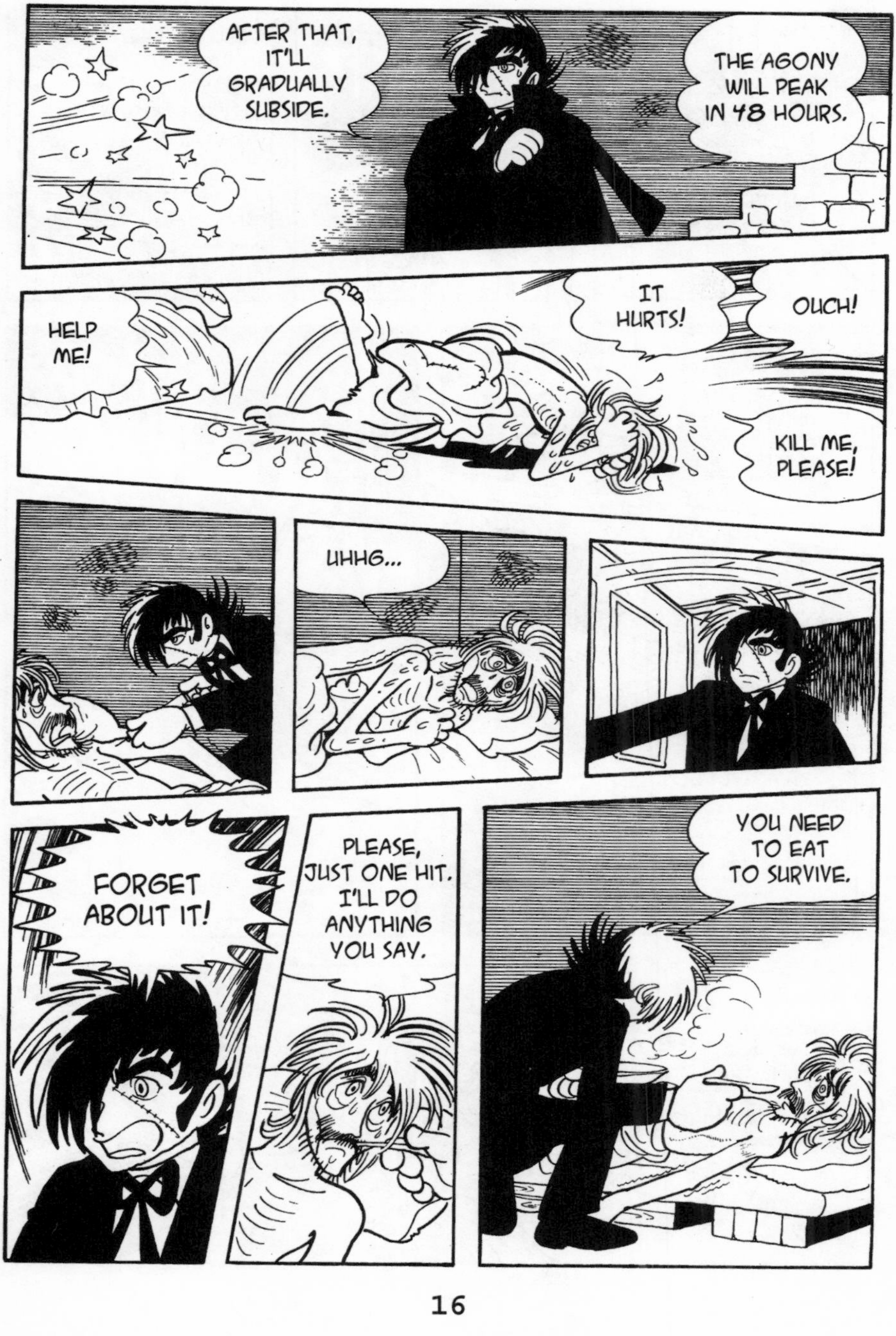
THE AGONY WILL PEAK IN 48 HOURS.
AFTER THAT, IT'LL GRADUALLY SUBSIDE.
OUCH!
IT HURTS!
KILL ME, PLEASE!
HELP ME!
UHHG...
YOU NEED TO EAT TO SURVIVE.
PLEASE, JUST ONE HIT. I'LL DO ANYTHING YOU SAY.
FORGET ABOUT IT!

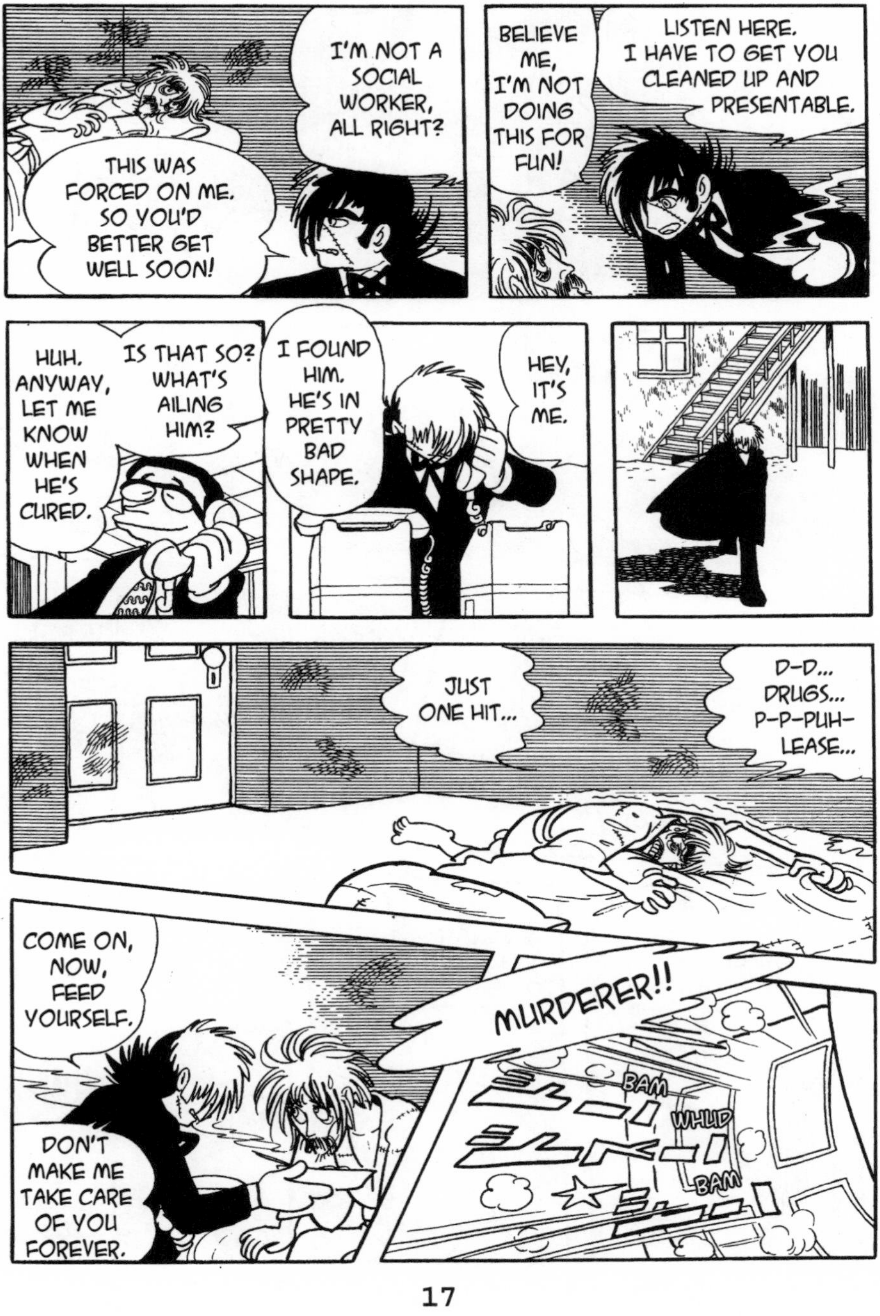
LISTEN HERE. I HAVE TO GET YOU CLEANED UP AND PRESENTABLE.
BELIEVE ME, I'M NOT DOING THIS FOR FUN!
I'M NOT A SOCIAL WORKER, ALL RIGHT?
THIS WAS FORCED ON ME. SO YOU'D BETTER GET WELL SOON!
HEY, IT'S ME.
I FOUND HIM. HE'S IN PRETTY BAD SHAPE.
IS THAT SO? WHAT'S AILING HIM?
HUH. ANYWAY, LET ME KNOW WHEN HE'S CURED.
D-D... DRUGS... P-P-PUH-LEASE...
JUST ONE HIT...
MURDERER!!
BAM
WHUD
BAM
COME ON, NOW, FEED YOURSELF.
DON'T MAKE ME TAKE CARE OF YOU FOREVER.

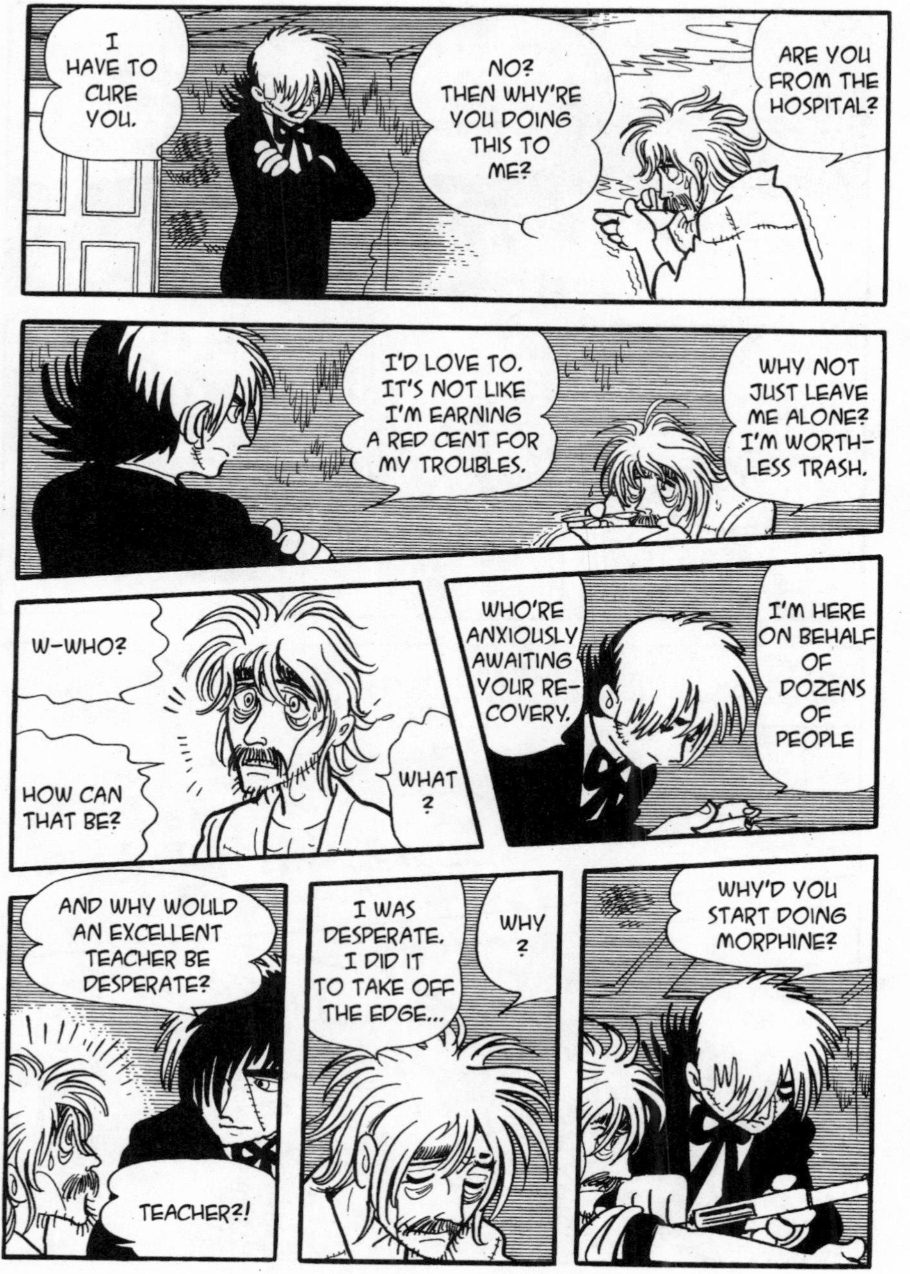
ARE YOU FROM THE HOSPITAL?
NO? THEN WHY'RE YOU DOING THIS TO ME?
I HAVE TO CURE YOU.
WHY NOT JUST LEAVE ME ALONE? I'M WORTHLESS TRASH.
I'D LOVE TO. IT'S NOT LIKE I'M EARNING A RED CENT FOR MY TROUBLES.
I'M HERE ON BEHALF OF DOZENS OF PEOPLE
WHO'RE ANXIOUSLY AWAITING YOUR RECOVERY.
WHAT?
W-WHO?
HOW CAN THAT BE?
WHY'D YOU START DOING MORPHINE?
WHY?
I WAS DESPERATE. I DID IT TO TAKE OFF THE EDGE...
AND WHY WOULD AN EXCELLENT TEACHER BE DESPERATE?
TEACHER?!

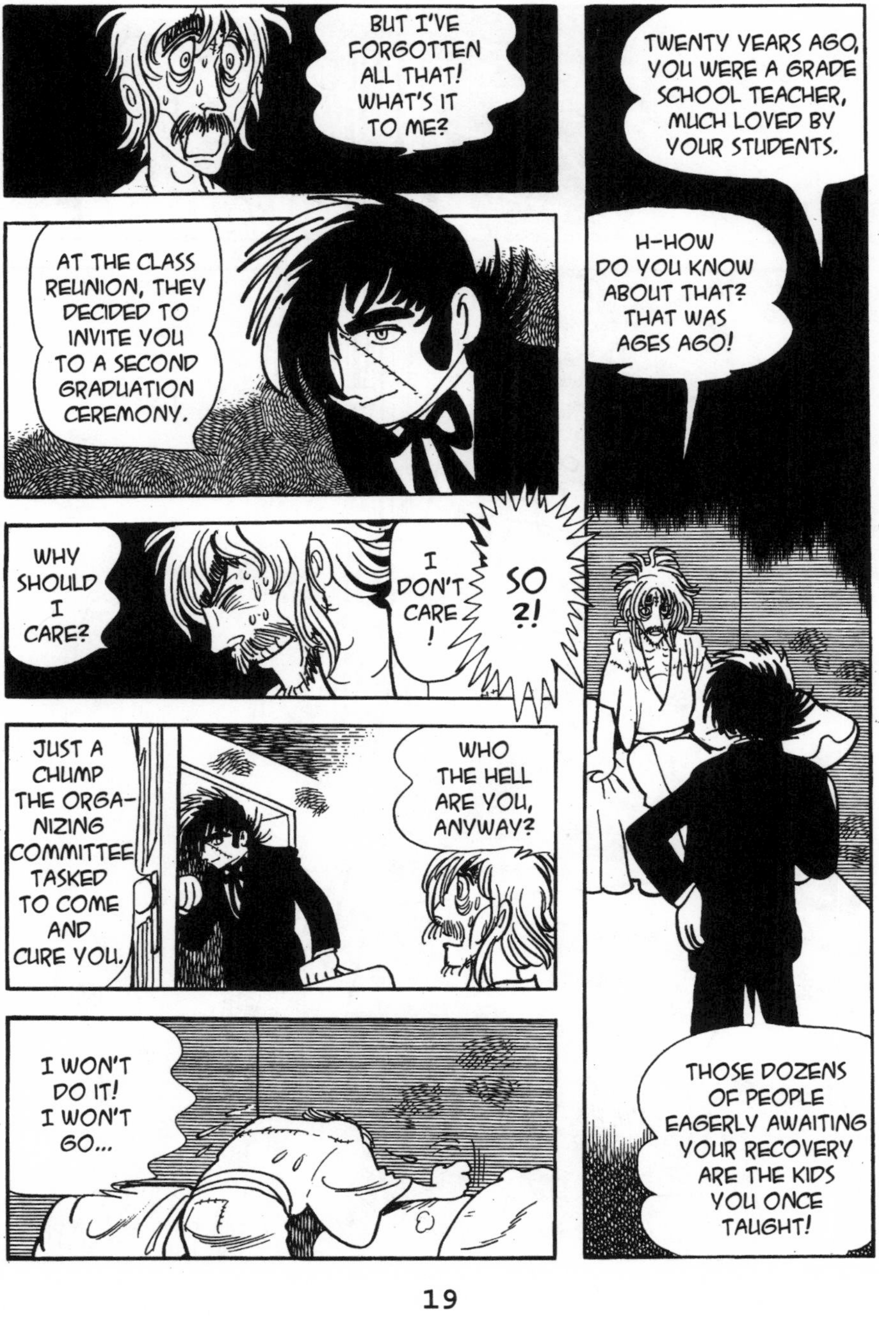
TWENTY YEARS AGO, YOU WERE A GRADE SCHOOL TEACHER, MUCH LOVED BY YOUR STUDENTS.
H-HOW DO YOU KNOW ABOUT THAT? THAT WAS AGES AGO!
THOSE DOZENS OF PEOPLE EAGERLY AWAITING YOUR RECOVERY ARE THE KIDS YOU ONCE TAUGHT!
BUT I'VE FORGOTTEN ALL THAT! WHAT'S IT TO ME?
AT THE CLASS REUNION, THEY DECIDED TO INVITE YOU TO A SECOND GRADUATION CEREMONY.
SO ?!
I DON'T CARE!
WHY SHOULD I CARE?
WHO THE HELL ARE YOU, ANYWAY?
JUST A CHUMP THE ORGA-NIZING COMMITTEE TASKED TO COME AND CURE YOU.
I WON'T DO IT! I WON'T GO...

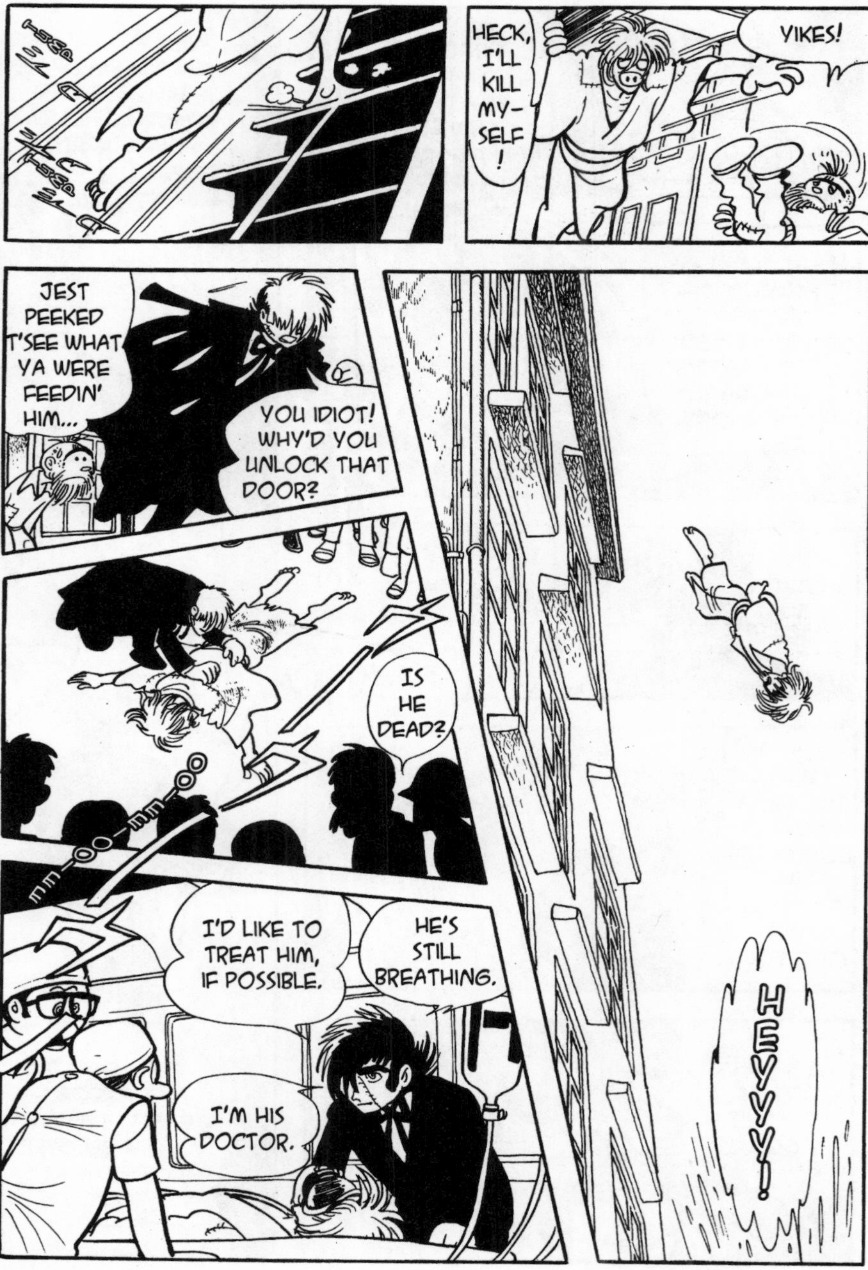
YIKES!
HECK, I'LL KILL MY-SELF!
HEYYY!
YOU IDIOT! WHY'D YOU UNLOCK THAT DOOR?
JEST PEEKED T'SEE WHAT YA WERE FEEDIN' HIM...
IS HE DEAD?
EE-OO-EE-OO
HE'S STILL BREATHING.
I'D LIKE TO TREAT HIM, IF POSSIBLE.
I'M HIS DOCTOR.

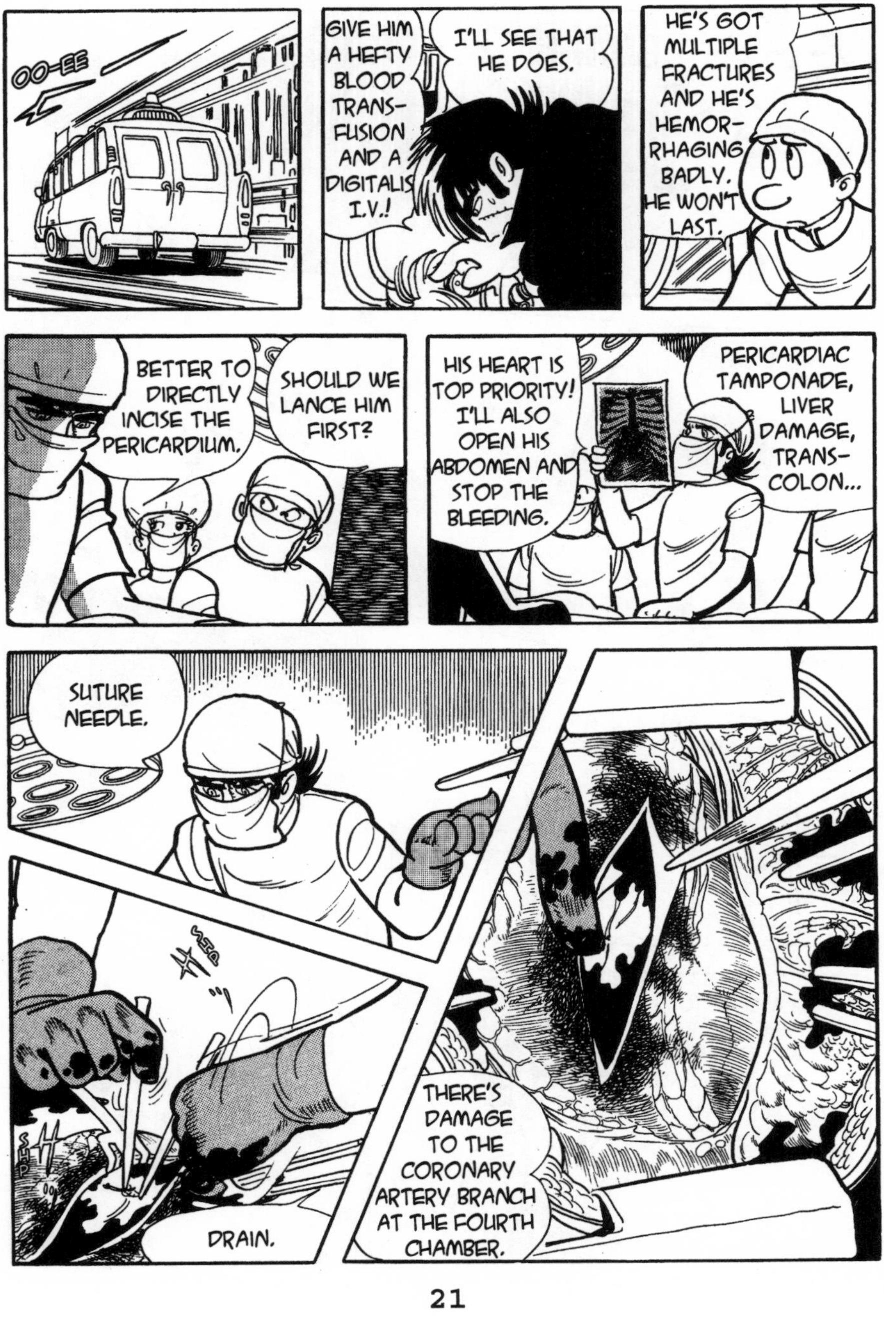
HE'S GOT MULTIPLE FRACTURES AND HE'S HEMOR-RHAGING BADLY. HE WON'T LAST.
GIVE HIM A HEFTY BLOOD TRANS-FUSION AND A DIGITALIS I.V.!
I'LL SEE THAT HE DOES.
OO-EE
PERICARDIAC TAMPONADE, LIVER DAMAGE, TRANS-COLON...
HIS HEART IS TOP PRIORITY! I'LL ALSO OPEN HIS ABDOMEN AND STOP THE BLEEDING.
SHOULD WE LANCE HIM FIRST?
BETTER TO DIRECTLY INCISE THE PERICARDIUM.
THERE'S DAMAGE TO THE CORONARY ARTERY BRANCH AT THE FOURTH CHAMBER.
SUTURE NEEDLE.
DRAIN.

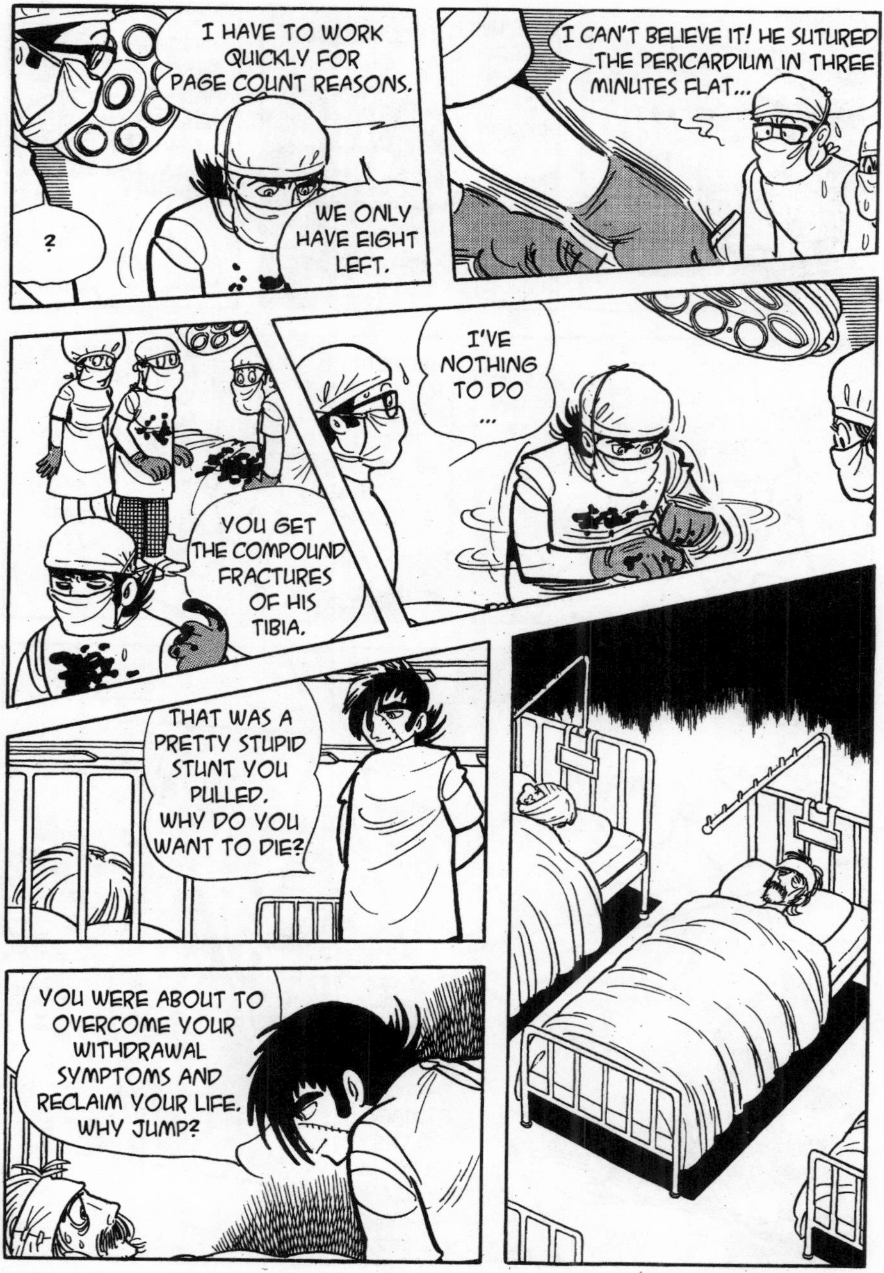
I CAN'T BELIEVE IT! HE SUTURED THE PERICARDIUM IN THREE MINUTES FLAT...
I HAVE TO WORK QUICKLY FOR PAGE COUNT REASONS.
WE ONLY HAVE EIGHT LEFT.
?
I'VE NOTHING TO DO ...
YOU GET THE COMPOUND FRACTURES OF HIS TIBIA.
THAT WAS A PRETTY STUPID STUNT YOU PULLED. WHY DO YOU WANT TO DIE?
YOU WERE ABOUT TO OVERCOME YOUR WITHDRAWAL SYMPTOMS AND RECLAIM YOUR LIFE. WHY JUMP?

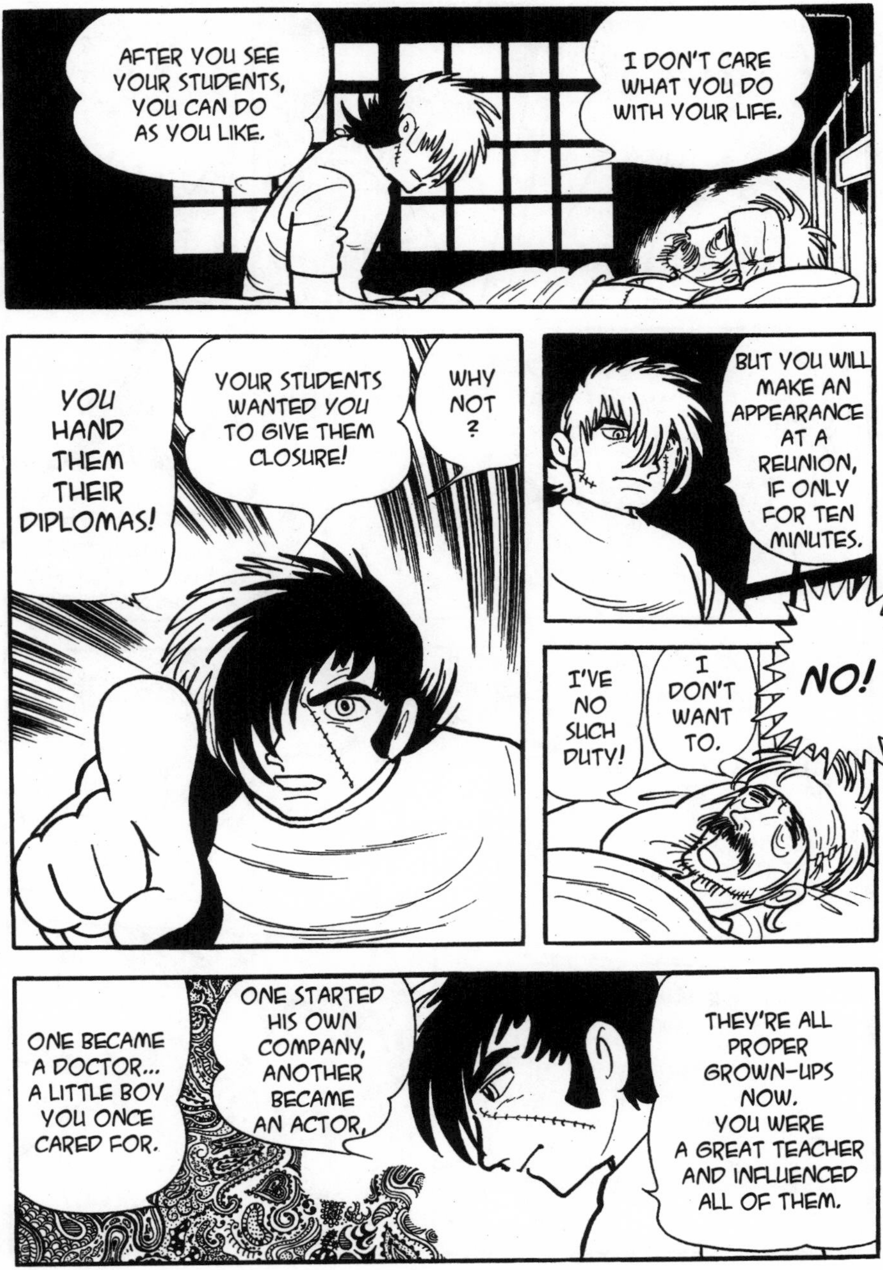
I DON'T CARE WHAT YOU DO WITH YOUR LIFE.
AFTER YOU SEE YOUR STUDENTS, YOU CAN DO AS YOU LIKE.
BUT YOU WILL MAKE AN APPEARANCE AT A REUNION, IF ONLY FOR TEN MINUTES.
NO!
I DON'T WANT TO.
I'VE NO SUCH DUTY!
WHY NOT?
YOUR STUDENTS WANTED YOU TO GIVE THEM CLOSURE!
YOU HAND THEM THEIR DIPLOMAS!
THEY'RE ALL PROPER GROWN-UPS NOW. YOU WERE A GREAT TEACHER AND INFLUENCED ALL OF THEM.
ONE STARTED HIS OWN COMPANY, ANOTHER BECAME AN ACTOR,
ONE BECAME A DOCTOR... A LITTLE BOY YOU ONCE CARED FOR.

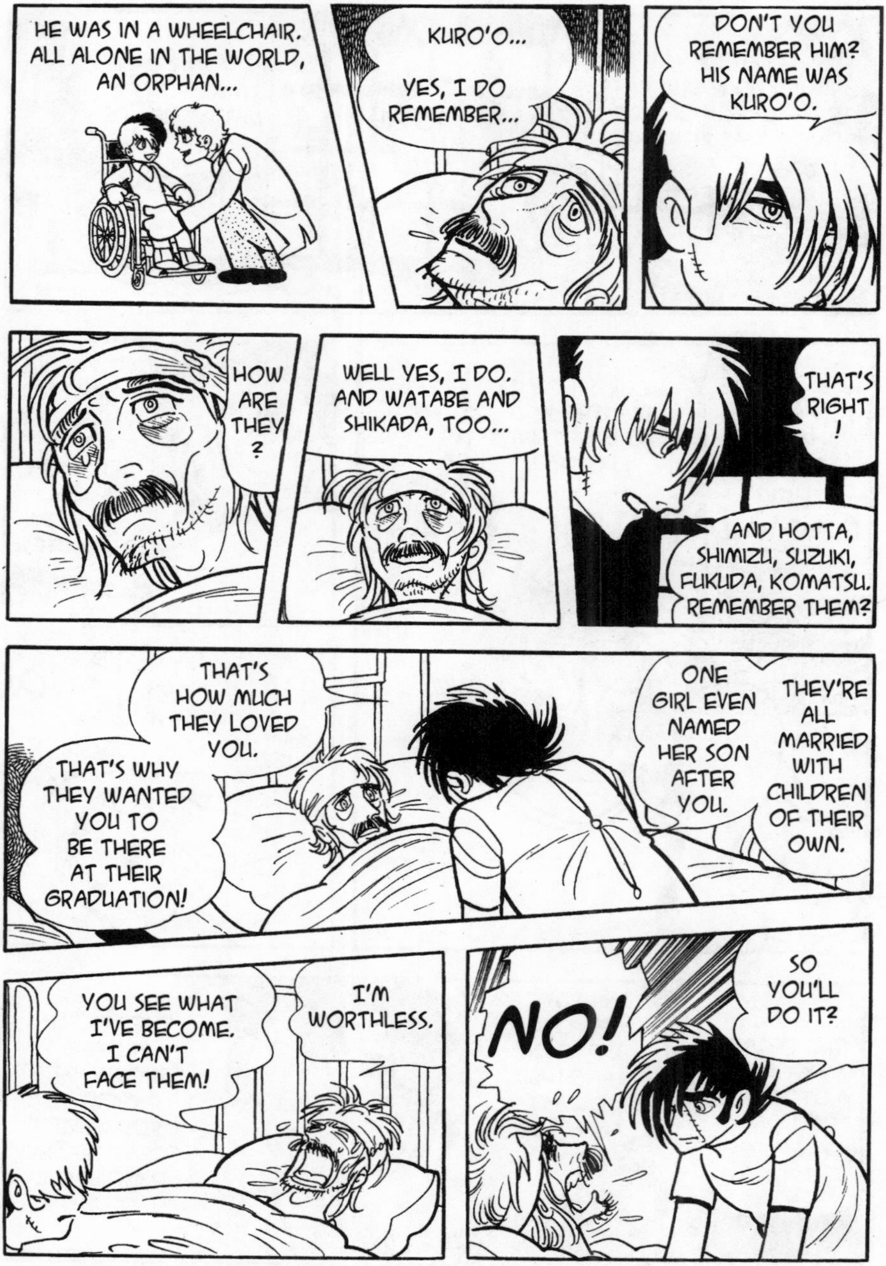
DON'T YOU REMEMBER HIM? HIS NAME WAS KURO'O.
KURO'O...
YES, I DO REMEMBER...
HE WAS IN A WHEELCHAIR. ALL ALONE IN THE WORLD, AN ORPHAN...
THAT'S RIGHT!
AND HOTTA, SHIMIZU, SUZUKI, FUKUDA, KOMATSU. REMEMBER THEM?
WELL YES, I DO. AND WATABE AND SHIKADA, TOO...
HOW ARE THEY?
THEY'RE ALL MARRIED WITH CHILDREN OF THEIR OWN.
ONE GIRL EVEN NAMED HER SON AFTER YOU.
THAT'S HOW MUCH THEY LOVED YOU.
THAT'S WHY THEY WANTED YOU TO BE THERE AT THEIR GRADUATION!
SO YOU'LL DO IT?
NO!
I'M WORTHLESS.
YOU SEE WHAT I'VE BECOME. I CAN'T FACE THEM!

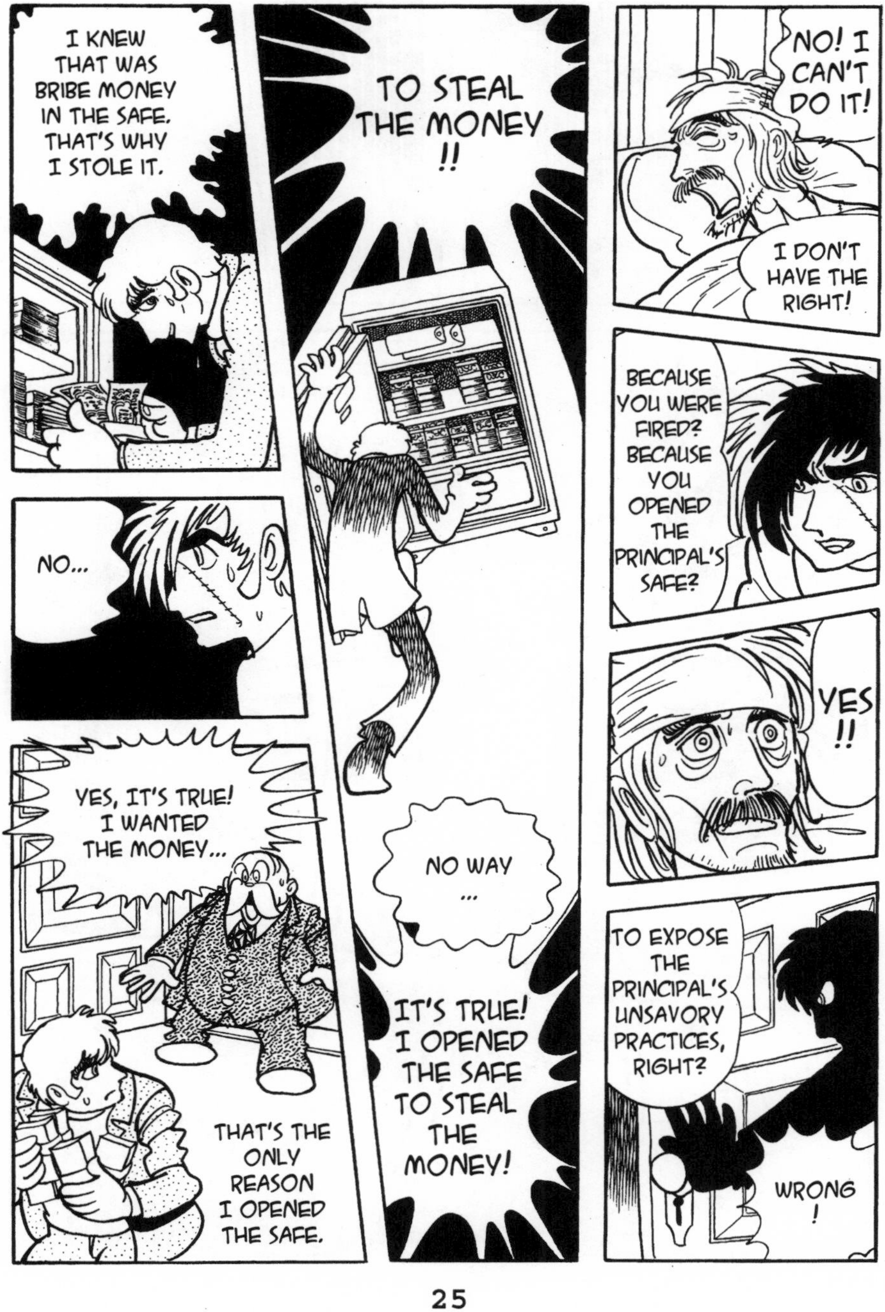

NO! I CAN'T DO IT!
I DON'T HAVE THE RIGHT!
BECAUSE YOU WERE FIRED? BECAUSE YOU OPENED THE PRINCIPAL'S SAFE?
YES !!
TO EXPOSE THE PRINCIPAL'S UNSAVORY PRACTICES, RIGHT?
WRONG !
TO STEAL THE MONEY !!
NO WAY ...
IT'S TRUE! I OPENED THE SAFE TO STEAL THE MONEY!
I KNEW THAT WAS BRIBE MONEY IN THE SAFE. THAT'S WHY I STOLE IT.
NO...
YES, IT'S TRUE! I WANTED THE MONEY...
THAT'S THE ONLY REASON I OPENED THE SAFE.

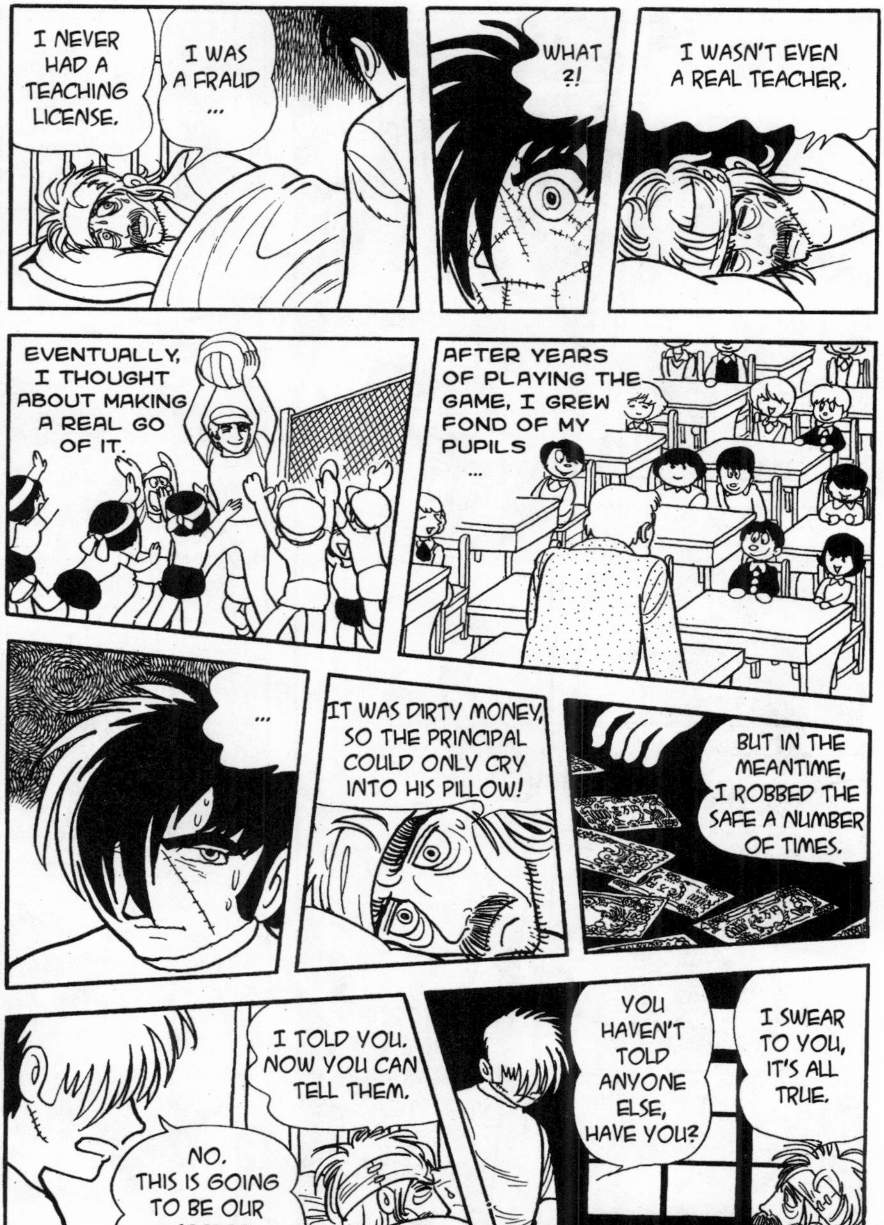
I WASN'T EVEN A REAL TEACHER.
WHAT ?!
I WAS A FRAUD ...
I NEVER HAD A TEACHING LICENSE.
AFTER YEARS OF PLAYING THE GAME, I GREW FOND OF MY PUPILS ...
EVENTUALLY, I THOUGHT ABOUT MAKING A REAL GO OF IT.
BUT IN THE MEANTIME, I ROBBED THE SAFE A NUMBER OF TIMES.
IT WAS DIRTY MONEY, SO THE PRINCIPAL COULD ONLY CRY INTO HIS PILLOW!
...
I SWEAR TO YOU, IT'S ALL TRUE.
YOU HAVEN'T TOLD ANYONE ELSE, HAVE YOU?
I TOLD YOU. NOW YOU CAN TELL THEM.
NO. THIS IS GOING TO BE OUR SECRET.

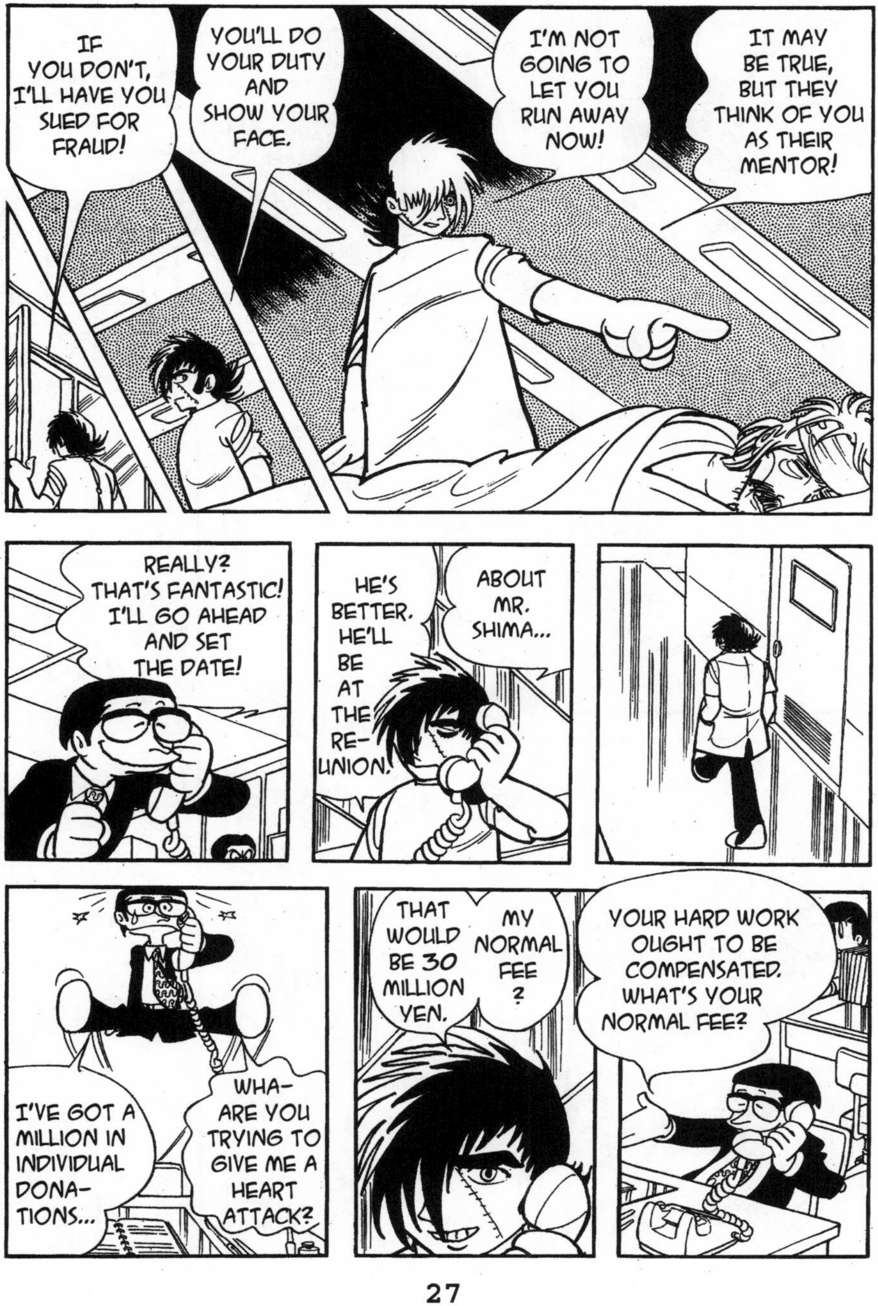
IT MAY BE TRUE, BUT THEY THINK OF YOU AS THEIR MENTOR!
I'M NOT GOING TO LET YOU RUN AWAY NOW!
YOU'LL DO YOUR DUTY AND SHOW YOUR FACE.
IF YOU DON'T, I'LL HAVE YOU SUED FOR FRAUD!
ABOUT MR. SHIMA...
HE'S BETTER. HE'LL BE AT THE RE-UNION.
REALLY? THAT'S FANTASTIC! I'LL GO AHEAD AND SET THE DATE!
YOUR HARD WORK OUGHT TO BE COMPENSATED. WHAT'S YOUR NORMAL FEE?
MY NORMAL FEE?
THAT WOULD BE 30 MILLION YEN.
WHA- ARE YOU TRYING TO GIVE ME A HEART ATTACK?
I'VE GOT A MILLION IN INDIVIDUAL DONA-TIONS...

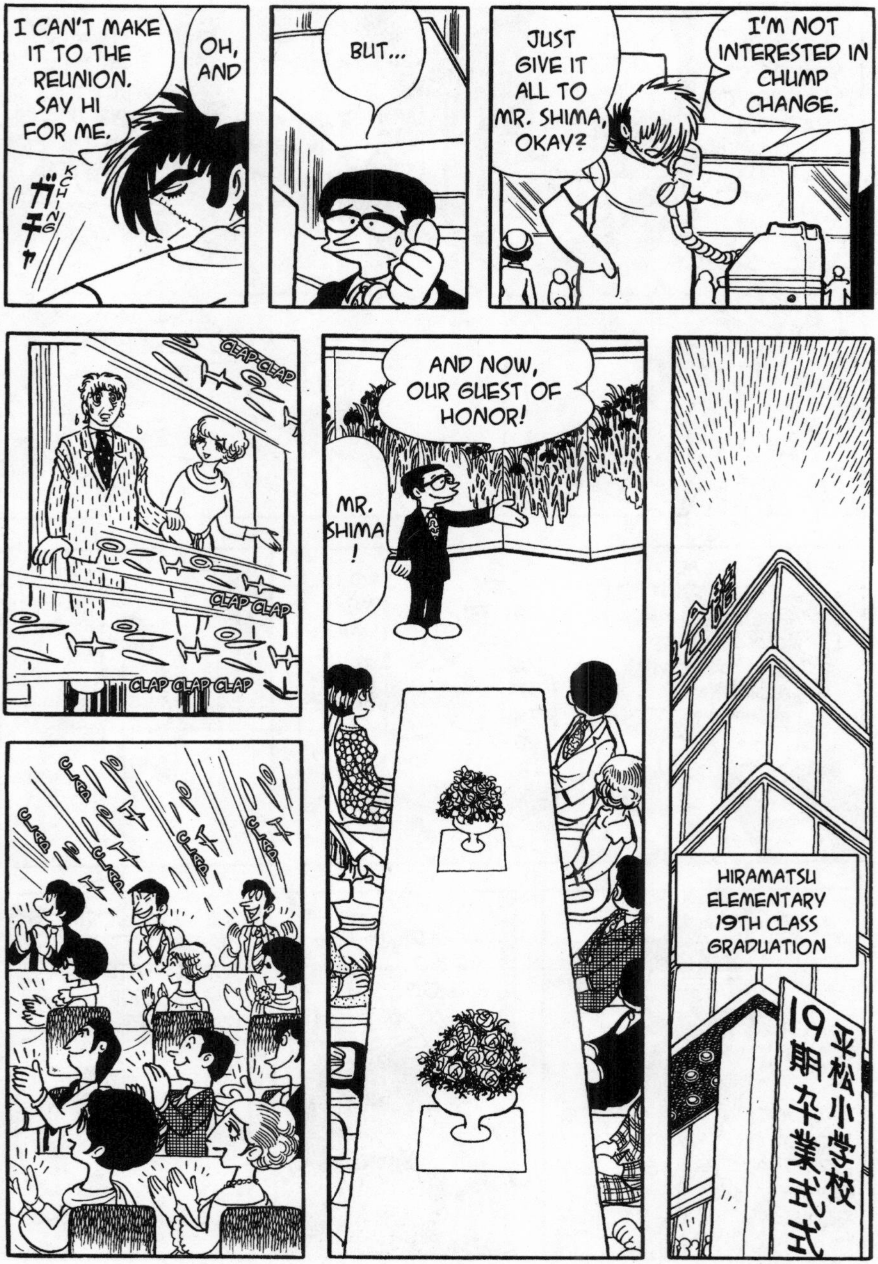
I'M NOT INTERESTED IN CHUMP CHANGE.
JUST GIVE IT ALL TO MR. SHIMA, OKAY?
BUT...
OH, AND
I CAN'T MAKE IT TO THE REUNION. SAY HI FOR ME.
KCHING
ガチャ
平松小学校
19期卒業式
HIRAMATSU ELEMENTARY 19TH CLASS GRADUATION
AND NOW, OUR GUEST OF HONOR!
MR. SHIMA!
CLAP CLAP
CLAP CLAP
CLAP CLAP CLAP

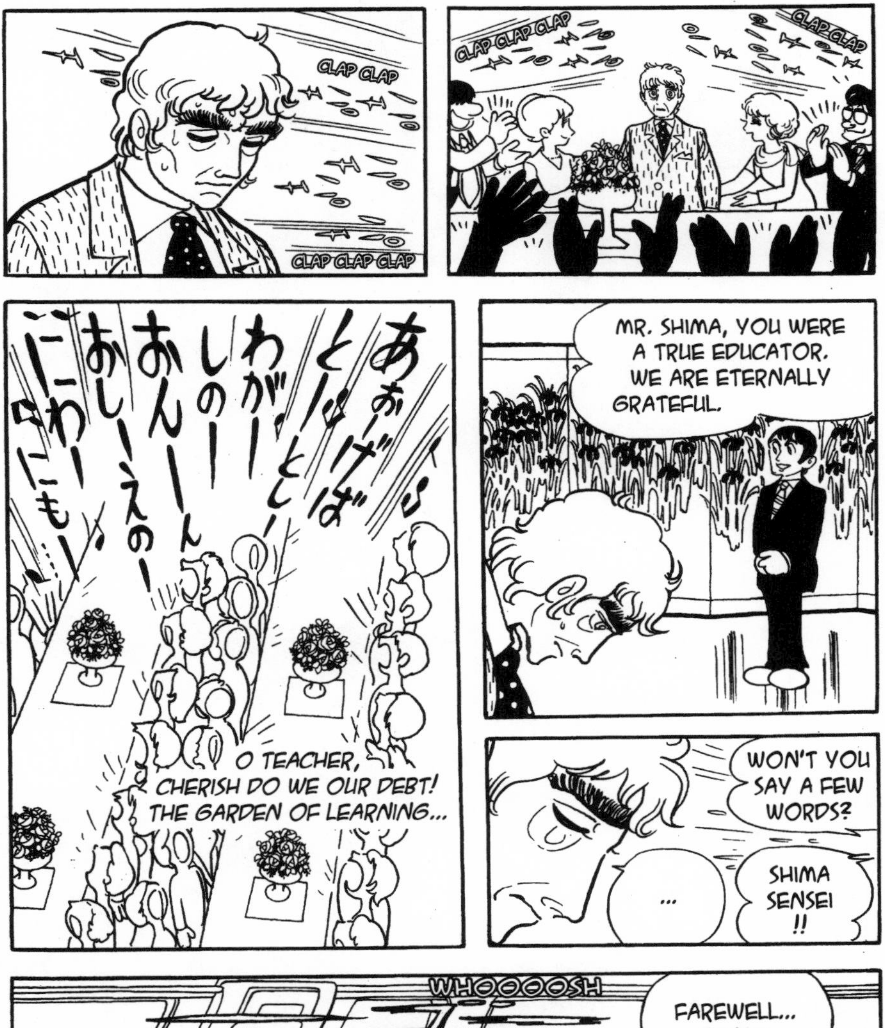
CLAP CLAP
CLAP CLAP
CLAP CLAP CLAP
CLAP CLAP
CLAP CLAP CLAP
MR. SHIMA, YOU WERE A TRUE EDUCATOR. WE ARE ETERNALLY GRATEFUL.
WON'T YOU SAY A FEW WORDS?
SHIMA SENSEI !!
...
あぉーげば とーとしー わがーしのー おんーん おしーえのー にーわーにもー
O TEACHER, CHERISH DO WE OUR DEBT! THE GARDEN OF LEARNING...
WHOOOOOSH
FAREWELL... SENSEI.

NOTE: "SENSEI," USUALLY TRANSLATED AS TEACHER, IS ALSO THE HONORIFIC FOR DOCTORS. IN THE ORIGINAL JAPANESE, DR. BLACK JACK IS ALWAYS "BURAKKU JAKKU SENSEI."

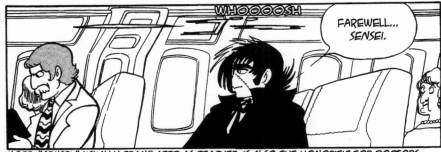

THE SCREAM

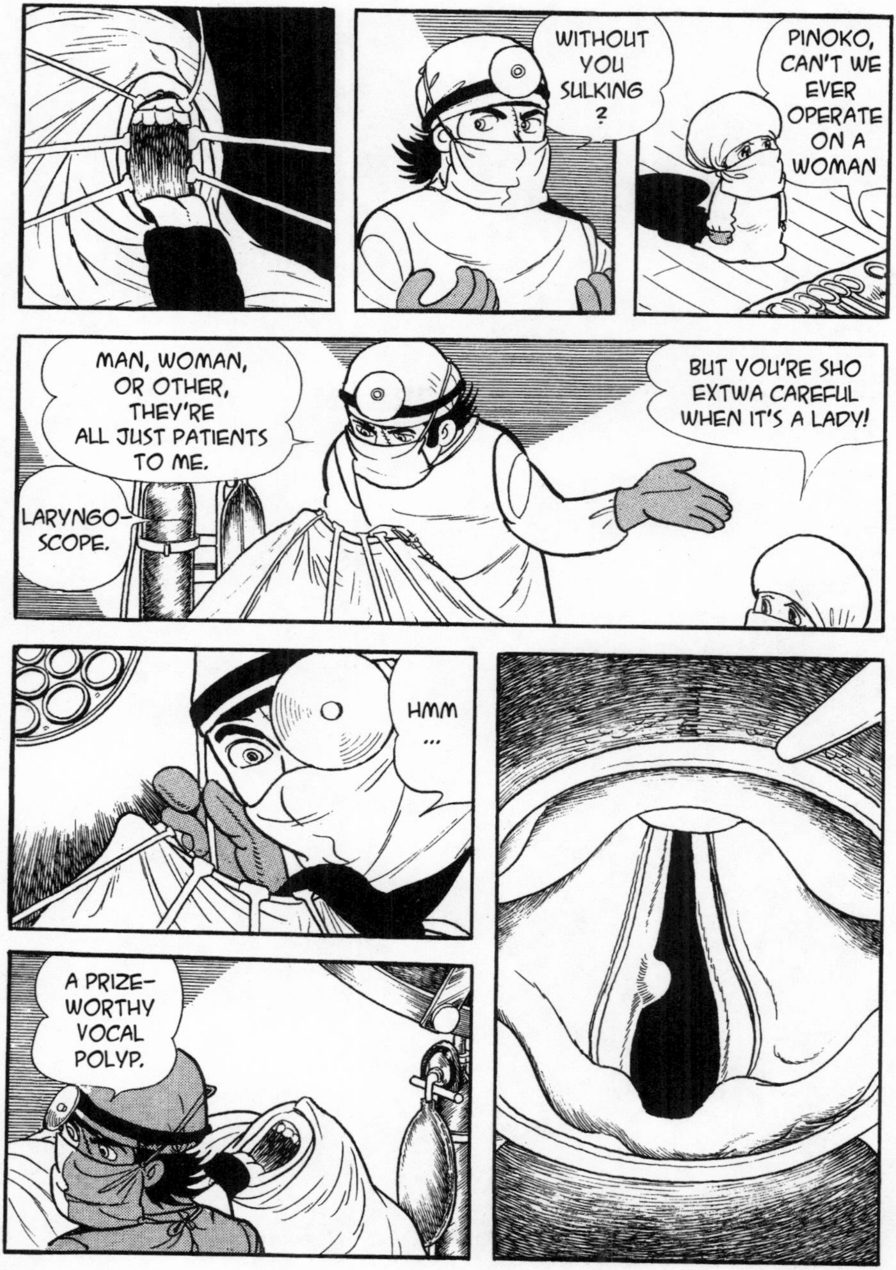
PINOKO, CAN'T WE EVER OPERATE ON A WOMAN
WITHOUT YOU SULKING ?
BUT YOU'RE SHO EXTWA CAREFUL WHEN IT'S A LADY!
MAN, WOMAN, OR OTHER, THEY'RE ALL JUST PATIENTS TO ME.
LARYNGO-SCOPE.
HMM ...
A PRIZE-WORTHY VOCAL POLYP.

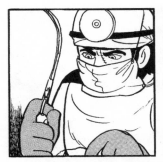
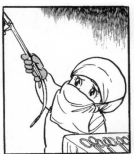
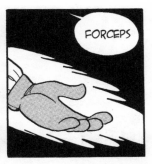

FORCEPS

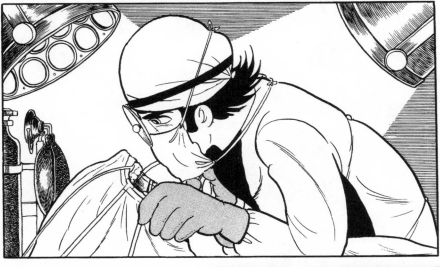

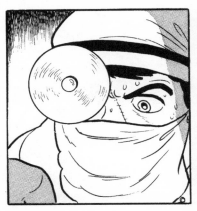
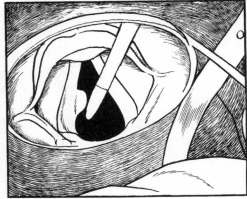

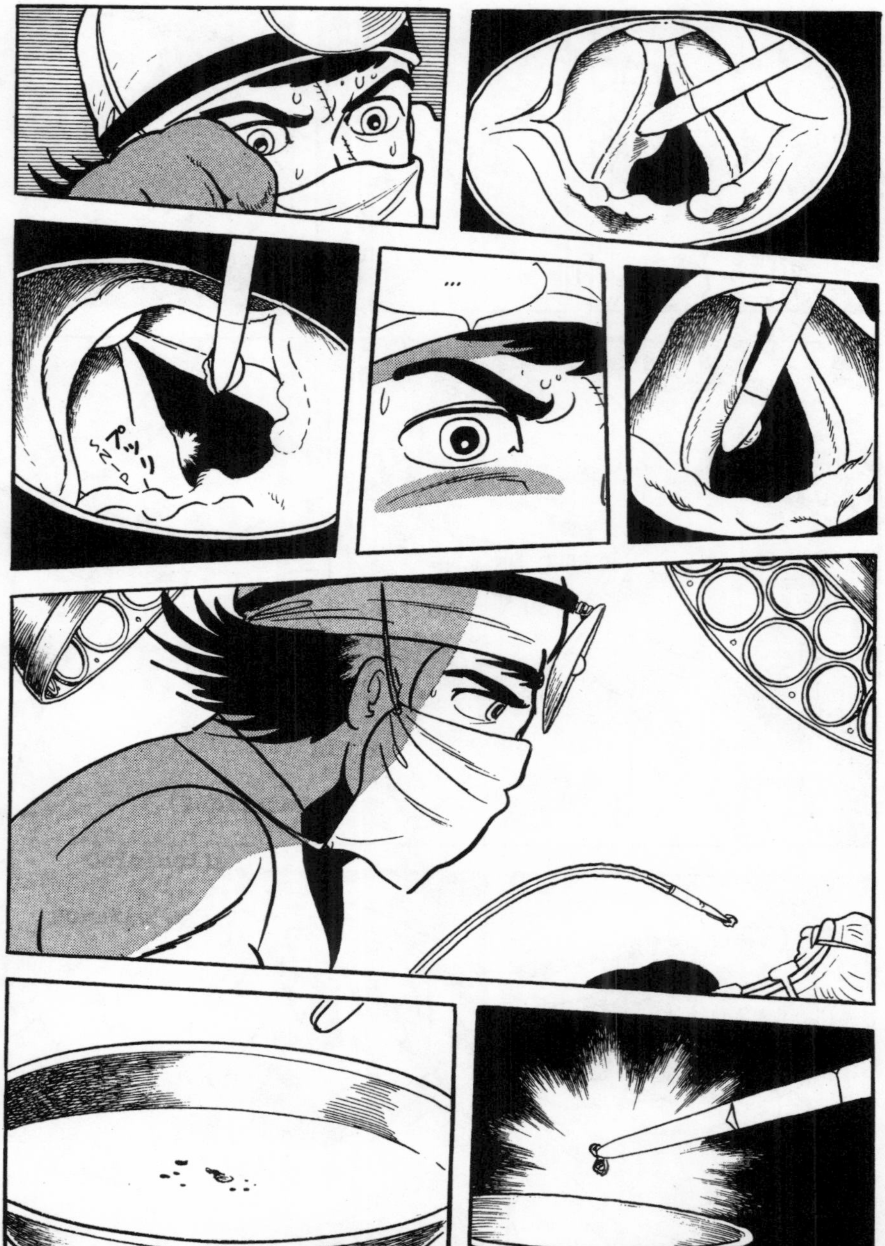
...
プッツリ
SNIP

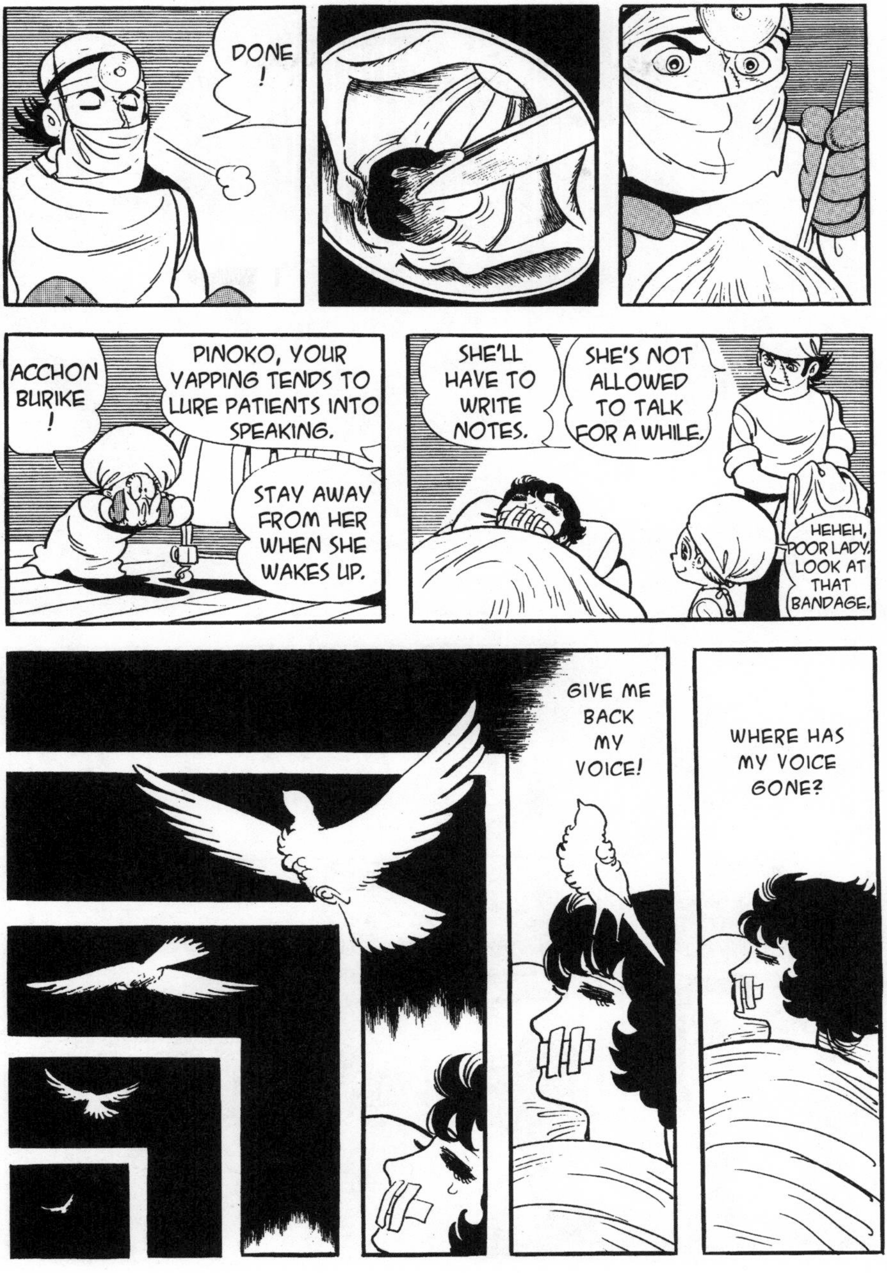
DONE!
SHE'S NOT ALLOWED TO TALK FOR A WHILE.
SHE'LL HAVE TO WRITE NOTES.
HEHEH, POOR LADY. LOOK AT THAT BANDAGE.
PINOKO, YOUR YAPPING TENDS TO LURE PATIENTS INTO SPEAKING.
STAY AWAY FROM HER WHEN SHE WAKES UP.
ACCHON BURIKE!
WHERE HAS MY VOICE GONE?
GIVE ME BACK MY VOICE!

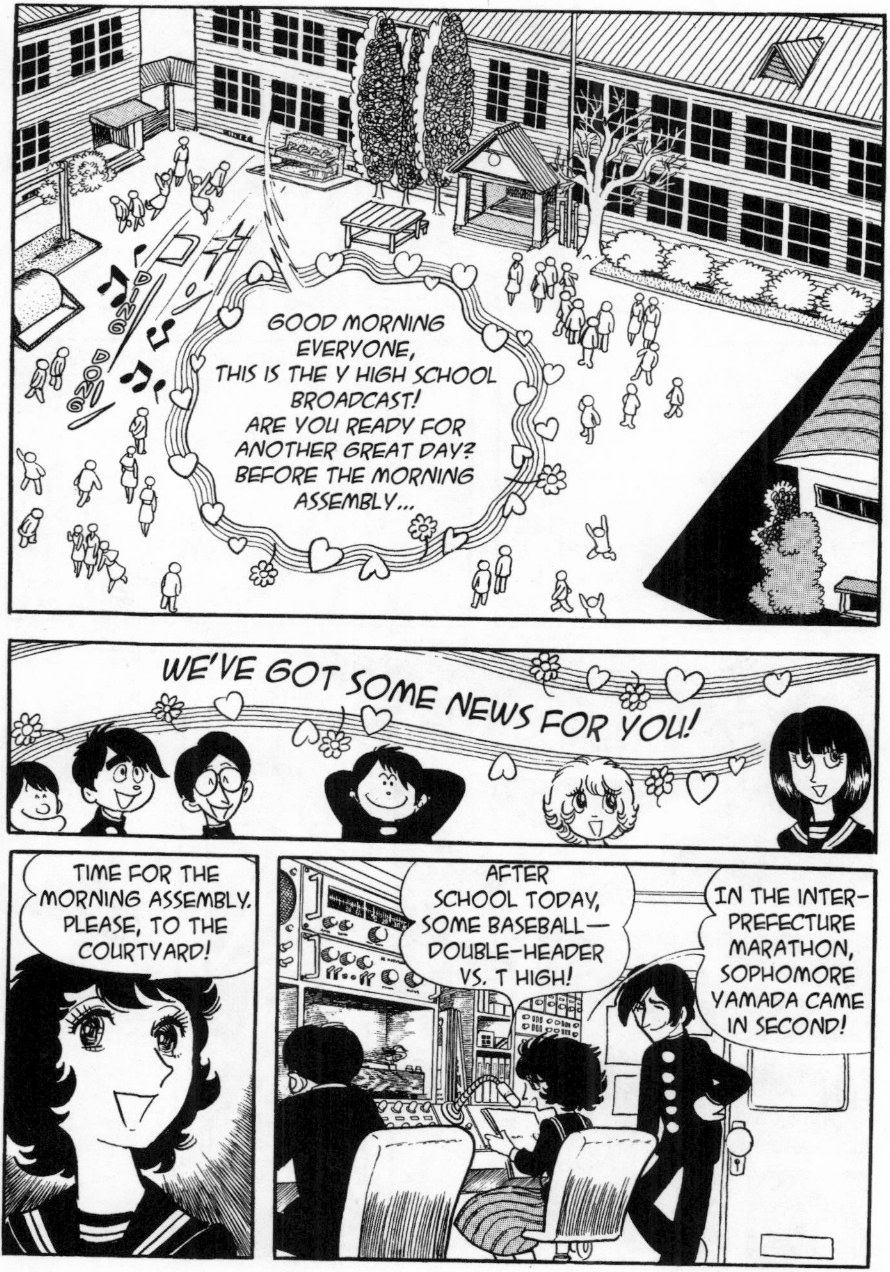
DING DONG
GOOD MORNING EVERYONE, THIS IS THE Y HIGH SCHOOL BROADCAST! ARE YOU READY FOR ANOTHER GREAT DAY? BEFORE THE MORNING ASSEMBLY...
WE'VE GOT SOME NEWS FOR YOU!
IN THE INTER-PREFECTURE MARATHON, SOPHOMORE YAMADA CAME IN SECOND!
AFTER SCHOOL TODAY, SOME BASEBALL— DOUBLE-HEADER VS. T HIGH!
TIME FOR THE MORNING ASSEMBLY. PLEASE, TO THE COURTYARD!

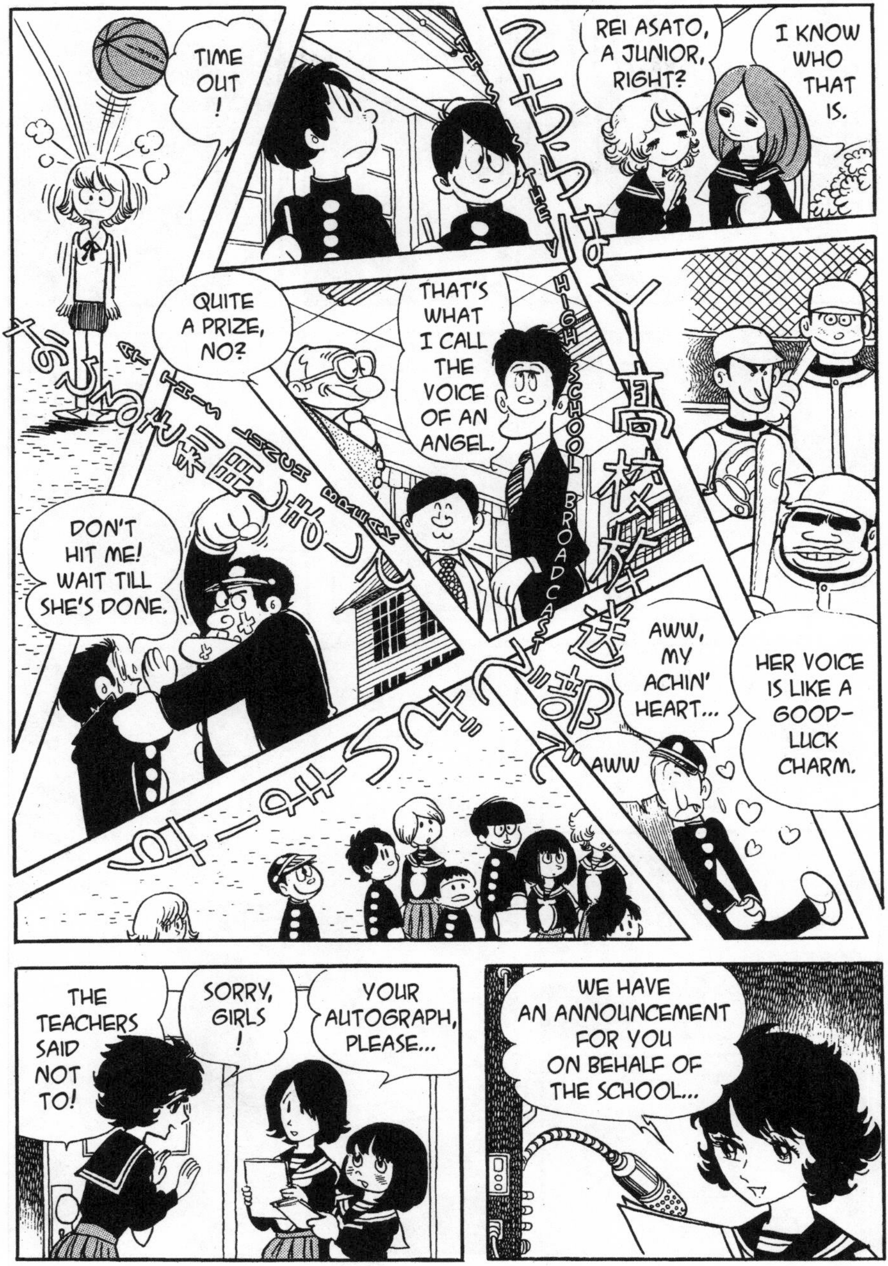
I KNOW WHO THAT IS.
REI ASATO, A JUNIOR, RIGHT?
こちらはY高校放送部で
HIGH SCHOOL BROADCAST
TIME OUT!
HER VOICE IS LIKE A GOOD-LUCK CHARM.
AWW, MY ACHIN' HEART...
AWW
THAT'S WHAT I CALL THE VOICE OF AN ANGEL.
QUITE A PRIZE, NO?
DON'T HIT ME! WAIT TILL SHE'S DONE.
WE HAVE AN ANNOUNCEMENT FOR YOU ON BEHALF OF THE SCHOOL...
YOUR AUTOGRAPH, PLEASE...
SORRY, GIRLS!
THE TEACHERS SAID NOT TO!

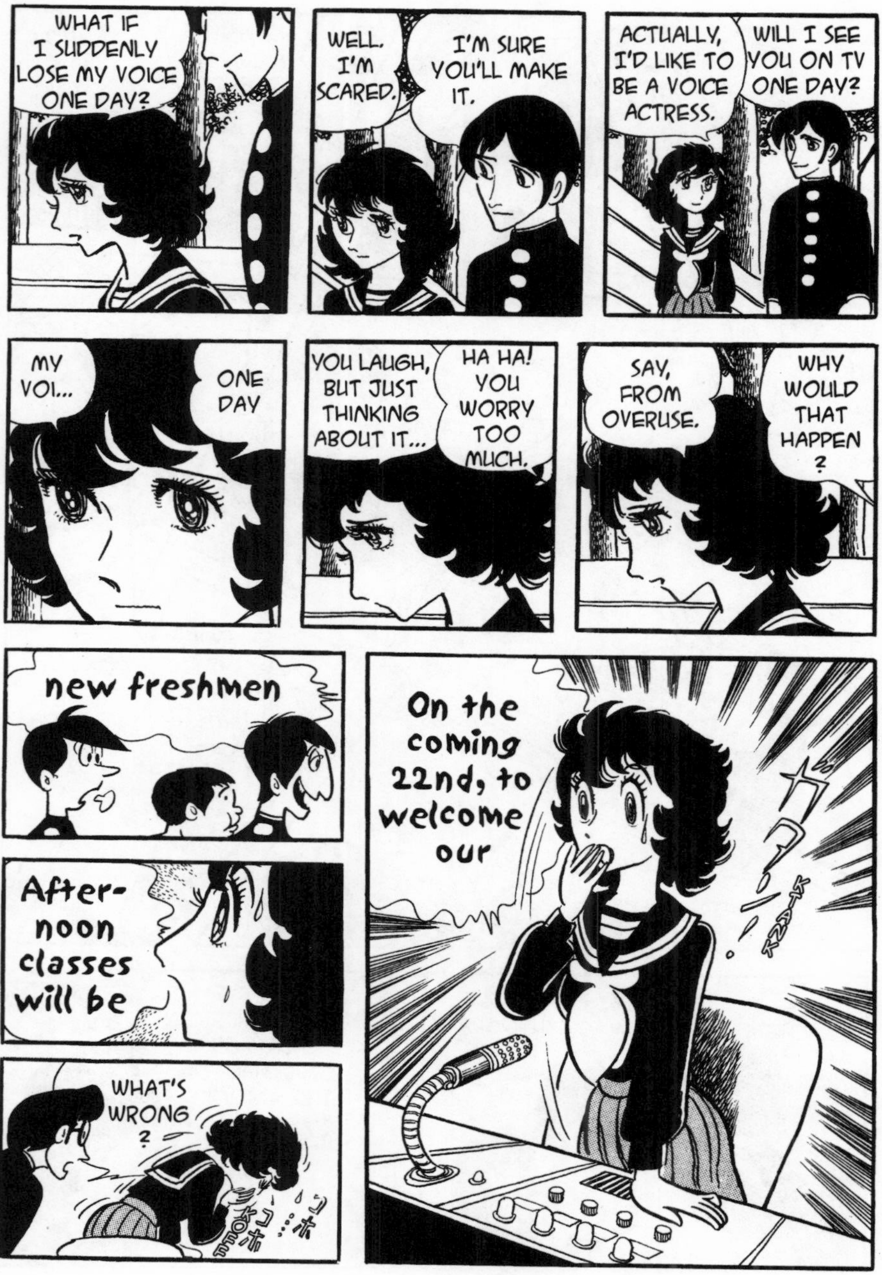
WILL I SEE YOU ON TV ONE DAY?
ACTUALLY, I'D LIKE TO BE A VOICE ACTRESS.
I'M SURE YOU'LL MAKE IT.
WELL. I'M SCARED.
WHAT IF I SUDDENLY LOSE MY VOICE ONE DAY?
WHY WOULD THAT HAPPEN?
SAY, FROM OVERUSE.
HA HA! YOU WORRY TOO MUCH.
YOU LAUGH, BUT JUST THINKING ABOUT IT...
ONE DAY
MY VOI...
On the coming 22nd, to welcome our
new freshmen
After-noon classes will be
WHAT'S WRONG?

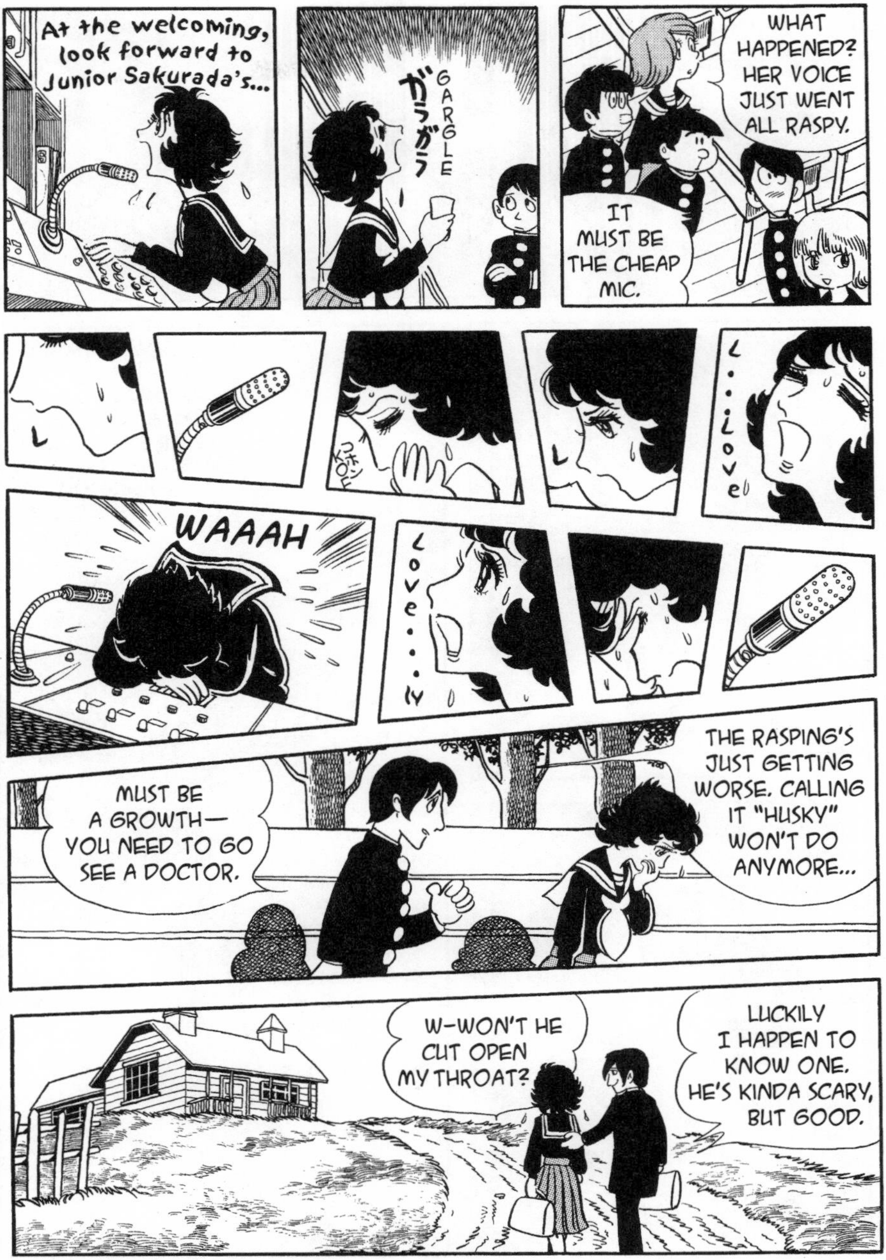
WHAT HAPPENED? HER VOICE JUST WENT ALL RASPY.
IT MUST BE THE CHEAP MIC.
ガラガラ
GARGLE
At the welcoming, look forward to Junior Sakurada's...
L...Love
L
L
Love....ly
WAAAH
THE RASPING'S JUST GETTING WORSE. CALLING IT "HUSKY" WON'T DO ANYMORE...
MUST BE A GROWTH— YOU NEED TO GO SEE A DOCTOR.
LUCKILY I HAPPEN TO KNOW ONE. HE'S KINDA SCARY, BUT GOOD.
W-WON'T HE CUT OPEN MY THROAT?

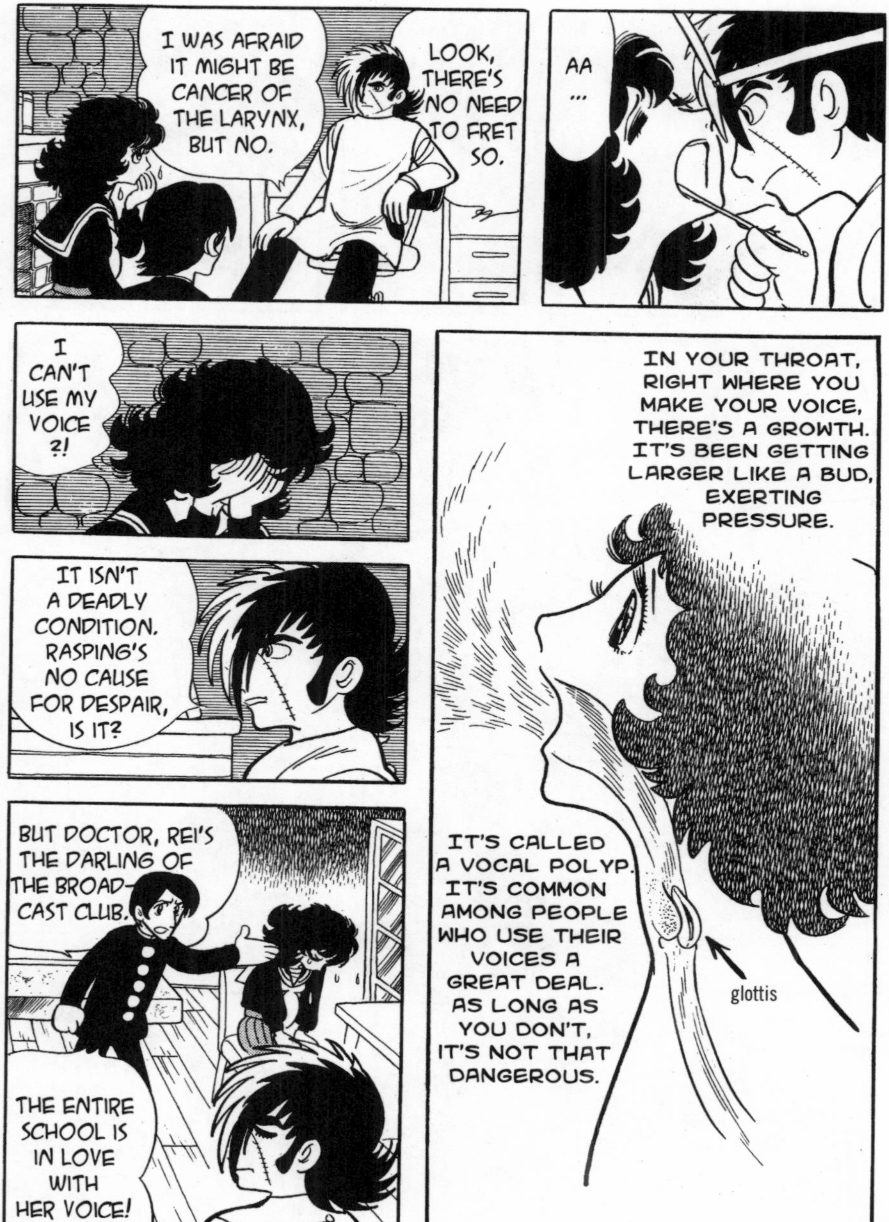
AA ...
LOOK, THERE'S NO NEED TO FRET SO.
I WAS AFRAID IT MIGHT BE CANCER OF THE LARYNX, BUT NO.
IN YOUR THROAT, RIGHT WHERE YOU MAKE YOUR VOICE, THERE'S A GROWTH. IT'S BEEN GETTING LARGER LIKE A BUD, EXERTING PRESSURE.
IT'S CALLED A VOCAL POLYP. IT'S COMMON AMONG PEOPLE WHO USE THEIR VOICES A GREAT DEAL. AS LONG AS YOU DON'T, IT'S NOT THAT DANGEROUS.
glottis
I CAN'T USE MY VOICE ?!
IT ISN'T A DEADLY CONDITION. RASPING'S NO CAUSE FOR DESPAIR, IS IT?
BUT DOCTOR, REI'S THE DARLING OF THE BROAD-CAST CLUB.
THE ENTIRE SCHOOL IS IN LOVE WITH HER VOICE!

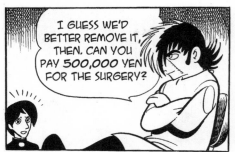

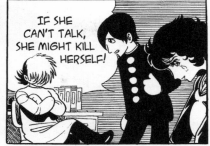

IF SHE CAN'T TALK, SHE MIGHT KILL HERSELF!
I GUESS WE'D BETTER REMOVE IT, THEN. CAN YOU PAY 500,000 YEN FOR THE SURGERY?
AH, BUT YOUR GRANDFATHER WAS MY MENTOR ...
AND I'M NO INGRATE. I'D LOVE TO CHARGE THE FULL FEE, BUT I'LL GIVE YOU A DISCOUNT. 1000 YEN.
ARE YOU KIDDING ?
THIS IS ABSURD. LET'S GO.
PERHAPS YOU MISUNDERSTOOD?
I'M SAYING I'LL CHARGE YOU 1000 YEN INSTEAD OF 500,000.
DOWN TO 1000 YEN ?
ARE ALL DOCTORS' FEES SO ARBITRARY ?
LET ME SAY THIS, THOUGH.
AFTER SURGERY, YOU FOLLOW MY INSTRUCTIONS TO THE LETTER UNTIL YOU'RE BETTER. NO FOOLING AROUND!

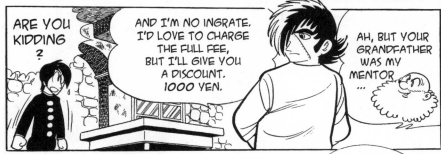

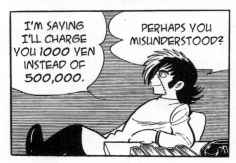

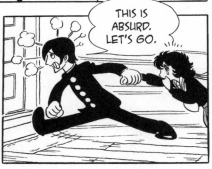

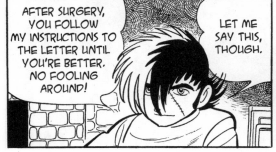

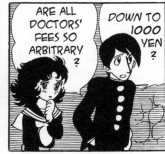

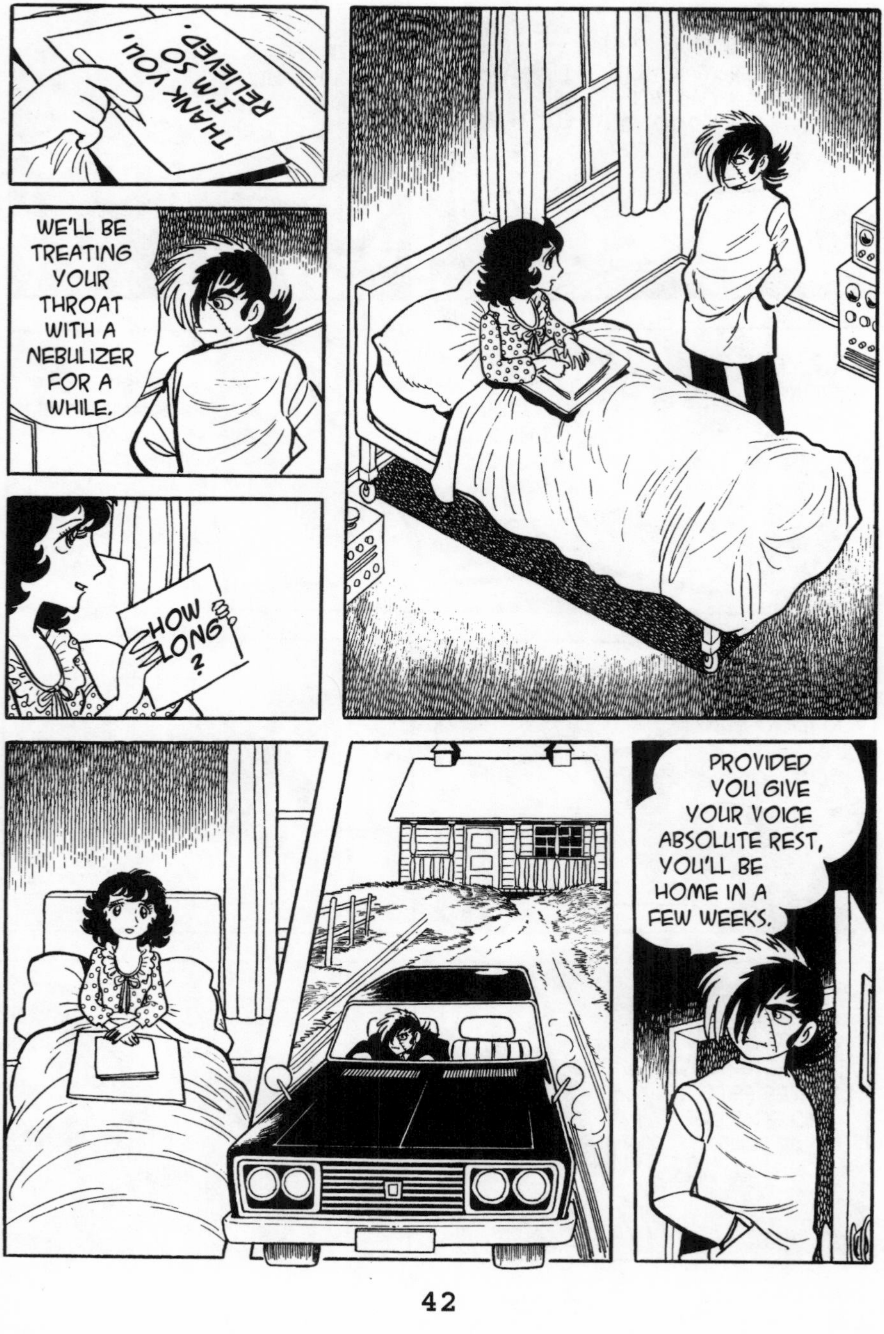
THANK YOU, I'M SO RELIEVED.
WE'LL BE TREATING YOUR THROAT WITH A NEBULIZER FOR A WHILE.
HOW LONG?
PROVIDED YOU GIVE YOUR VOICE ABSOLUTE REST, YOU'LL BE HOME IN A FEW WEEKS.

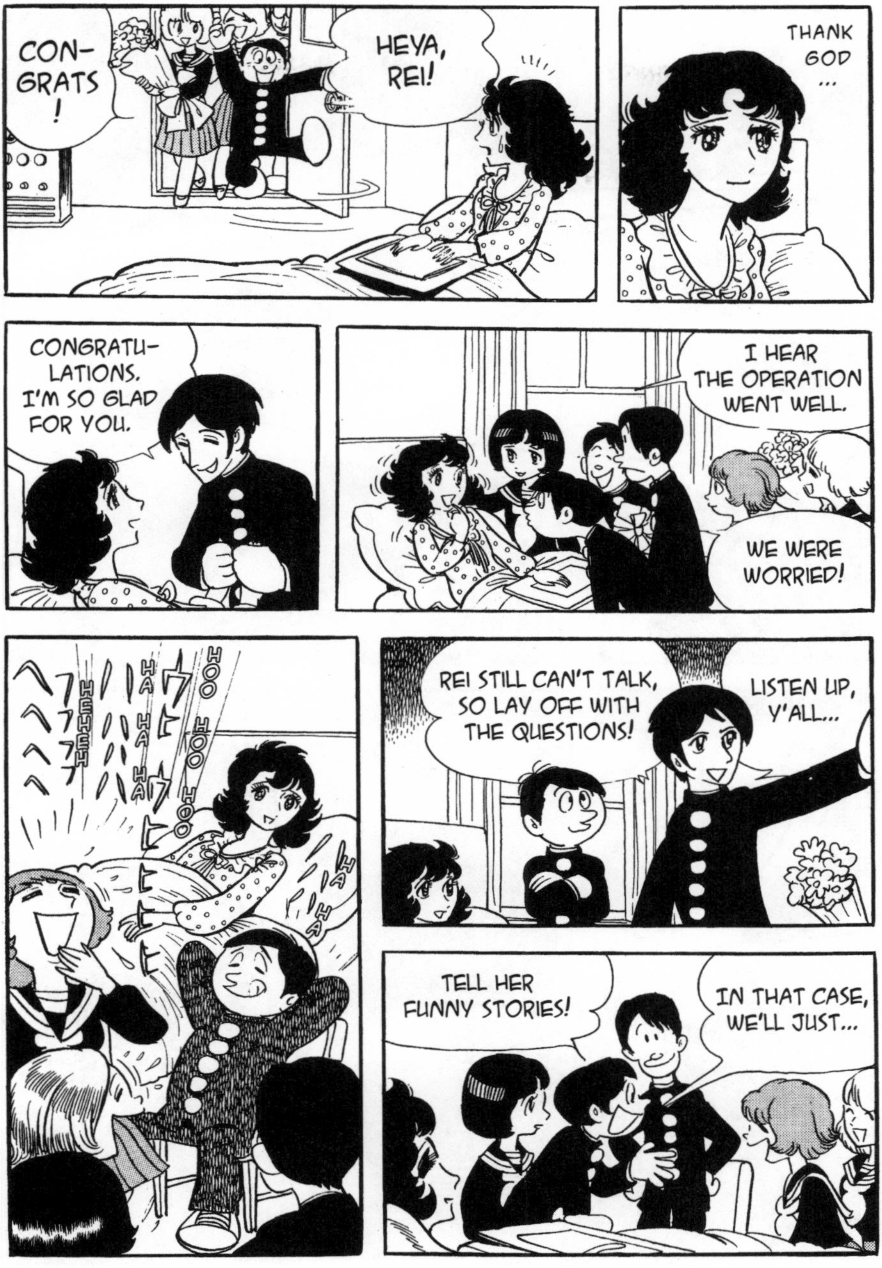
THANK GOD ...
HEYA, REI!
CON-GRATS!
I HEAR THE OPERATION WENT WELL.
WE WERE WORRIED!
CONGRATULATIONS. I'M SO GLAD FOR YOU.
LISTEN UP, Y'ALL...
REI STILL CAN'T TALK, SO LAY OFF WITH THE QUESTIONS!
IN THAT CASE, WE'LL JUST...
TELL HER FUNNY STORIES!
HOO HOO HOO HOO
HA HA HA HA
HEHEHEH
HA HA HA

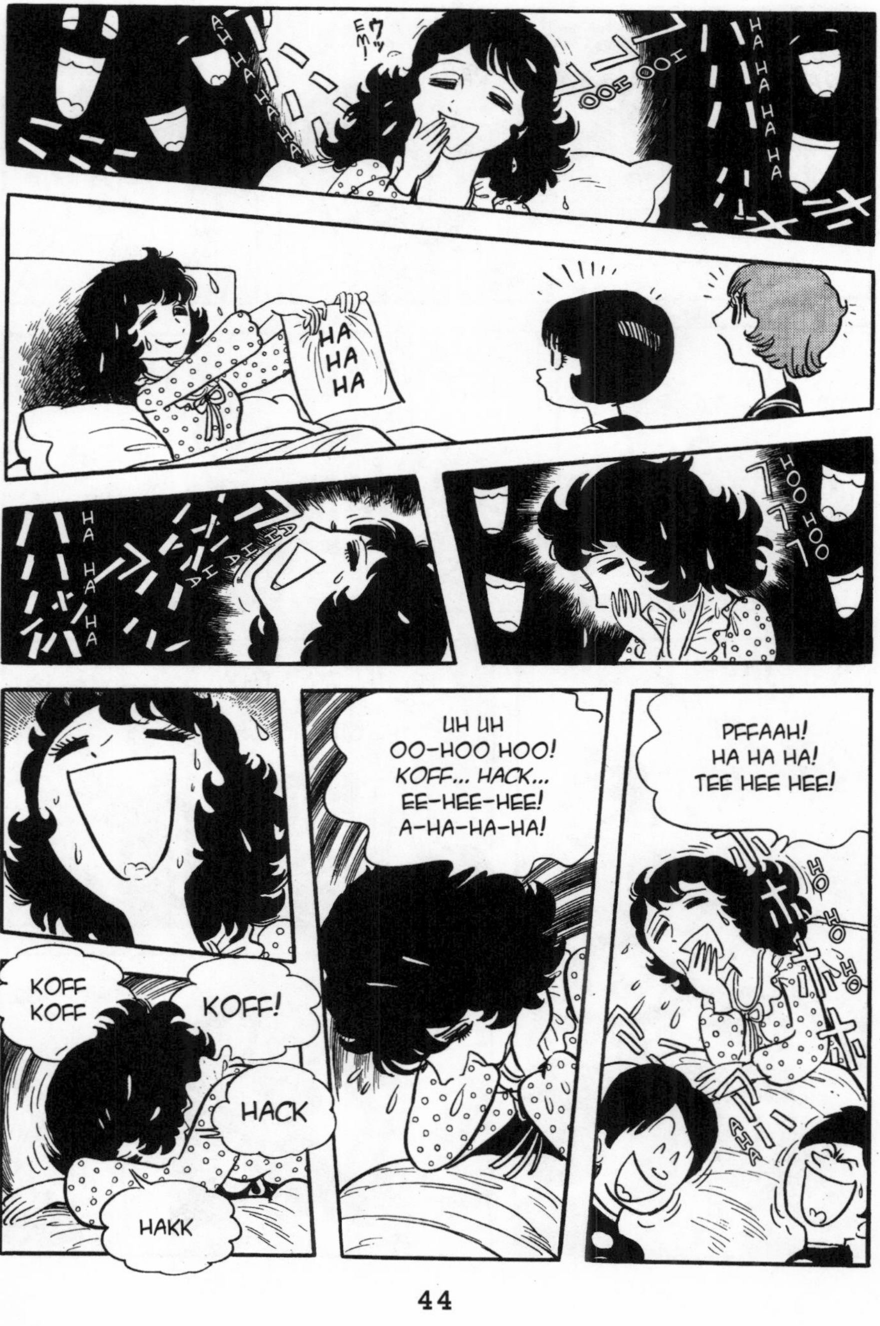
HA HA HA HA HA
HOO HOO
AH HA HA HA HA
HA
HA
HA
HOO HOO
HA HA HA HA
PFFAAH!
HA HA HA!
TEE HEE HEE!
HO HO HO HO
UH UH
OO-HOO HOO!
KOFF... HACK...
EE-HEE-HEE!
A-HA-HA-HA!
KOFF
KOFF
KOFF!
HACK
HAKK

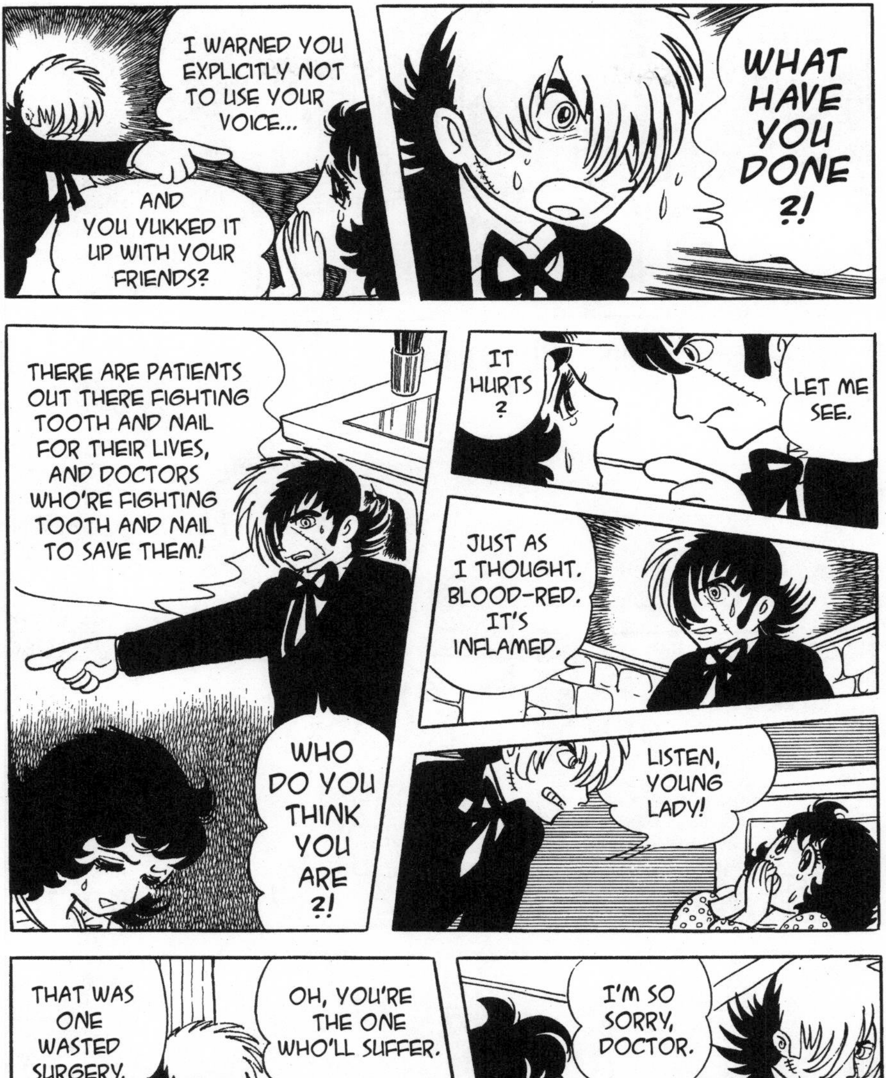
WHAT HAVE YOU DONE?!
I WARNED YOU EXPLICITLY NOT TO USE YOUR VOICE...
AND YOU YUKKED IT UP WITH YOUR FRIENDS?
LET ME SEE.
IT HURTS?
JUST AS I THOUGHT. BLOOD-RED. IT'S INFLAMED.
LISTEN, YOUNG LADY!
THERE ARE PATIENTS OUT THERE FIGHTING TOOTH AND NAIL FOR THEIR LIVES, AND DOCTORS WHO'RE FIGHTING TOOTH AND NAIL TO SAVE THEM!
WHO DO YOU THINK YOU ARE?!
I'M SO SORRY, DOCTOR.
YOU WERE TO FOLLOW MY INSTRUCTIONS.
OH, YOU'RE THE ONE WHO'LL SUFFER.
THAT WAS ONE WASTED SURGERY, THANK YOU.

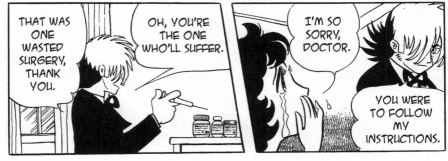

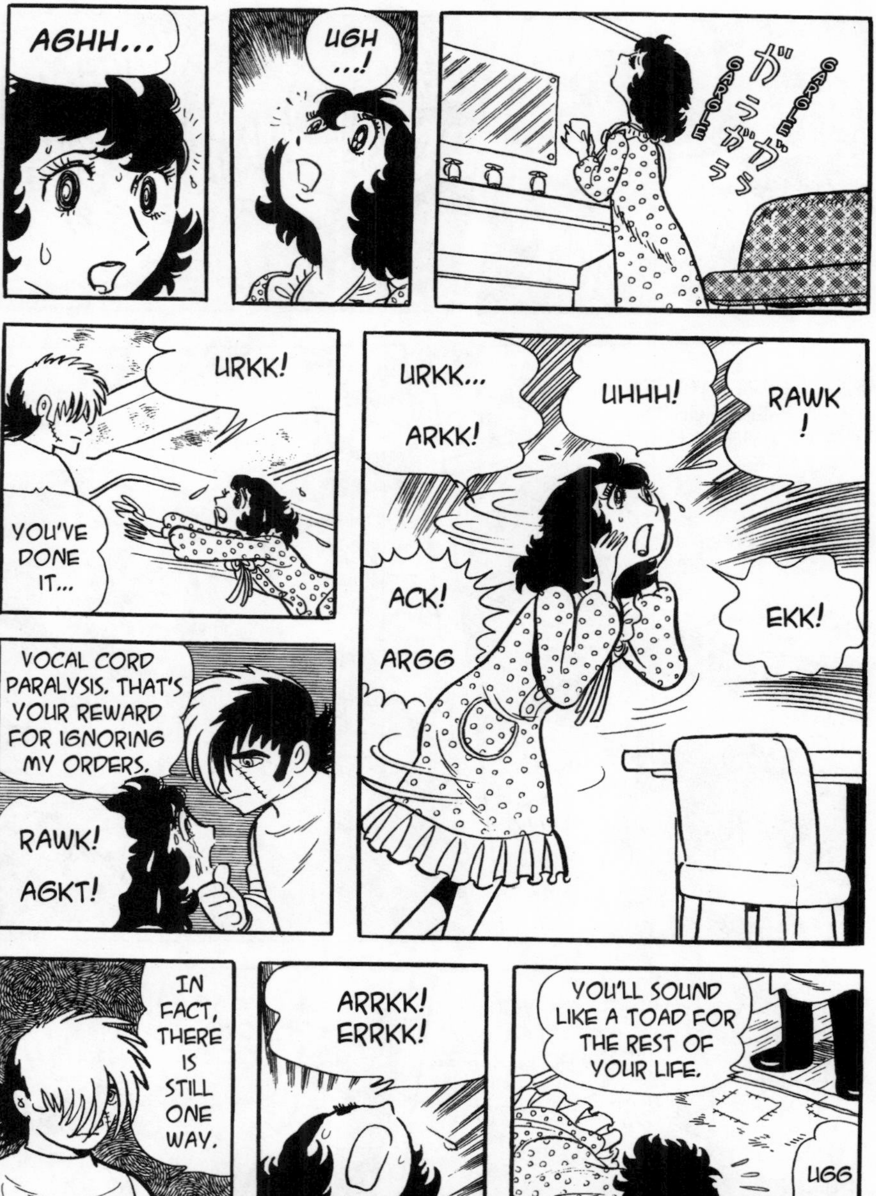
GARGLE
GARGLE
UGH ...!
AGHH...
RAWK !
UHHH!
URKK... ARKK!
EKK!
ACK! ARGG
URKK!
YOU'VE DONE IT...
VOCAL CORD PARALYSIS. THAT'S YOUR REWARD FOR IGNORING MY ORDERS.
RAWK! AGKT!
YOU'LL SOUND LIKE A TOAD FOR THE REST OF YOUR LIFE.
UGG UGG
ARRKK! ERRKK!
IN FACT, THERE IS STILL ONE WAY.

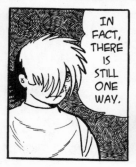

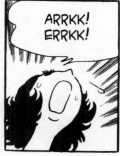

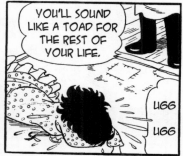

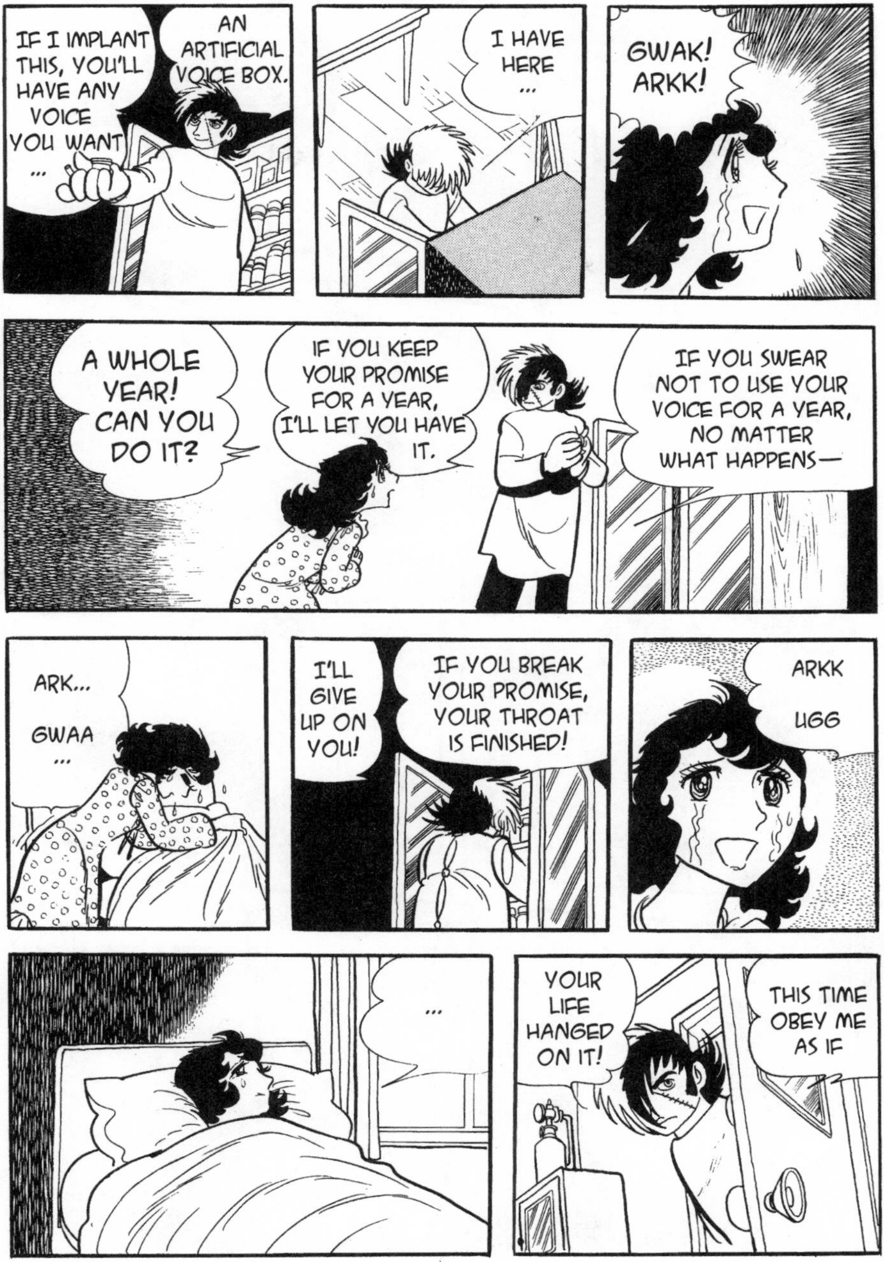
GWAK! ARKK!
I HAVE HERE ...
AN ARTIFICIAL VOICE BOX.
IF I IMPLANT THIS, YOU'LL HAVE ANY VOICE YOU WANT ...
IF YOU SWEAR NOT TO USE YOUR VOICE FOR A YEAR, NO MATTER WHAT HAPPENS—
IF YOU KEEP YOUR PROMISE FOR A YEAR, I'LL LET YOU HAVE IT.
A WHOLE YEAR! CAN YOU DO IT?
ARKK UGG
IF YOU BREAK YOUR PROMISE, YOUR THROAT IS FINISHED!
I'LL GIVE UP ON YOU!
ARK... GWAA ...
THIS TIME OBEY ME AS IF
YOUR LIFE HANGED ON IT!
...

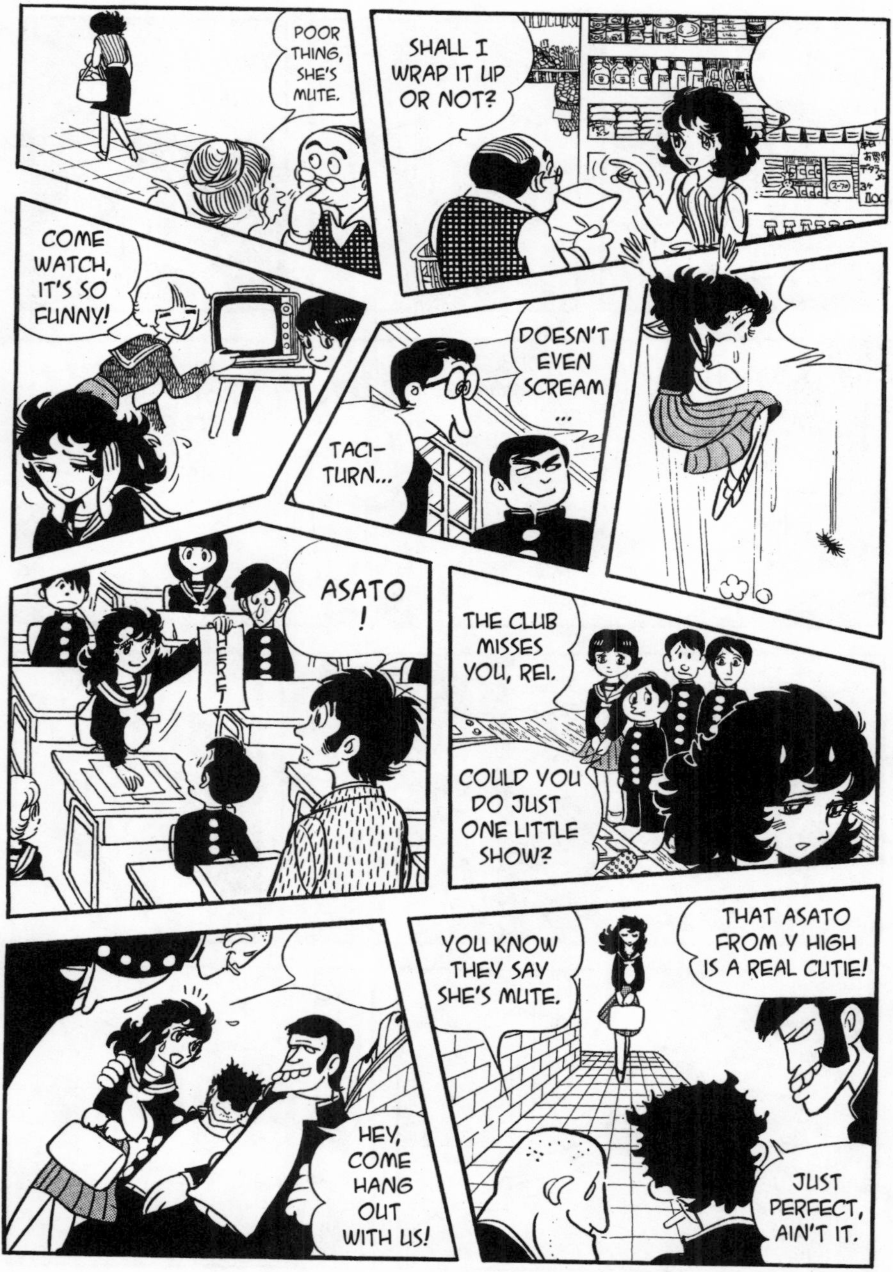
SHALL I WRAP IT UP OR NOT?
POOR THING, SHE'S MUTE.
DOESN'T EVEN SCREAM ...
TACI-TURN...
COME WATCH, IT'S SO FUNNY!
THE CLUB MISSES YOU, REI.
COULD YOU DO JUST ONE LITTLE SHOW?
ASATO !
HERE!
THAT ASATO FROM Y HIGH IS A REAL CUTIE!
YOU KNOW THEY SAY SHE'S MUTE.
JUST PERFECT, AIN'T IT.
HEY, COME HANG OUT WITH US!

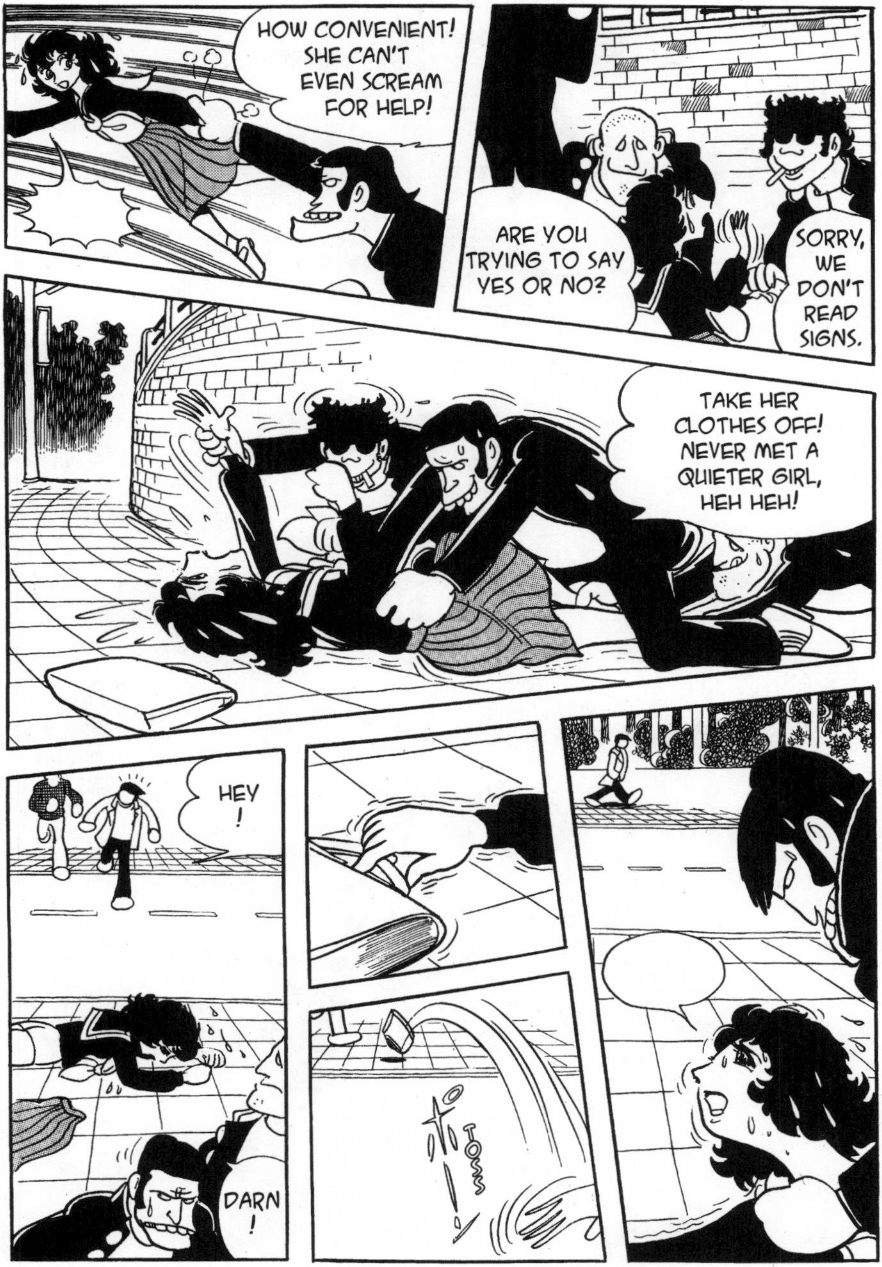
SORRY, WE DON'T READ SIGNS.
ARE YOU TRYING TO SAY YES OR NO?
HOW CONVENIENT! SHE CAN'T EVEN SCREAM FOR HELP!
TAKE HER CLOTHES OFF! NEVER MET A QUIETER GIRL, HEH HEH!
TOSS
HEY !
DARN !

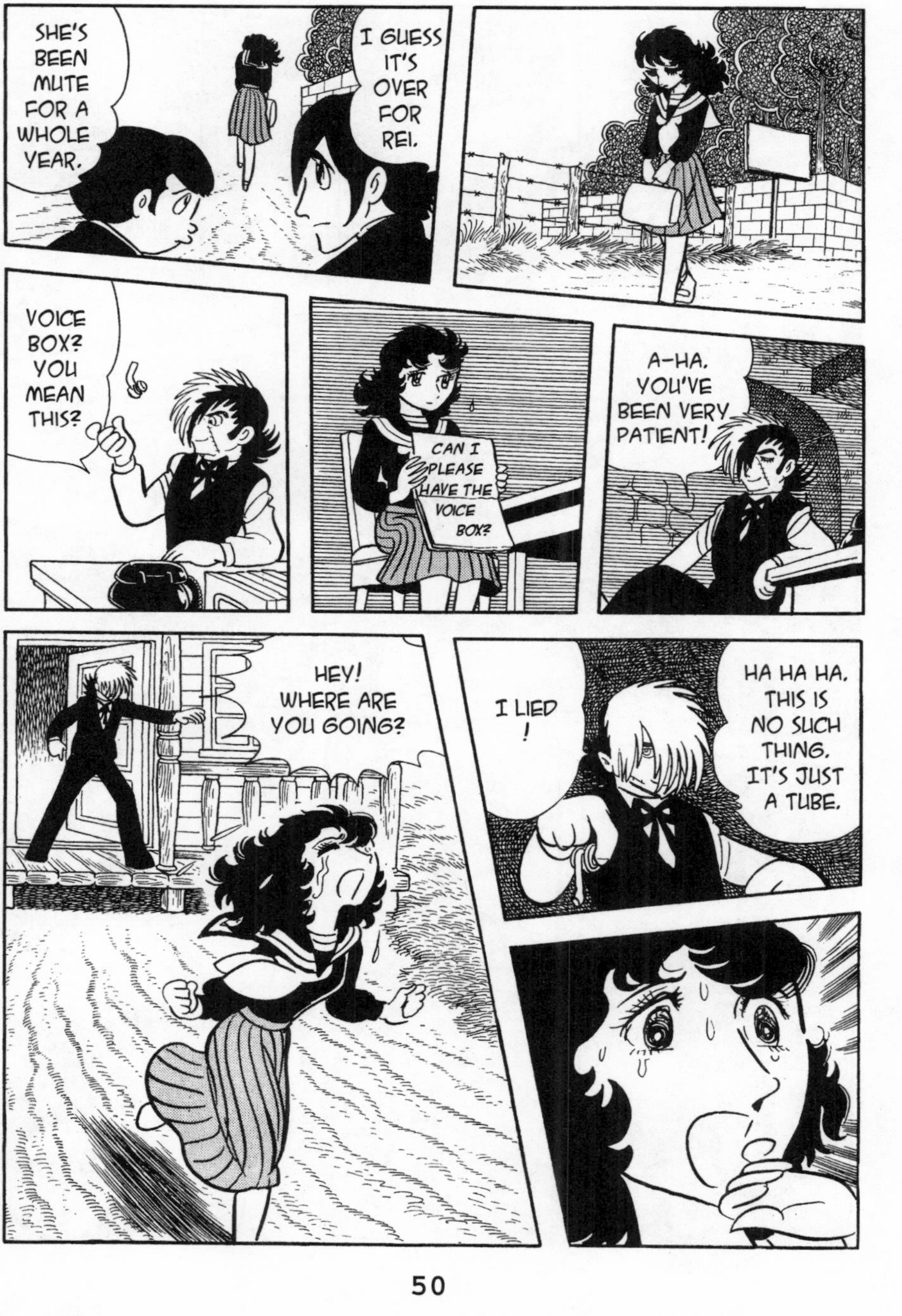
I GUESS IT'S OVER FOR REI.
SHE'S BEEN MUTE FOR A WHOLE YEAR.
A-HA. YOU'VE BEEN VERY PATIENT!
CAN I PLEASE HAVE THE VOICE BOX?
VOICE BOX? YOU MEAN THIS?
HA HA HA. THIS IS NO SUCH THING. IT'S JUST A TUBE.
I LIED!
HEY! WHERE ARE YOU GOING?

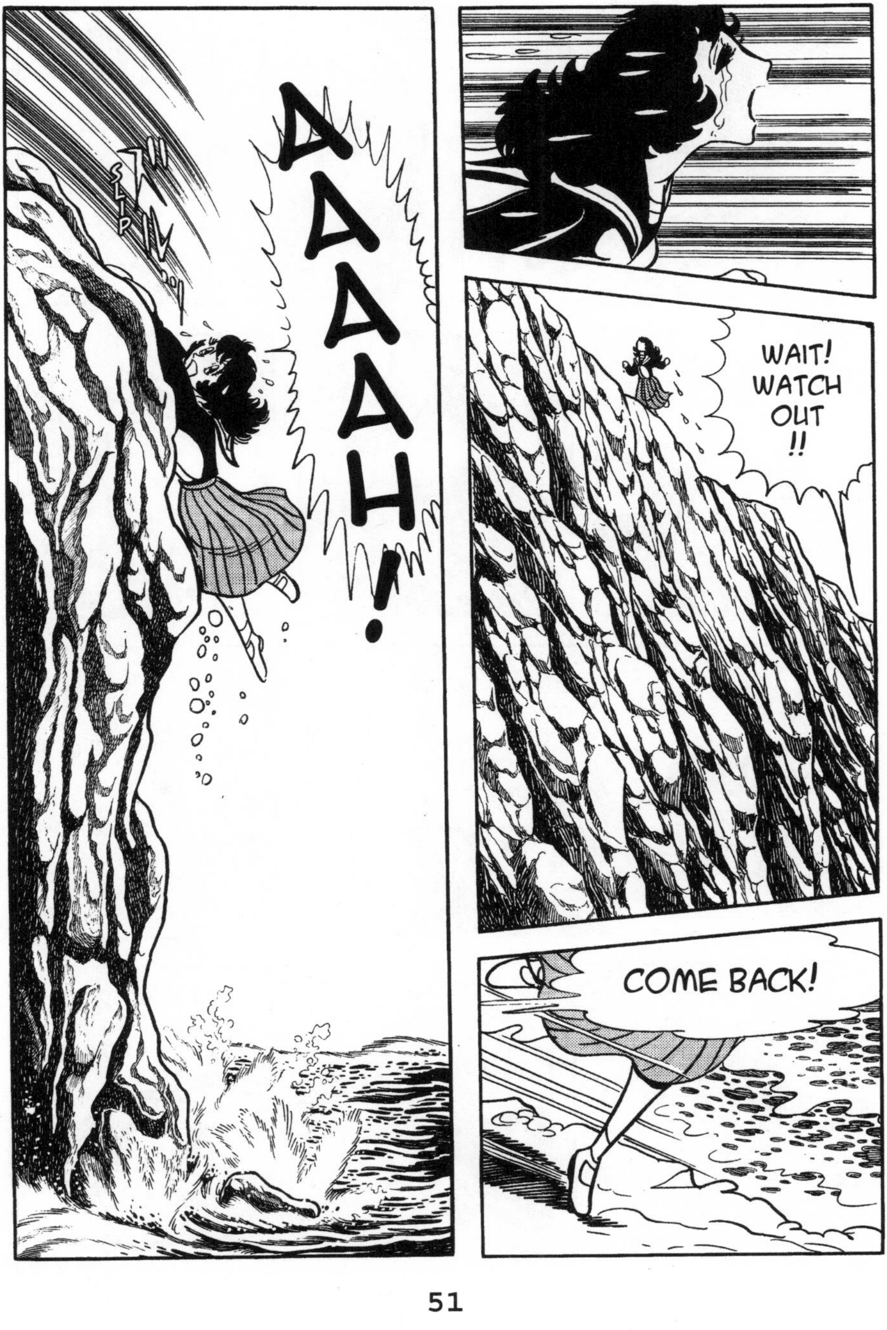
WAIT! WATCH OUT !!
COME BACK!
SLIP
AAAAH!

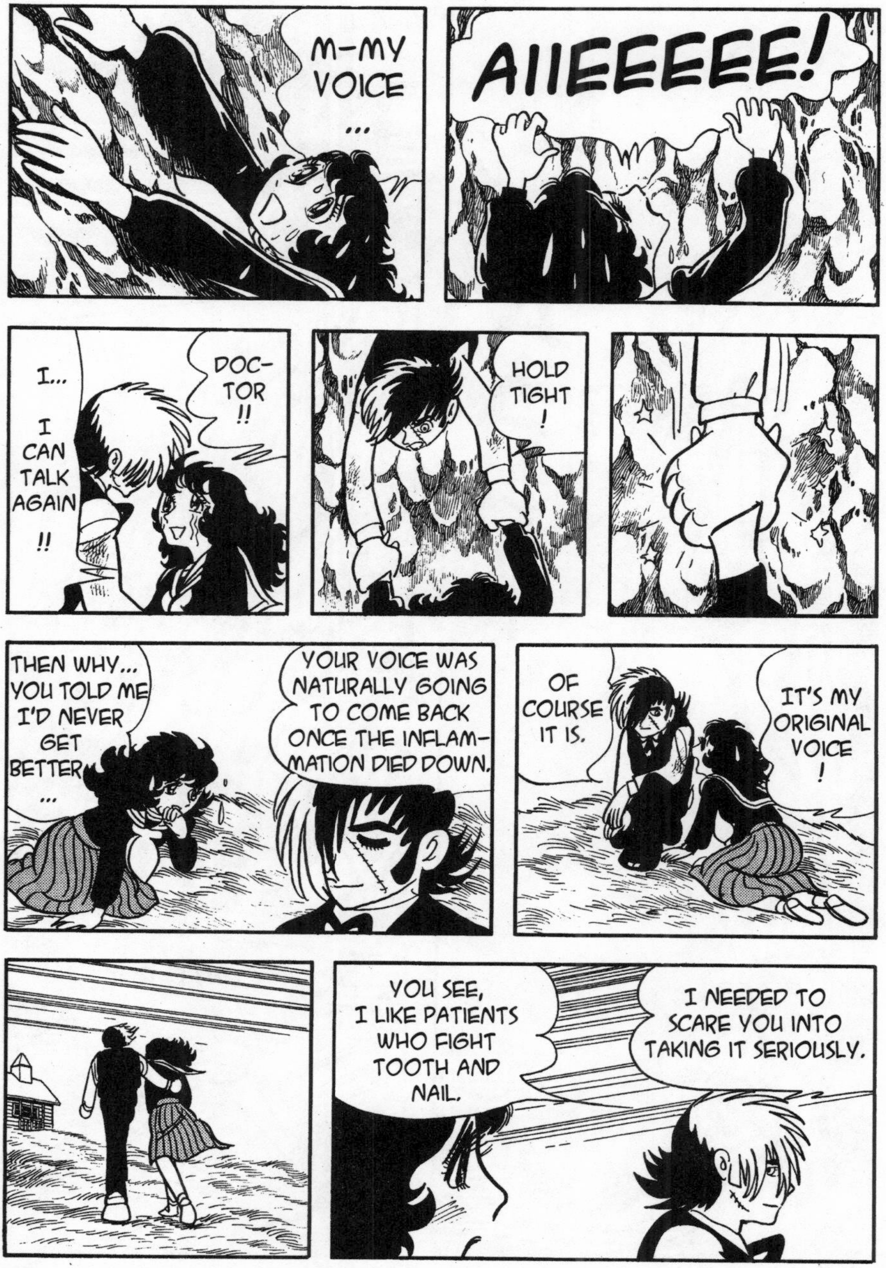
AIIEEEEE!
M-MY VOICE ...
HOLD TIGHT !
DOC-TOR !!
I... I CAN TALK AGAIN !!
IT'S MY ORIGINAL VOICE !
OF COURSE IT IS.
YOUR VOICE WAS NATURALLY GOING TO COME BACK ONCE THE INFLAM-MATION DIED DOWN.
THEN WHY... YOU TOLD ME I'D NEVER GET BETTER ...
I NEEDED TO SCARE YOU INTO TAKING IT SERIOUSLY.
YOU SEE, I LIKE PATIENTS WHO FIGHT TOOTH AND NAIL.

DRIFTER IN A GHOST TOWN

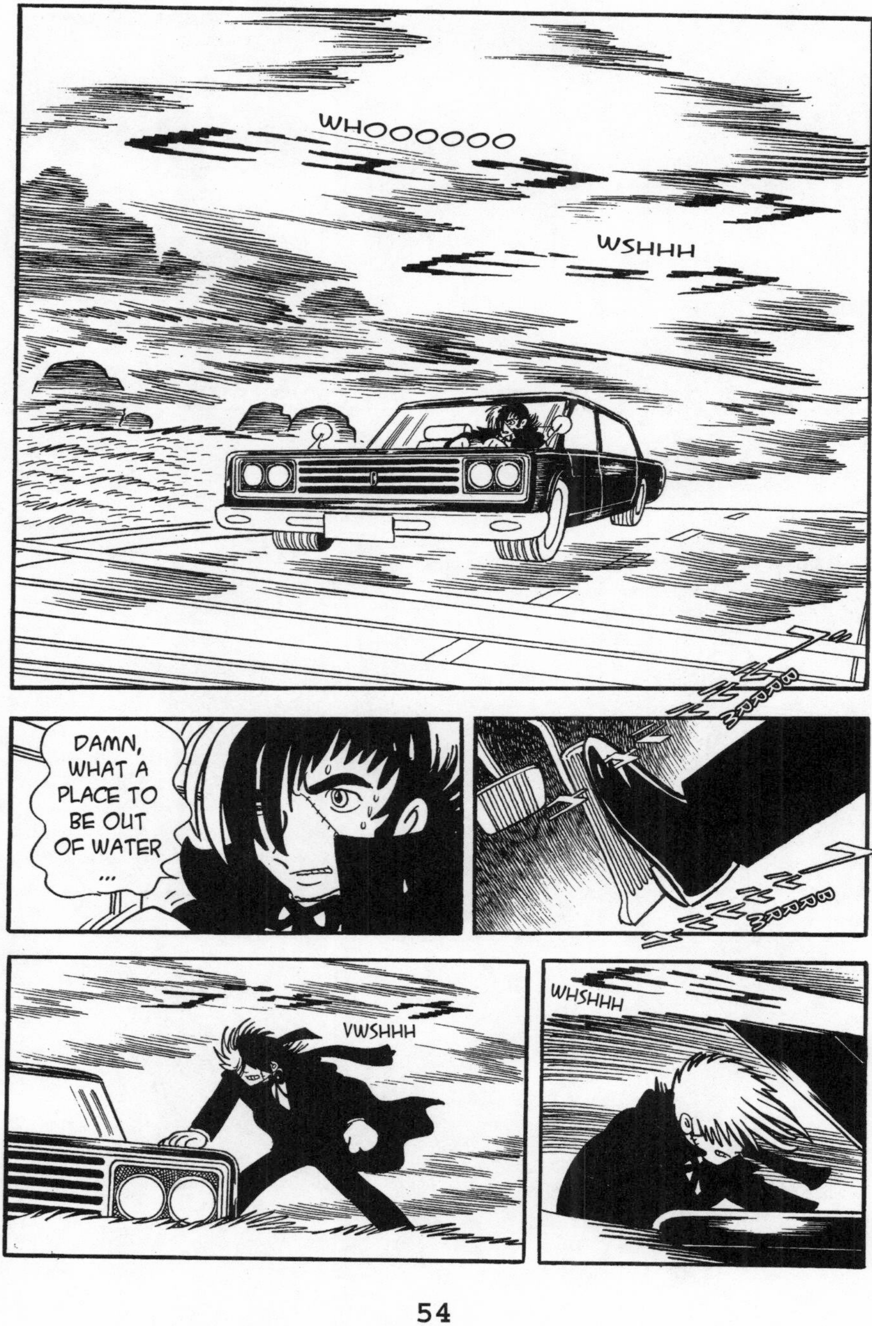
WHOOOOOO
WSHHH
BRRRRR
BRRRRR
DAMN, WHAT A PLACE TO BE OUT OF WATER ...
WHSHHH
VWSHHH

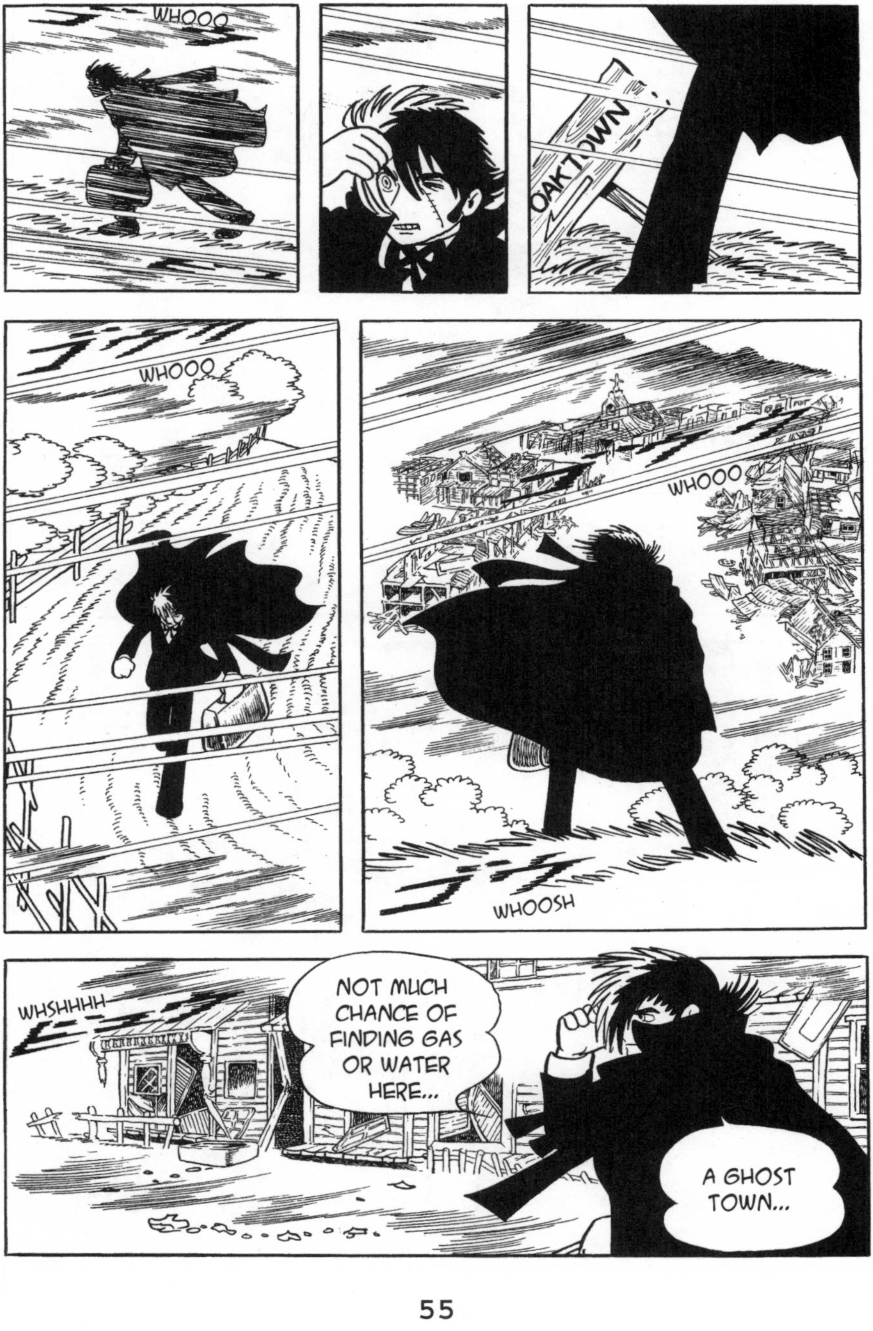
OAKTOWN
WHOOO
WHOOO
WHOOSH
WHOOO
A GHOST TOWN...
NOT MUCH CHANCE OF FINDING GAS OR WATER HERE...
WHSHHHH

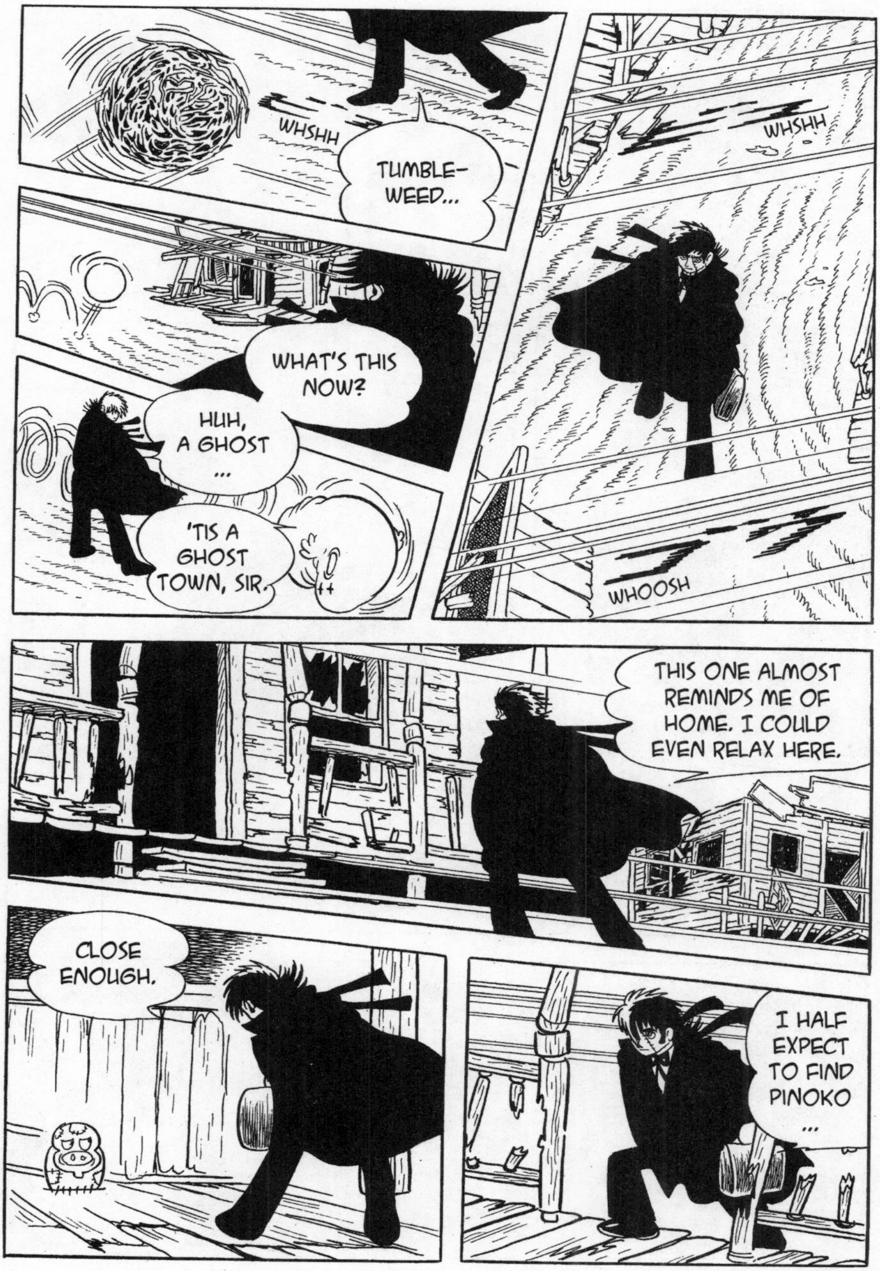
WHSHH
WHOOSH
WHSHH
TUMBLE-WEED...
WHAT'S THIS NOW?
HUH, A GHOST ...
'TIS A GHOST TOWN, SIR.
THIS ONE ALMOST REMINDS ME OF HOME. I COULD EVEN RELAX HERE.
I HALF EXPECT TO FIND PINOKO ...
CLOSE ENOUGH.

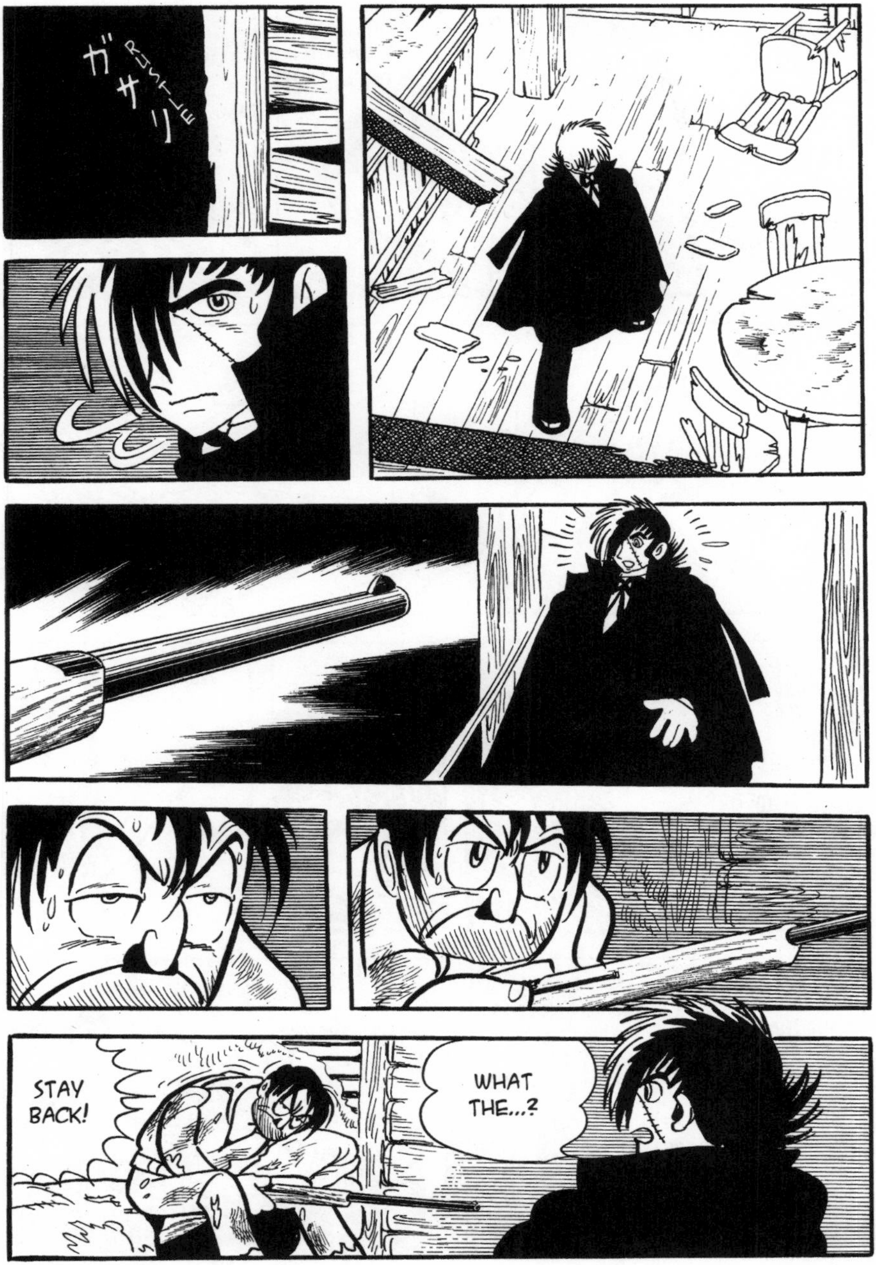
ガサリ
RUSTLE
WHAT THE...?
STAY BACK!

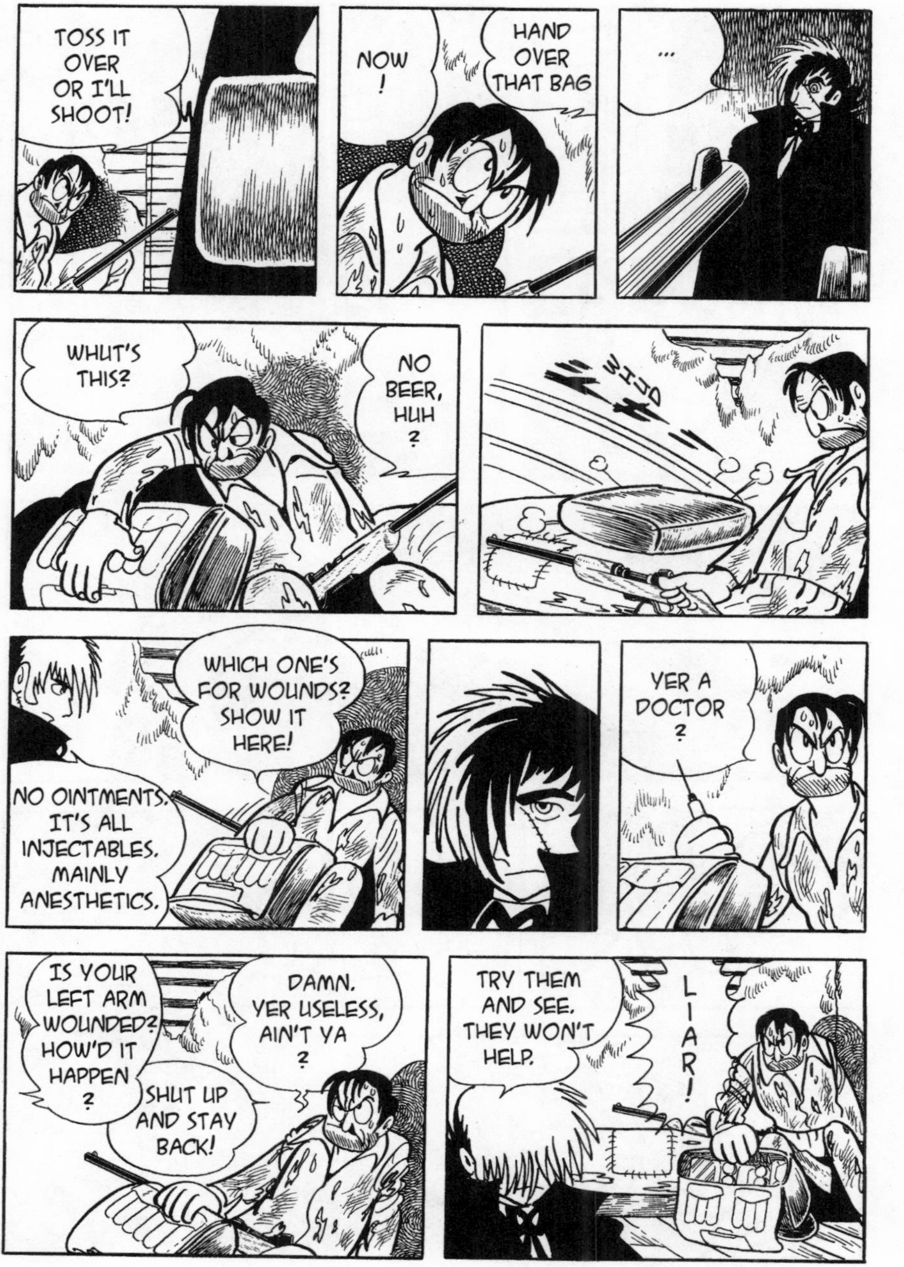
...
HAND OVER THAT BAG
NOW!
TOSS IT OVER OR I'LL SHOOT!
NO BEER, HUH?
WHUT'S THIS?
YER A DOCTOR?
WHICH ONE'S FOR WOUNDS? SHOW IT HERE!
NO OINTMENTS. IT'S ALL INJECTABLES. MAINLY ANESTHETICS.
LIAR!
TRY THEM AND SEE. THEY WON'T HELP.
DAMN. YER USELESS, AIN'T YA?
IS YOUR LEFT ARM WOUNDED? HOW'D IT HAPPEN?
SHUT UP AND STAY BACK!

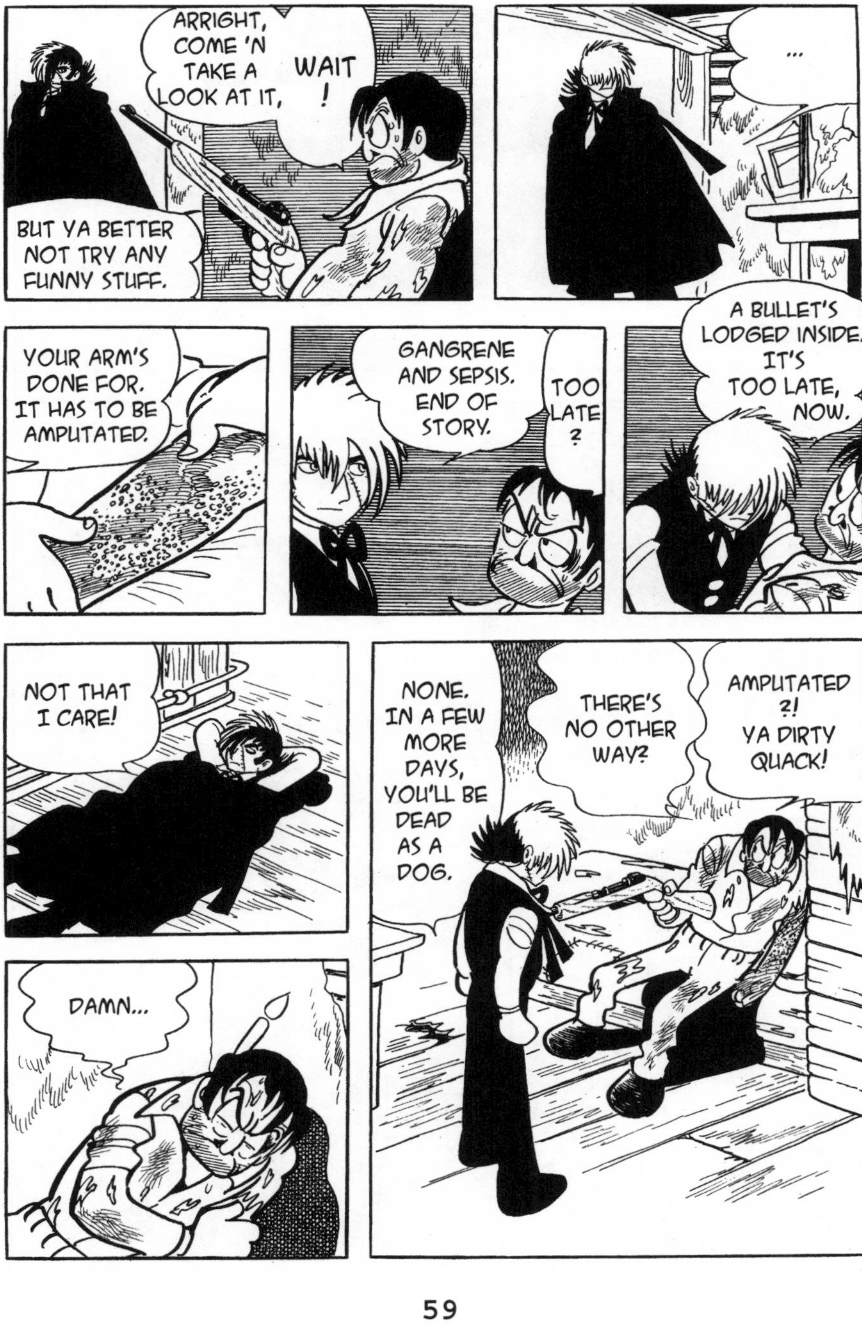
...
WAIT !
ARRIGHT, COME 'N TAKE A LOOK AT IT,
BUT YA BETTER NOT TRY ANY FUNNY STUFF.
A BULLET'S LODGED INSIDE. IT'S TOO LATE, NOW.
TOO LATE ?
GANGRENE AND SEPSIS. END OF STORY.
YOUR ARM'S DONE FOR. IT HAS TO BE AMPUTATED.
AMPUTATED ?! YA DIRTY QUACK!
THERE'S NO OTHER WAY?
NONE. IN A FEW MORE DAYS, YOU'LL BE DEAD AS A DOG.
NOT THAT I CARE!
DAMN...

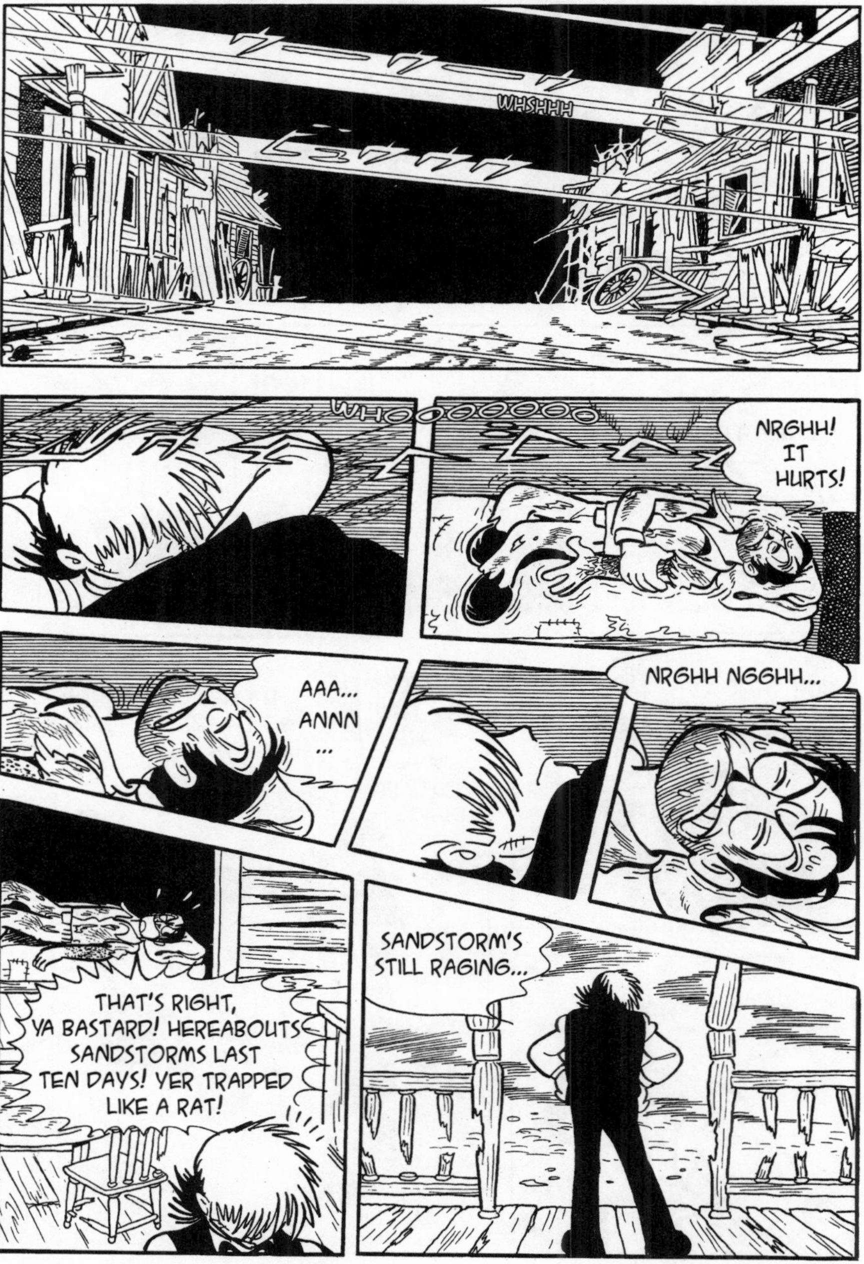
WHSHHH
WHOOOOOOOO
NRGHH! IT HURTS!
NRGHH NGGHH...
AAA... ANNN ...
SANDSTORM'S STILL RAGING...
THAT'S RIGHT, YA BASTARD! HEREABOUTS SANDSTORMS LAST TEN DAYS! YER TRAPPED LIKE A RAT!

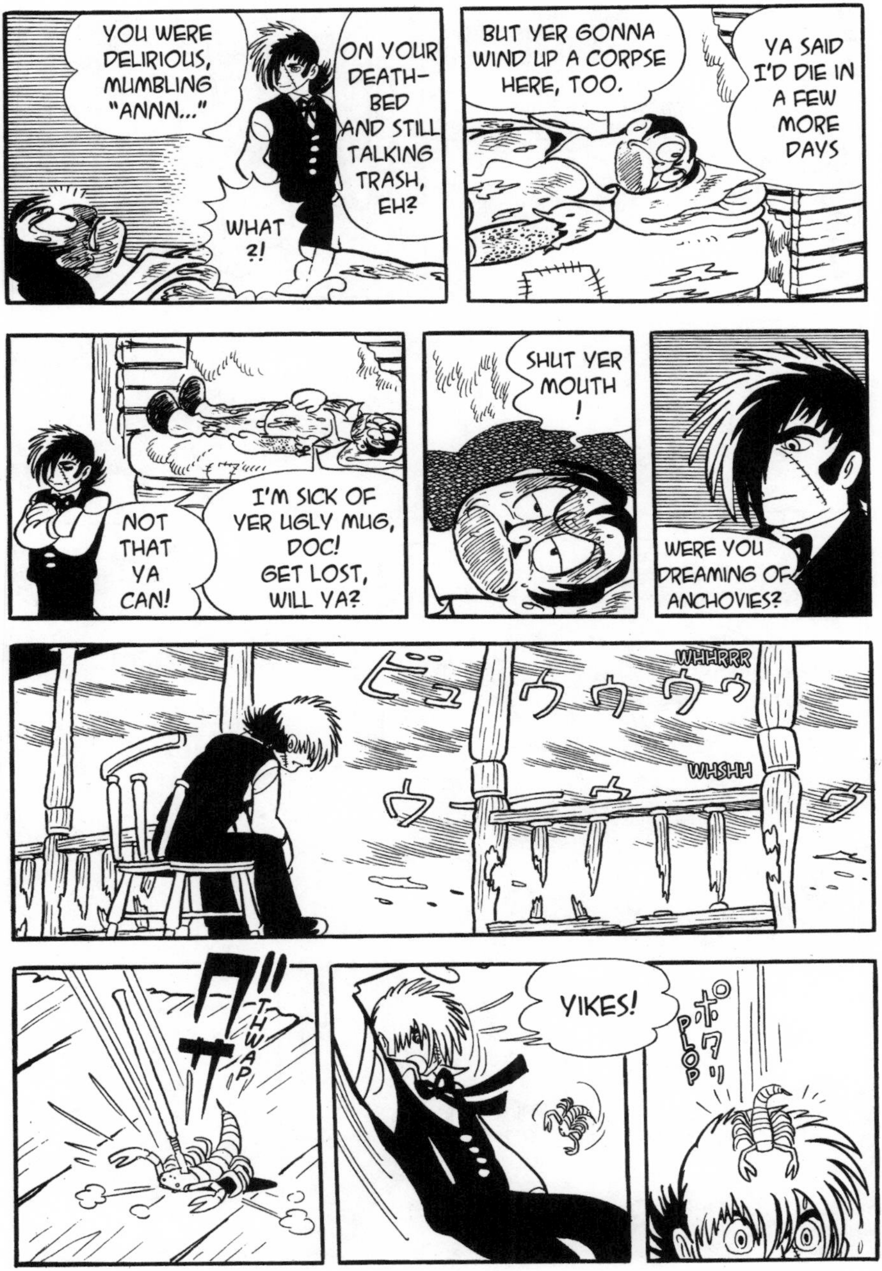
YA SAID I'D DIE IN A FEW MORE DAYS
BUT YER GONNA WIND UP A CORPSE HERE, TOO.
ON YOUR DEATH-BED AND STILL TALKING TRASH, EH?
YOU WERE DELIRIOUS, MUMBLING "ANNN..."
WHAT?!
WERE YOU DREAMING OF ANCHOVIES?
SHUT YER MOUTH!
I'M SICK OF YER UGLY MUG, DOC! GET LOST, WILL YA?
NOT THAT YA CAN!
WHHRRR
ビュウウウウ
WHSHH
YIKES!
ポタリ
PLOP
THWAP

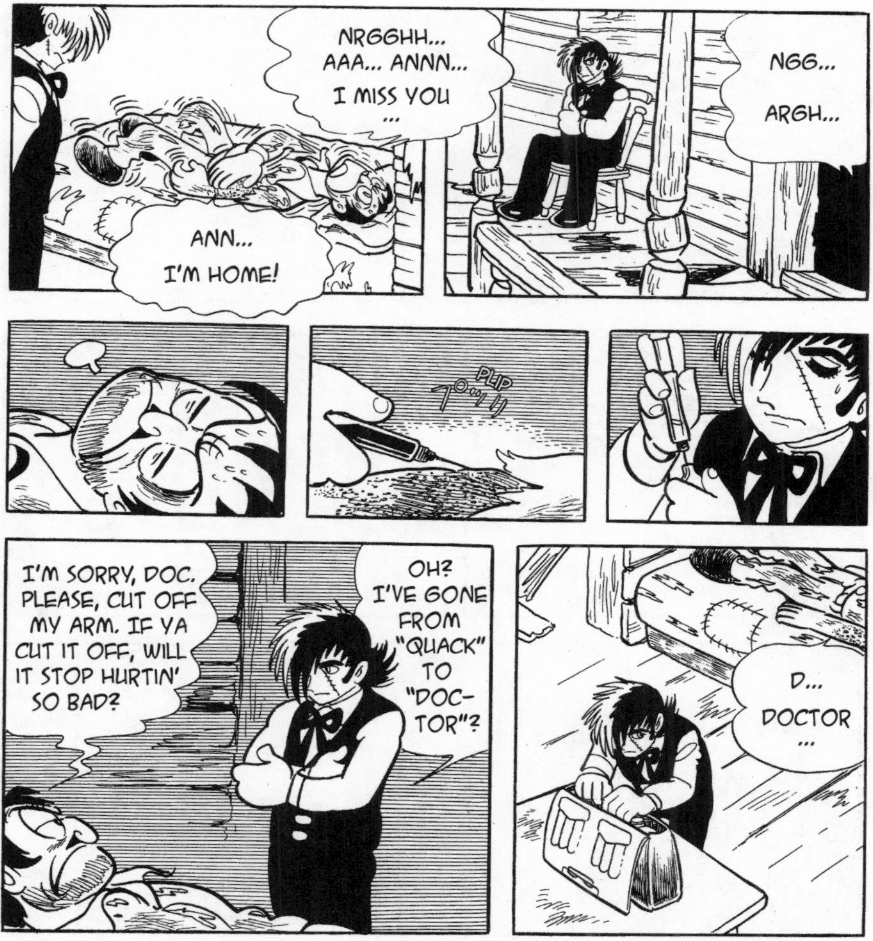
NGG... ARGH...
NRGGHH... AAA... ANNN... I MISS YOU ...
ANN... I'M HOME!
PLIP
D... DOCTOR ...
OH? I'VE GONE FROM "QUACK" TO "DOC-TOR"?
I'M SORRY, DOC. PLEASE, CUT OFF MY ARM. IF YA CUT IT OFF, WILL IT STOP HURTIN' SO BAD?
PLEASE OPERATE ON ME!
NOT ON YOUR LIFE. FOR ONE THING, I DON'T WORK FOR CHEAP!
I-IF YA DO IT, I'LL TELL YA... HOW TO LEAVE THIS TOWN!

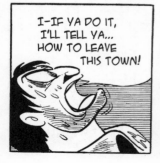

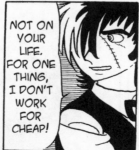

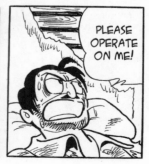

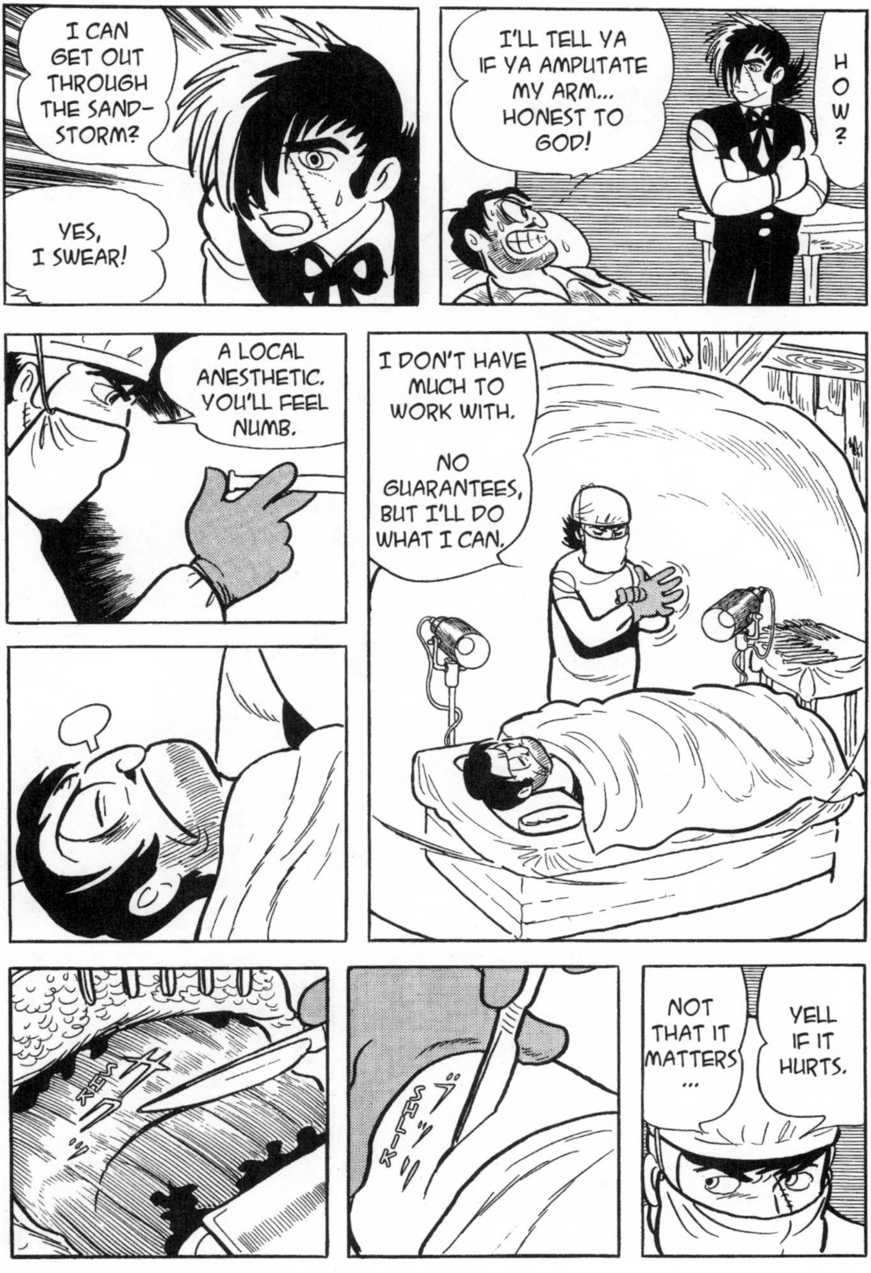
HOW?
I'LL TELL YA IF YA AMPUTATE MY ARM... HONEST TO GOD!
I CAN GET OUT THROUGH THE SAND-STORM?
YES, I SWEAR!
I DON'T HAVE MUCH TO WORK WITH.
NO GUARANTEES, BUT I'LL DO WHAT I CAN.
A LOCAL ANESTHETIC. YOU'LL FEEL NUMB.
YELL IF IT HURTS.
NOT THAT IT MATTERS ...

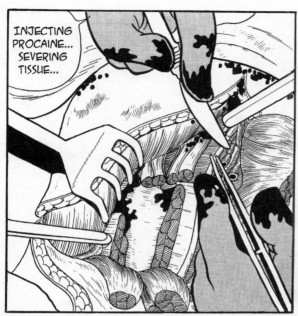

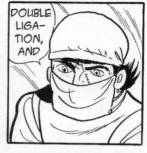

DOUBLE LIGA- TION, AND
ブチリ
SHIK
INJECTING PROCAINE... SEVERING TISSUE...
FINISHED.
WANT TO SEE YOUR SEVERED ARM?
HEH HEH. HE PASSED OUT.

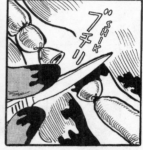

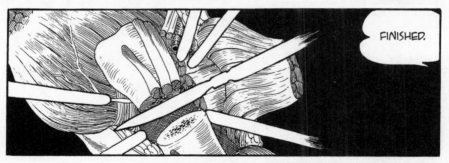

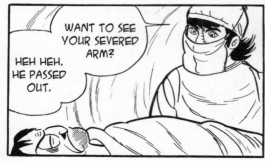

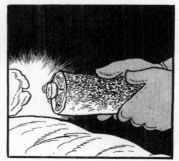

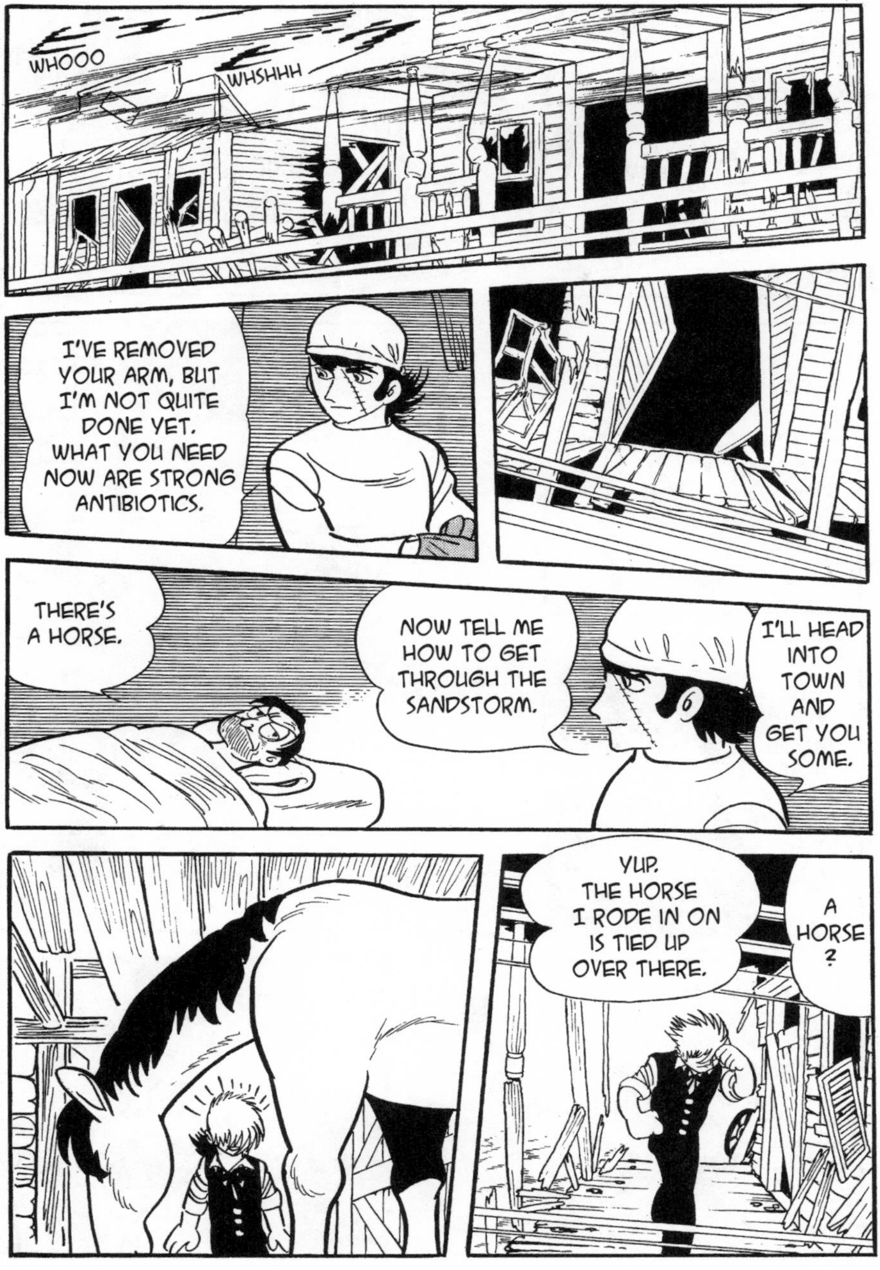
WHOOO
WHSHHH
I'VE REMOVED YOUR ARM, BUT I'M NOT QUITE DONE YET. WHAT YOU NEED NOW ARE STRONG ANTIBIOTICS.
I'LL HEAD INTO TOWN AND GET YOU SOME.
NOW TELL ME HOW TO GET THROUGH THE SANDSTORM.
THERE'S A HORSE.
A HORSE?
YUP. THE HORSE I RODE IN ON IS TIED UP OVER THERE.

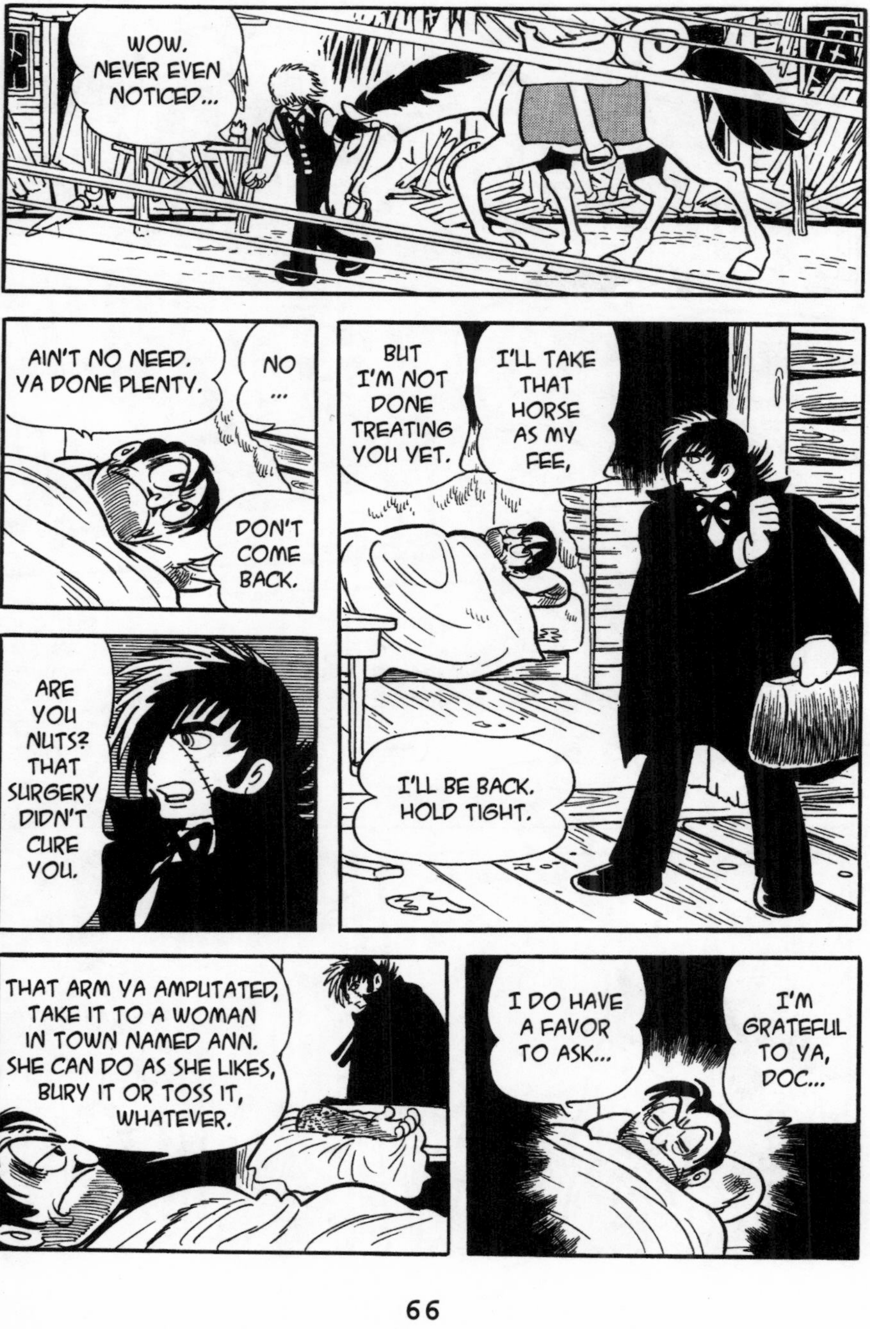
WOW. NEVER EVEN NOTICED...
I'LL TAKE THAT HORSE AS MY FEE,
BUT I'M NOT DONE TREATING YOU YET.
I'LL BE BACK. HOLD TIGHT.
NO ...
AIN'T NO NEED. YA DONE PLENTY.
DON'T COME BACK.
ARE YOU NUTS? THAT SURGERY DIDN'T CURE YOU.
I'M GRATEFUL TO YA, DOC...
I DO HAVE A FAVOR TO ASK...
THAT ARM YA AMPUTATED, TAKE IT TO A WOMAN IN TOWN NAMED ANN. SHE CAN DO AS SHE LIKES, BURY IT OR TOSS IT, WHATEVER.

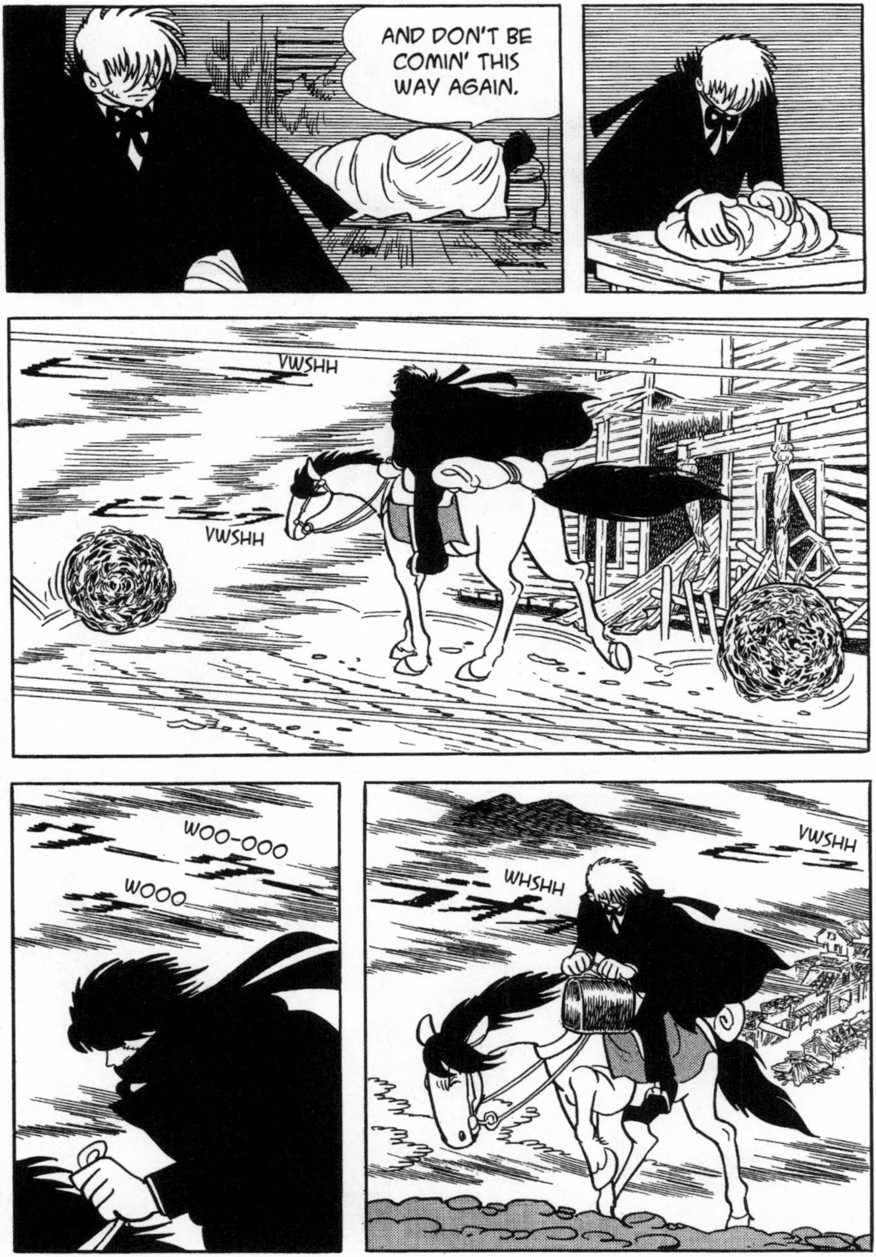
AND DON'T BE COMIN' THIS WAY AGAIN.
VWSHH
VWSHH
VWSHH
WHSHH
WOO-OOO
WOOO

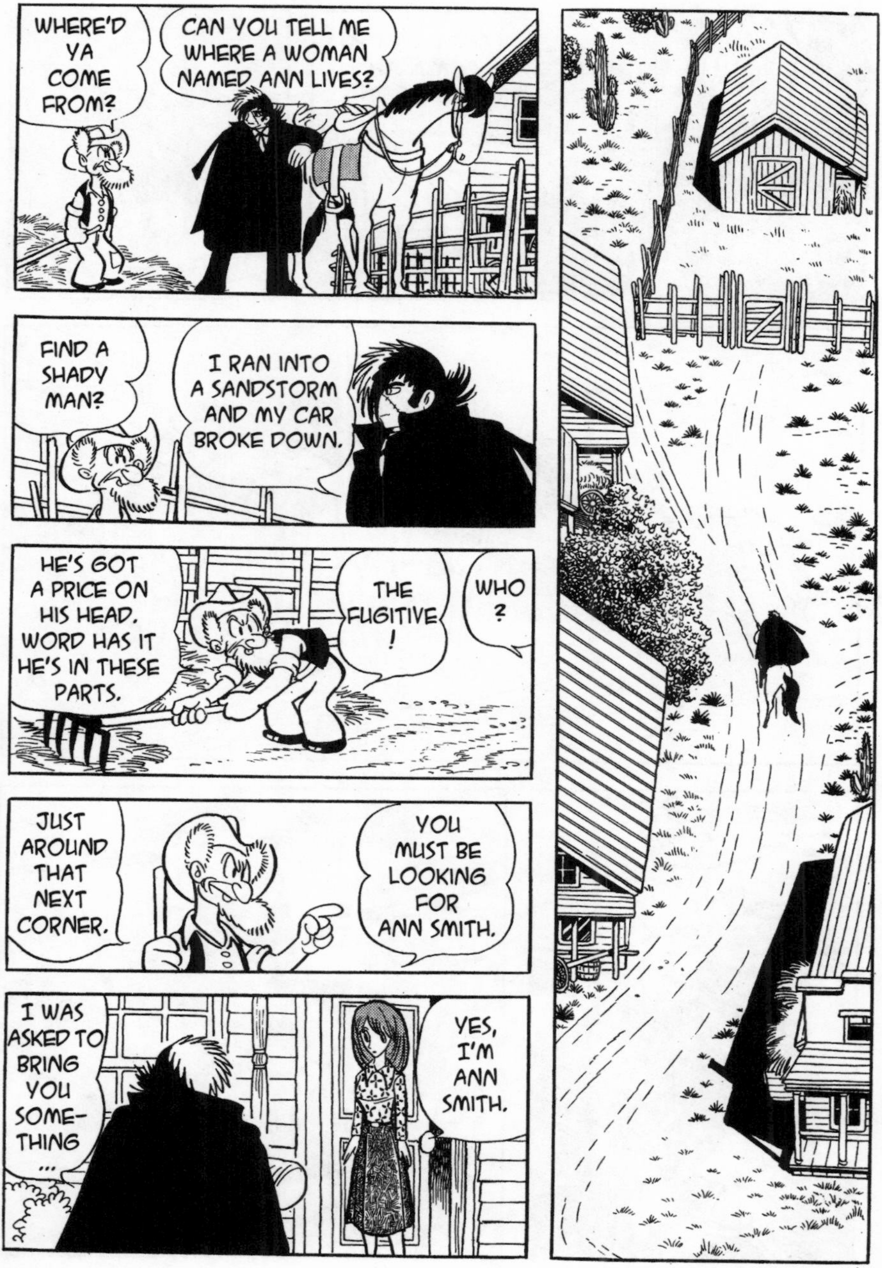
CAN YOU TELL ME WHERE A WOMAN NAMED ANN LIVES?
WHERE'D YA COME FROM?
I RAN INTO A SANDSTORM AND MY CAR BROKE DOWN.
FIND A SHADY MAN?
WHO?
THE FUGITIVE!
HE'S GOT A PRICE ON HIS HEAD. WORD HAS IT HE'S IN THESE PARTS.
YOU MUST BE LOOKING FOR ANN SMITH.
JUST AROUND THAT NEXT CORNER.
YES, I'M ANN SMITH.
I WAS ASKED TO BRING YOU SOME-THING ...

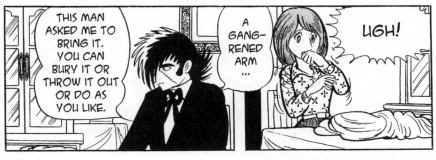

UGH!
A GANG-RENED ARM ...
THIS MAN ASKED ME TO BRING IT. YOU CAN BURY IT OR THROW IT OUT OR DO AS YOU LIKE.
...
THERE'S A LARGE MOLE ON THE UPPER ARM.
IT'S... IT'S TOM'S ...
HE WAS MY SWEETHEART, FIFTEEN YEARS AGO.
WE WERE ENGAGED. BUT HE HAD TO GO AWAY TO FIGHT IN THE WAR. HE... KILLED SOMEONE IN A TOWN THERE AND WAS SENTENCED TO LIFE IN PRISON.
APPARENTLY, HE ESCAPED.
YES. SO I HEAR. AND NOW HE'S A WANTED MAN.
HE WAS SHOT. THE WOUND FESTERED AND NEARLY KILLED HIM.

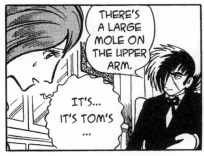

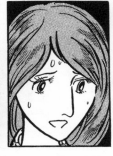

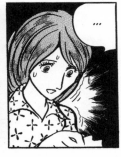

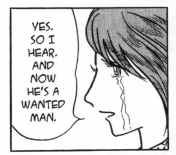

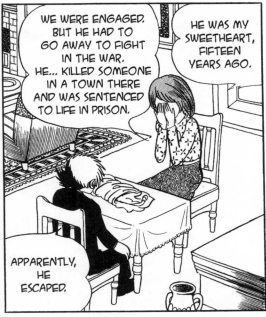

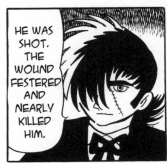

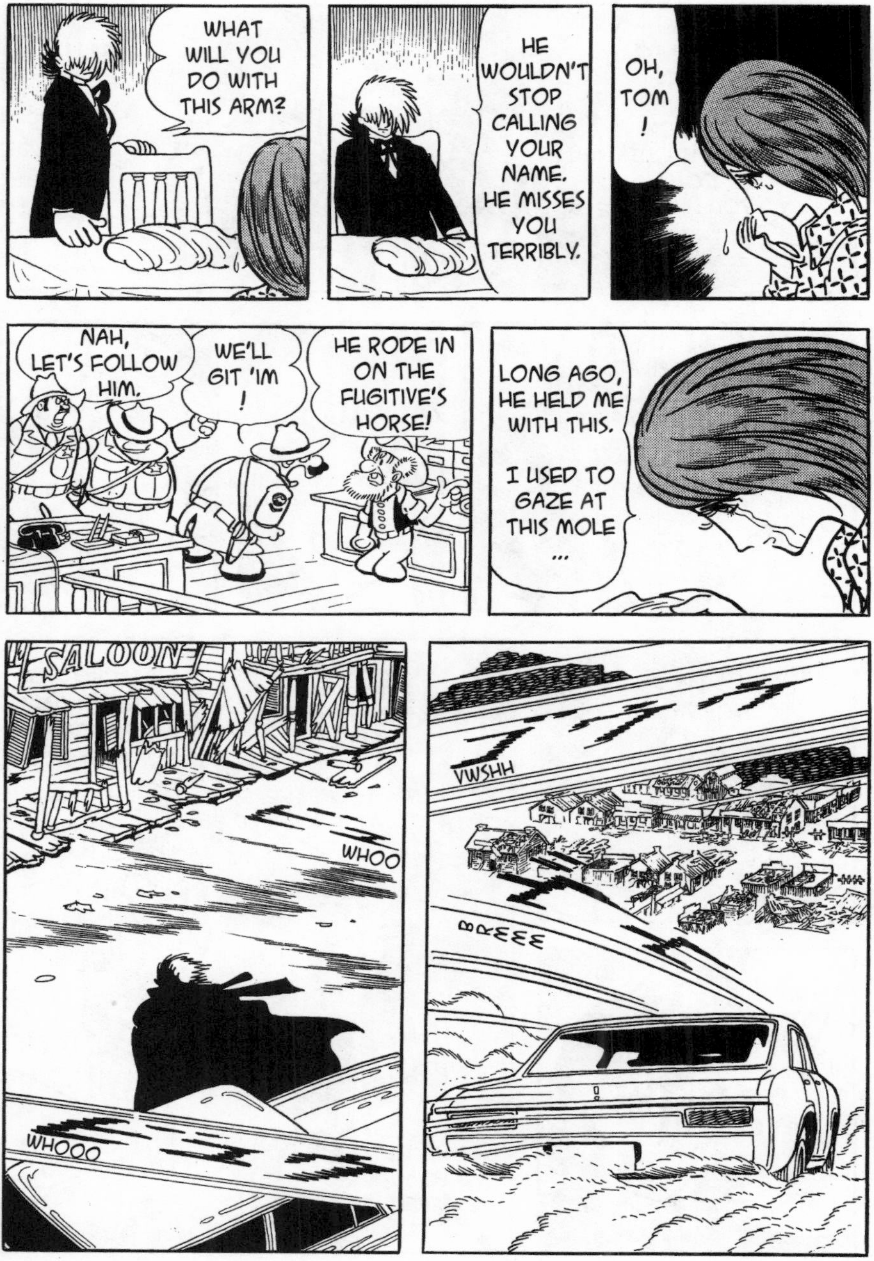
OH, TOM !
HE WOULDN'T STOP CALLING YOUR NAME. HE MISSES YOU TERRIBLY.
WHAT WILL YOU DO WITH THIS ARM?
LONG AGO, HE HELD ME WITH THIS.
I USED TO GAZE AT THIS MOLE ...
HE RODE IN ON THE FUGITIVE'S HORSE!
WE'LL GIT 'IM !
NAH, LET'S FOLLOW HIM.
VWSHH
BREEE
SALOON
WHOO
WHOOO

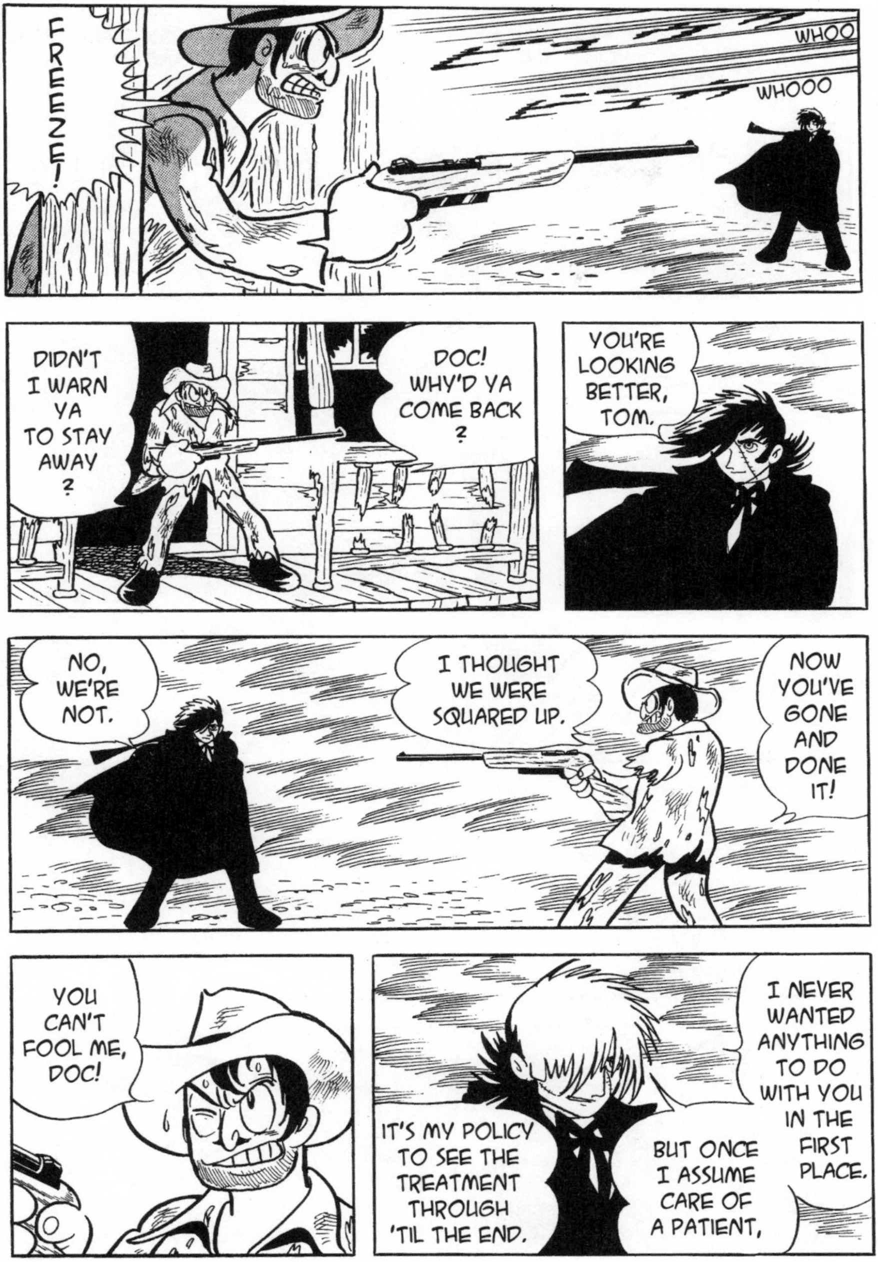
WHOO
WHOOO
FREEZE!
YOU'RE LOOKING BETTER, TOM.
DOC! WHY'D YA COME BACK ?
DIDN'T I WARN YA TO STAY AWAY ?
NOW YOU'VE GONE AND DONE IT!
I THOUGHT WE WERE SQUARED UP.
NO, WE'RE NOT.
I NEVER WANTED ANYTHING TO DO WITH YOU IN THE FIRST PLACE.
BUT ONCE I ASSUME CARE OF A PATIENT,
IT'S MY POLICY TO SEE THE TREATMENT THROUGH 'TIL THE END.
YOU CAN'T FOOL ME, DOC!

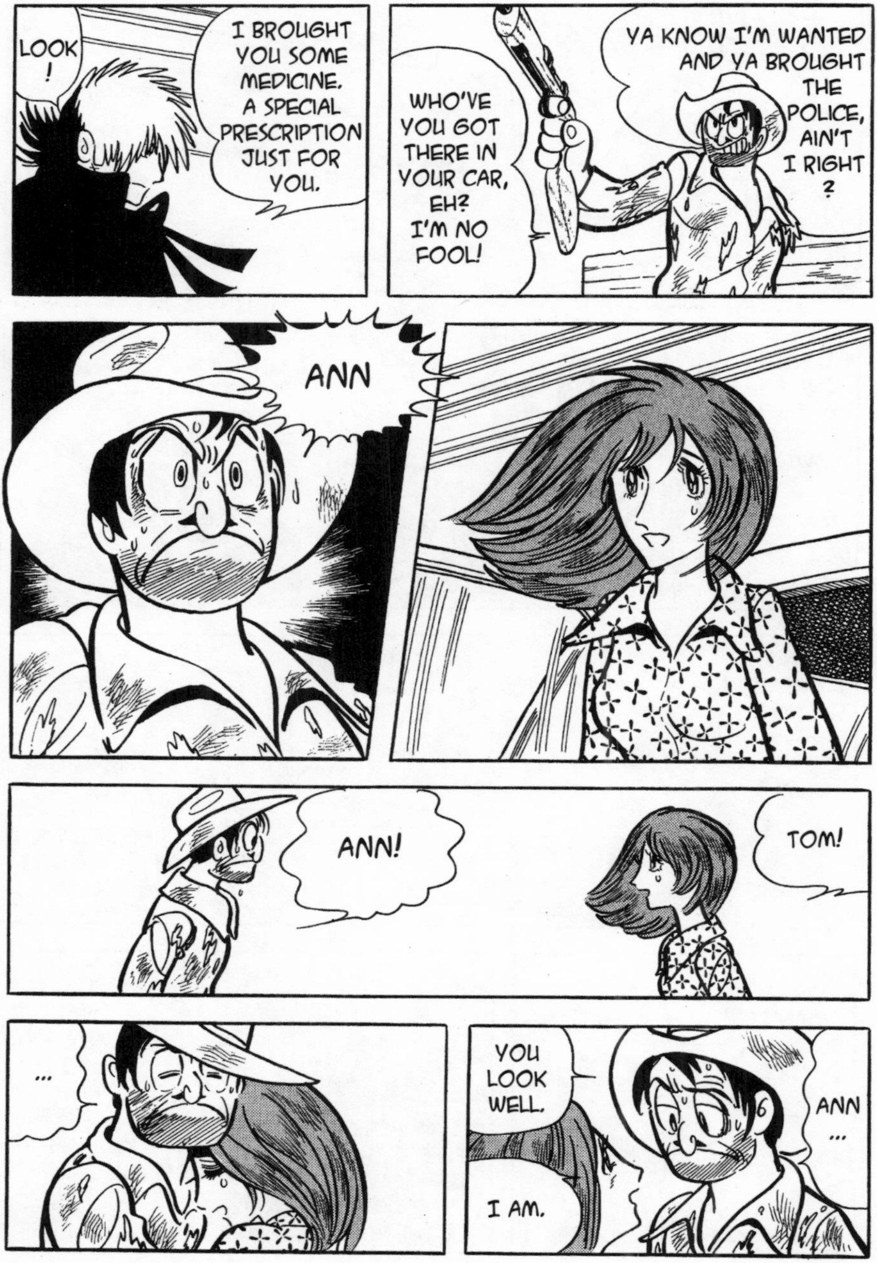

YA KNOW I'M WANTED AND YA BROUGHT THE POLICE, AIN'T I RIGHT?
WHO'VE YOU GOT THERE IN YOUR CAR, EH? I'M NO FOOL!
I BROUGHT YOU SOME MEDICINE. A SPECIAL PRESCRIPTION JUST FOR YOU.
LOOK!
ANN
TOM!
ANN!
ANN ...
YOU LOOK WELL.
I AM.
...

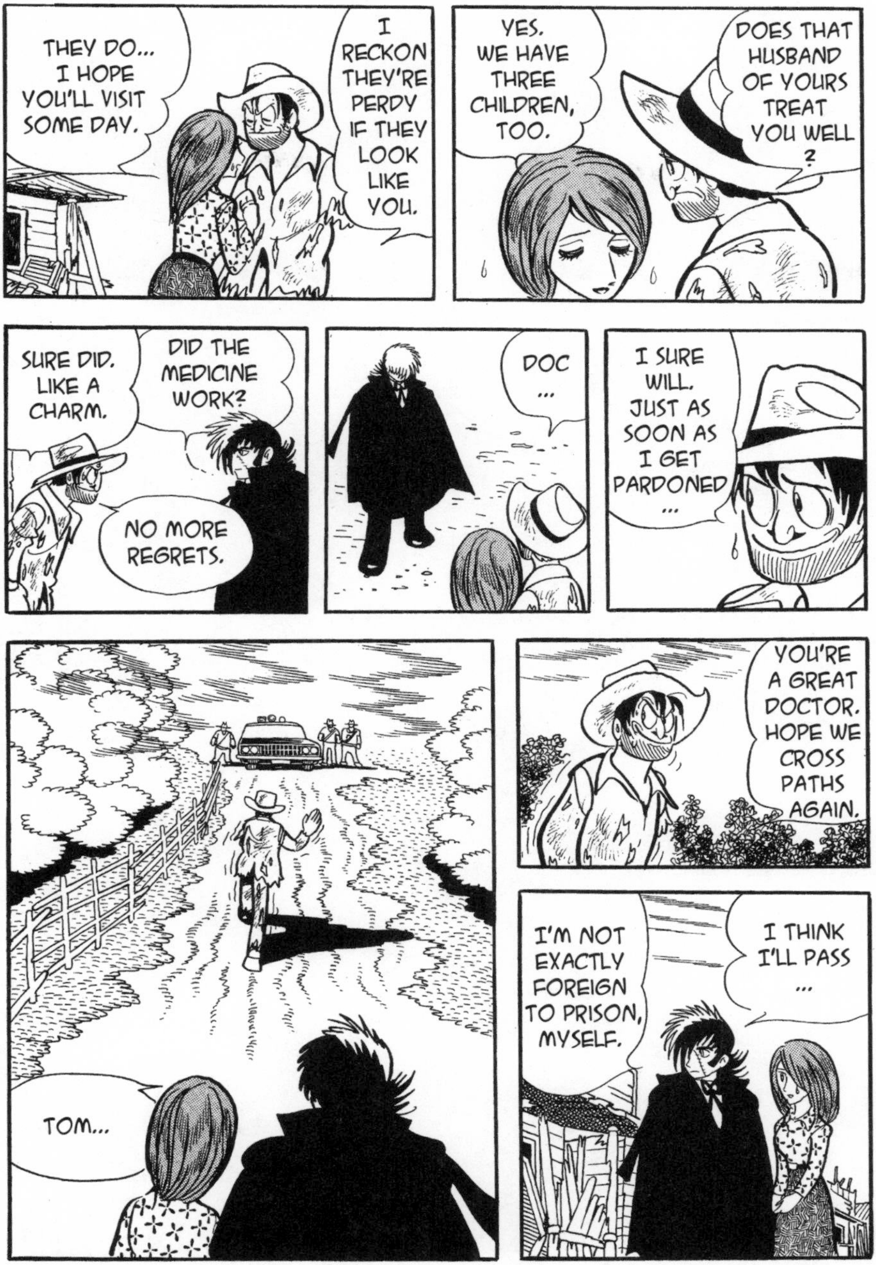
DOES THAT HUSBAND OF YOURS TREAT YOU WELL?
YES. WE HAVE THREE CHILDREN, TOO.
I RECKON THEY'RE PERDY IF THEY LOOK LIKE YOU.
THEY DO... I HOPE YOU'LL VISIT SOME DAY.
I SURE WILL. JUST AS SOON AS I GET PARDONED ...
DOC ...
DID THE MEDICINE WORK?
SURE DID. LIKE A CHARM.
NO MORE REGRETS.
YOU'RE A GREAT DOCTOR. HOPE WE CROSS PATHS AGAIN.
I THINK I'LL PASS ...
I'M NOT EXACTLY FOREIGN TO PRISON, MYSELF.
TOM...

PINOKO LOVE STORY

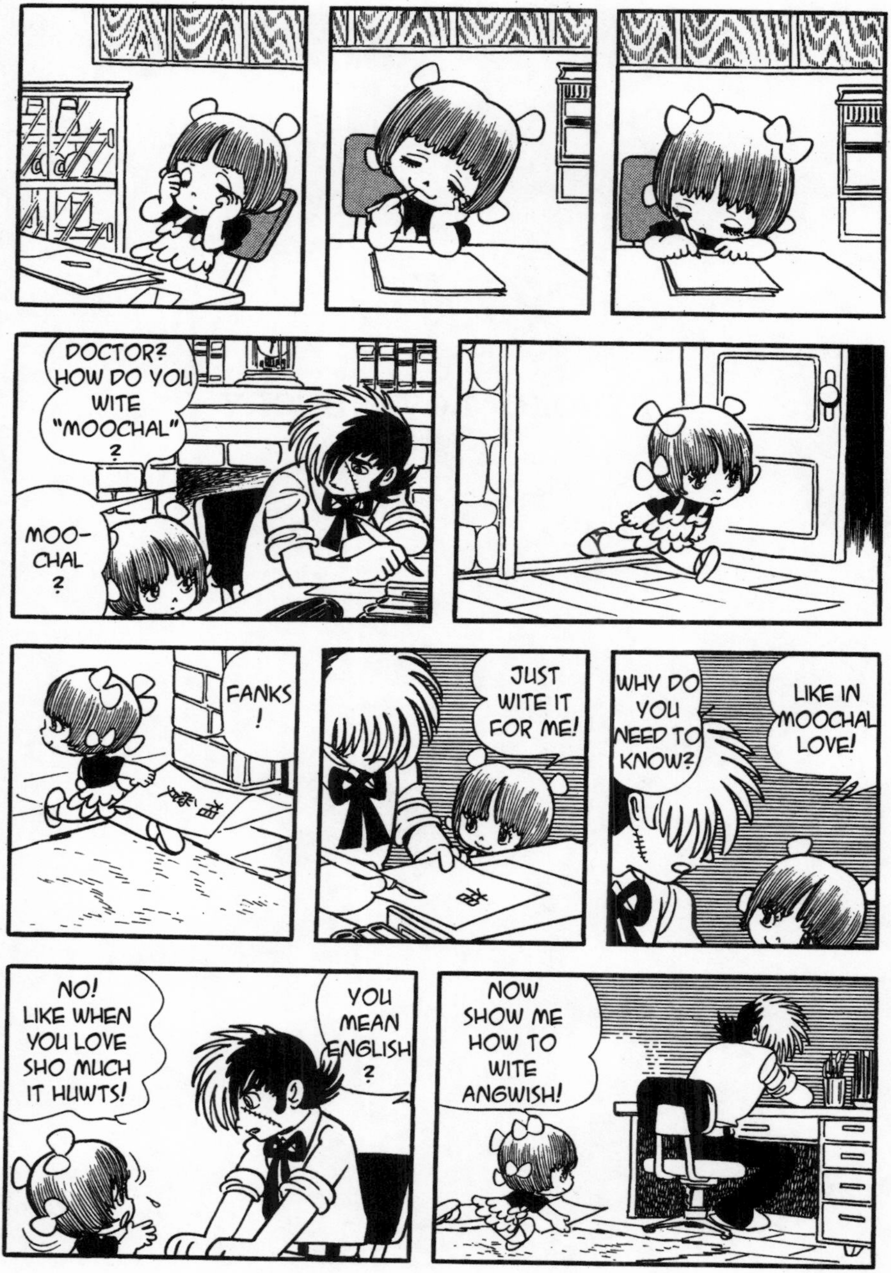
DOCTOR? HOW DO YOU WITE "MOOCHAL" ?
MOO-CHAL ?
WHY DO YOU NEED TO KNOW?
LIKE IN MOOCHAL LOVE!
JUST WITE IT FOR ME!
FANKS !
NOW SHOW ME HOW TO WITE ANGWISH!
YOU MEAN ENGLISH ?
NO! LIKE WHEN YOU LOVE SHO MUCH IT HUWTS!

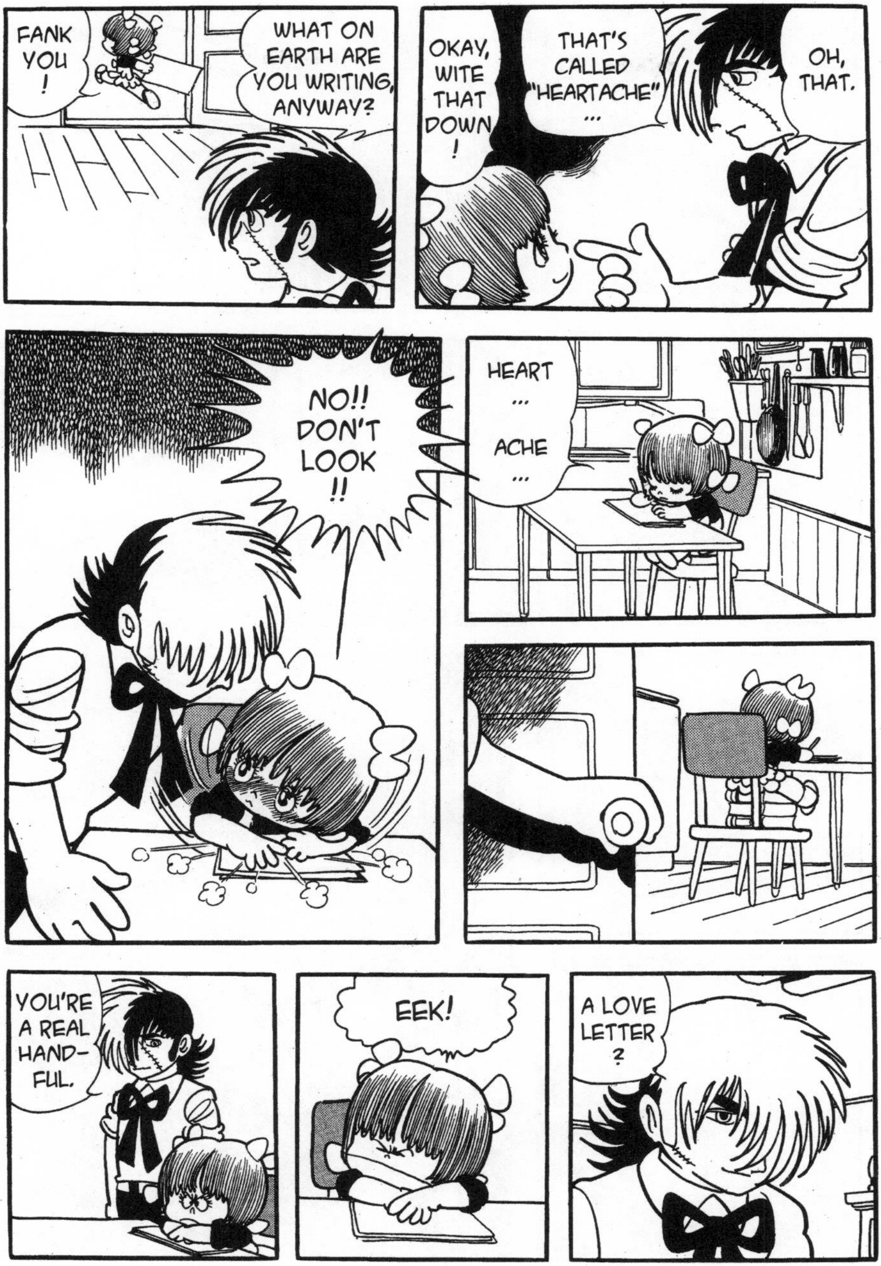
OH, THAT.
THAT'S CALLED "HEARTACHE" ...
OKAY, WITE THAT DOWN!
WHAT ON EARTH ARE YOU WRITING, ANYWAY?
FANK YOU!
HEART ... ACHE ...
NO!! DON'T LOOK !!
A LOVE LETTER?
EEK!
YOU'RE A REAL HAND-FUL.

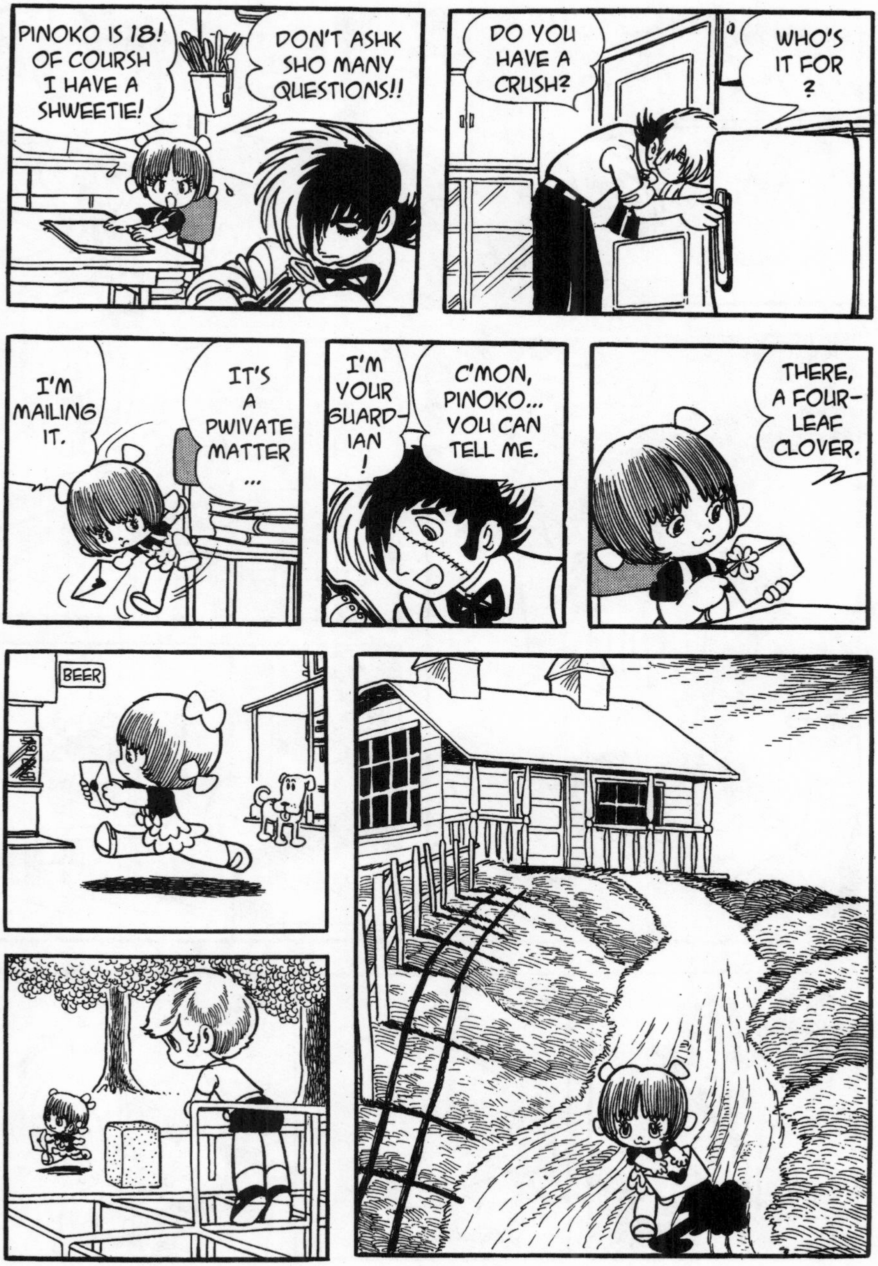
WHO'S IT FOR ?
DO YOU HAVE A CRUSH?
DON'T ASHK SHO MANY QUESTIONS!!
PINOKO IS 18! OF COURSH I HAVE A SHWEETIE!
THERE, A FOUR-LEAF CLOVER.
C'MON, PINOKO... YOU CAN TELL ME.
I'M YOUR GUARD-IAN!
IT'S A PWIVATE MATTER...
I'M MAILING IT.
BEER

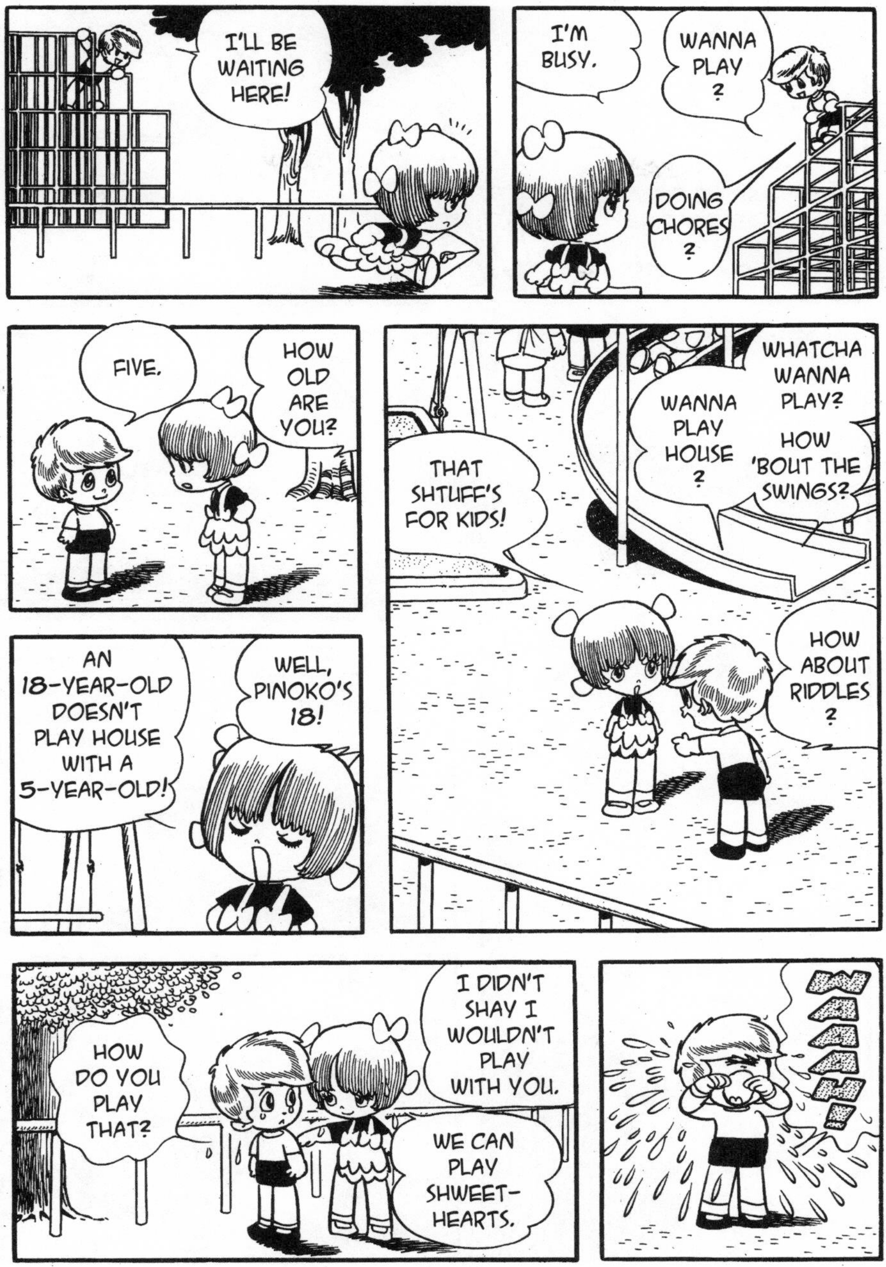
WANNA PLAY ?
I'M BUSY.
DOING CHORES ?
I'LL BE WAITING HERE!
WHATCHA WANNA PLAY?
HOW 'BOUT THE SWINGS?
WANNA PLAY HOUSE ?
THAT SHTUFF'S FOR KIDS!
HOW ABOUT RIDDLES ?
HOW OLD ARE YOU?
FIVE.
WELL, PINOKO'S 18!
AN 18-YEAR-OLD DOESN'T PLAY HOUSE WITH A 5-YEAR-OLD!
WAAAH!
I DIDN'T SHAY I WOULDN'T PLAY WITH YOU.
WE CAN PLAY SHWEET-HEARTS.
HOW DO YOU PLAY THAT?

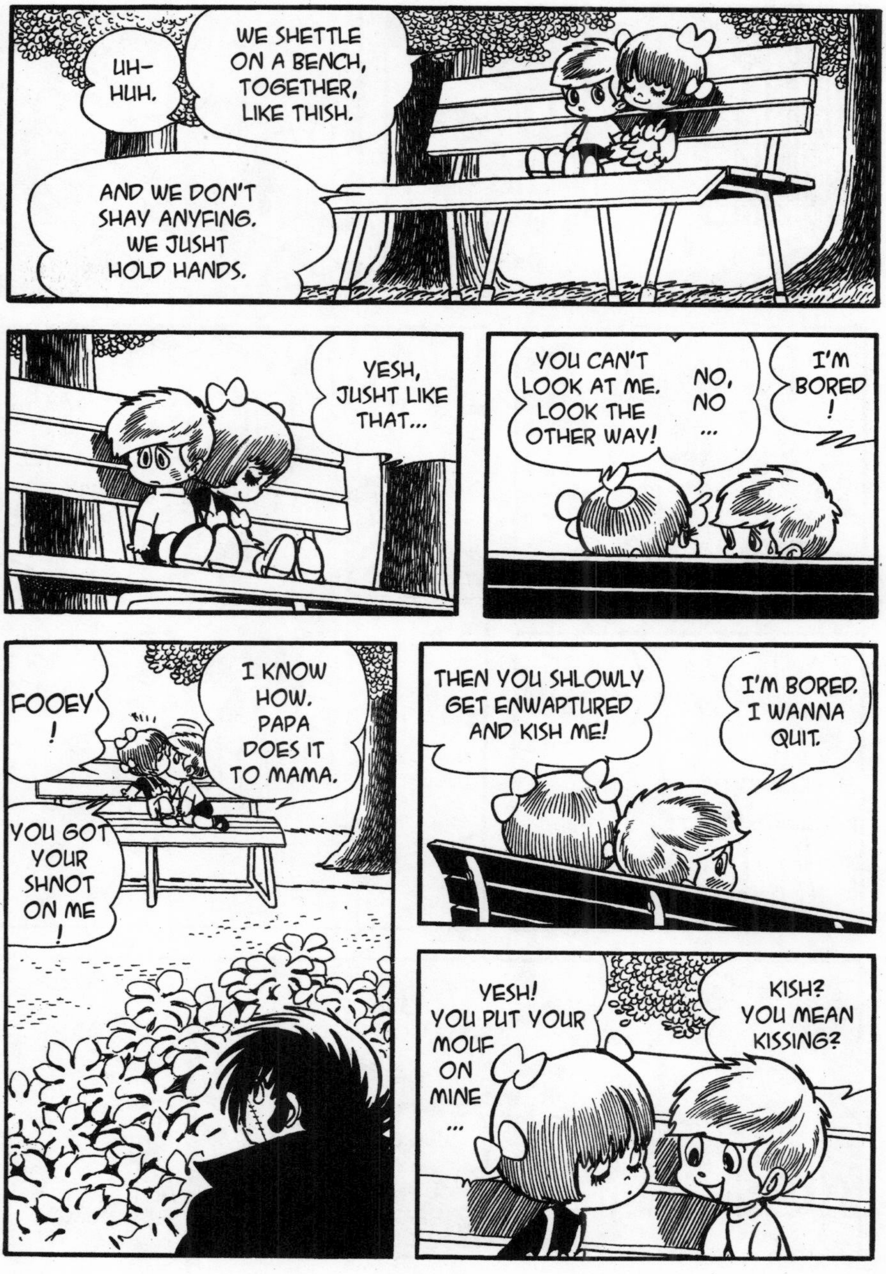
WE SHETTLE ON A BENCH, TOGETHER, LIKE THISH.
UH-HUH.
AND WE DON'T SHAY ANYFING. WE JUSHT HOLD HANDS.
I'M BORED!
NO, NO ...
YOU CAN'T LOOK AT ME. LOOK THE OTHER WAY!
YESH, JUSHT LIKE THAT...
I'M BORED. I WANNA QUIT.
THEN YOU SHLOWLY GET ENWAPTURED AND KISH ME!
KISH? YOU MEAN KISSING?
YESH! YOU PUT YOUR MOUF ON MINE ...
I KNOW HOW. PAPA DOES IT TO MAMA.
FOOEY!
YOU GOT YOUR SHNOT ON ME!

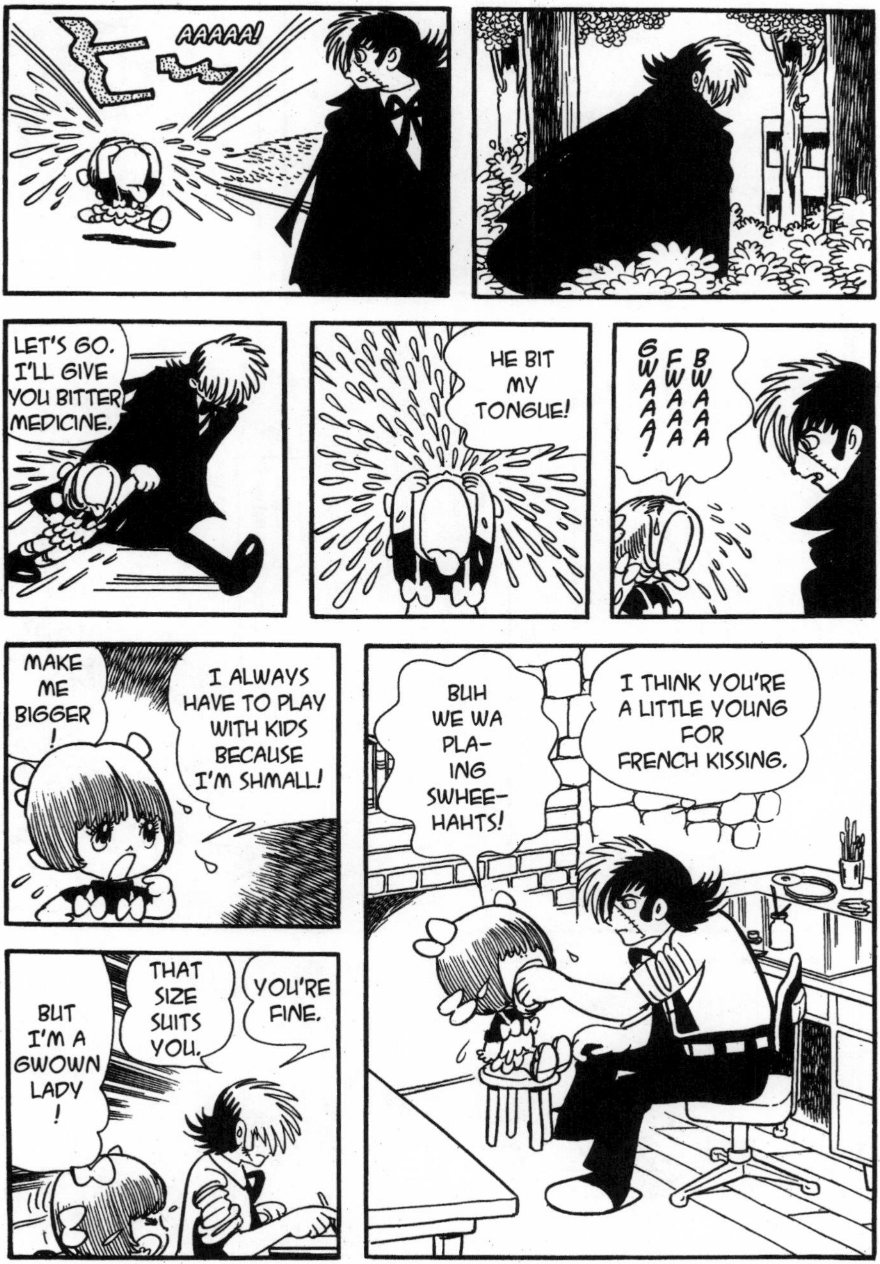
AAAAA!
BWAAAA FWAAAA GWAAA!
HE BIT MY TONGUE!
LET'S GO. I'LL GIVE YOU BITTER MEDICINE.
I THINK YOU'RE A LITTLE YOUNG FOR FRENCH KISSING.
BUH WE WA PLA-ING SWHEE-HAHTS!
I ALWAYS HAVE TO PLAY WITH KIDS BECAUSE I'M SHMALL!
MAKE ME BIGGER!
YOU'RE FINE.
THAT SIZE SUITS YOU.
BUT I'M A GWOWN LADY!

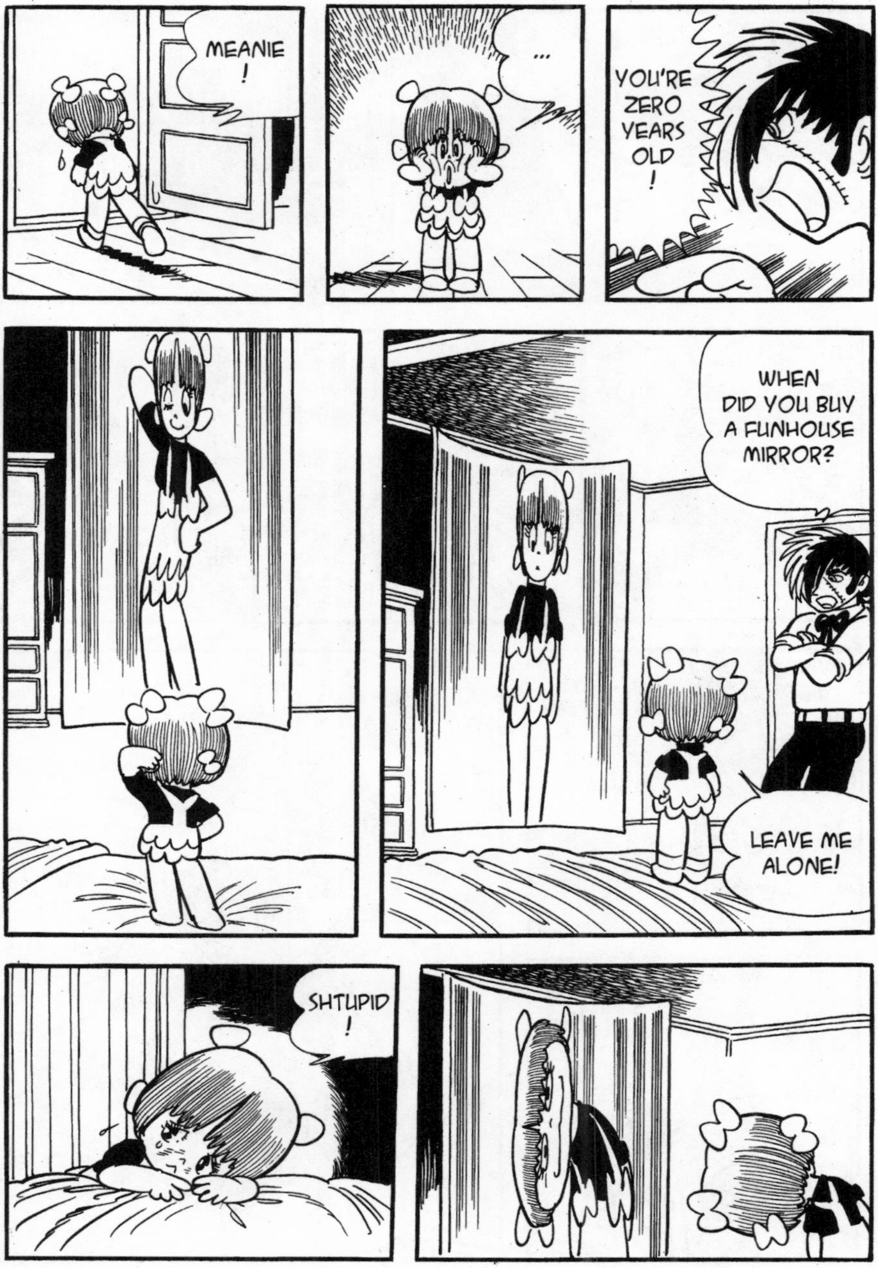
YOU'RE ZERO YEARS OLD !
...
MEANIE !
WHEN DID YOU BUY A FUNHOUSE MIRROR?
LEAVE ME ALONE!
SHTUPID !

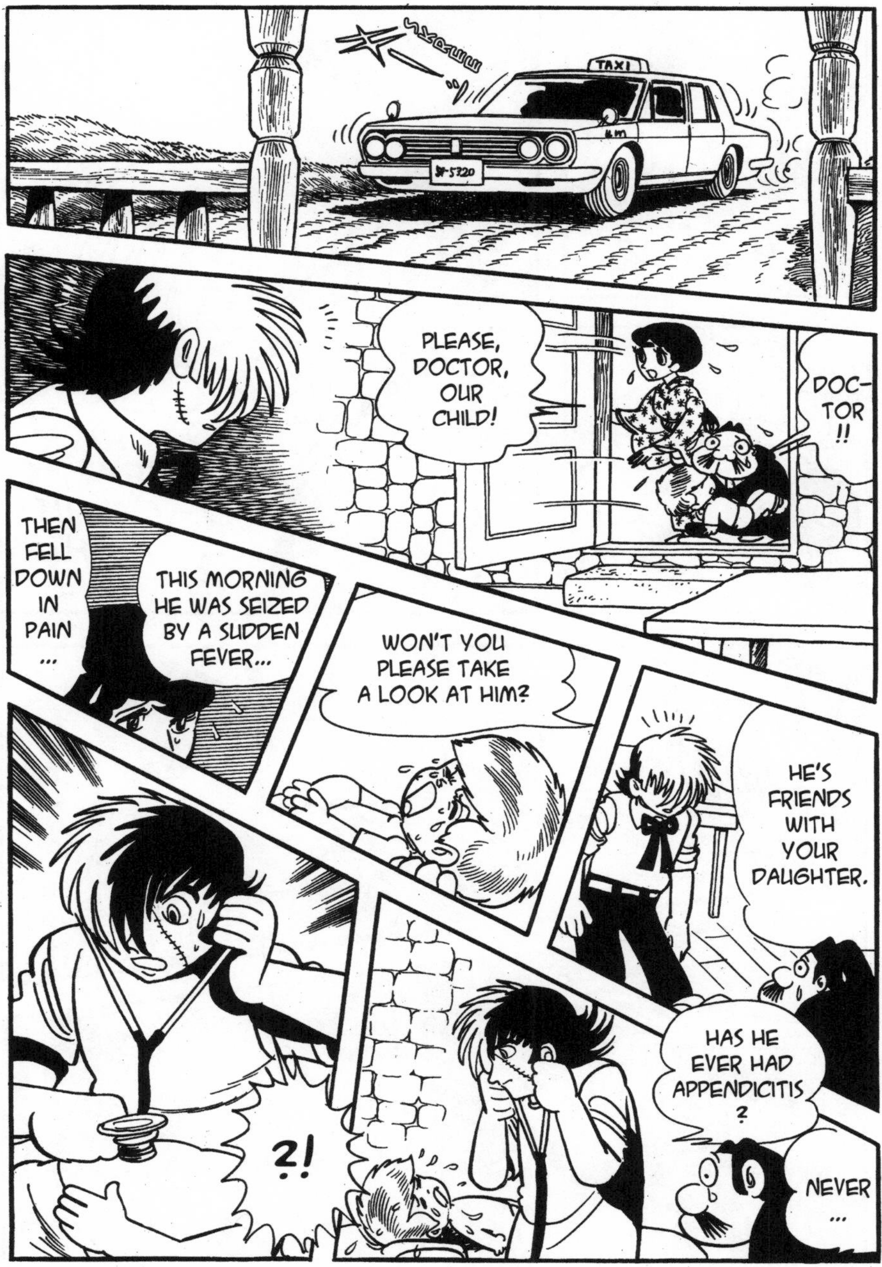
SKREEE
TAXI
DOC-TOR !!
PLEASE, DOCTOR, OUR CHILD!
THIS MORNING HE WAS SEIZED BY A SUDDEN FEVER...
THEN FELL DOWN IN PAIN ...
WON'T YOU PLEASE TAKE A LOOK AT HIM?
HE'S FRIENDS WITH YOUR DAUGHTER.
HAS HE EVER HAD APPENDICITIS ?
NEVER ...
?!

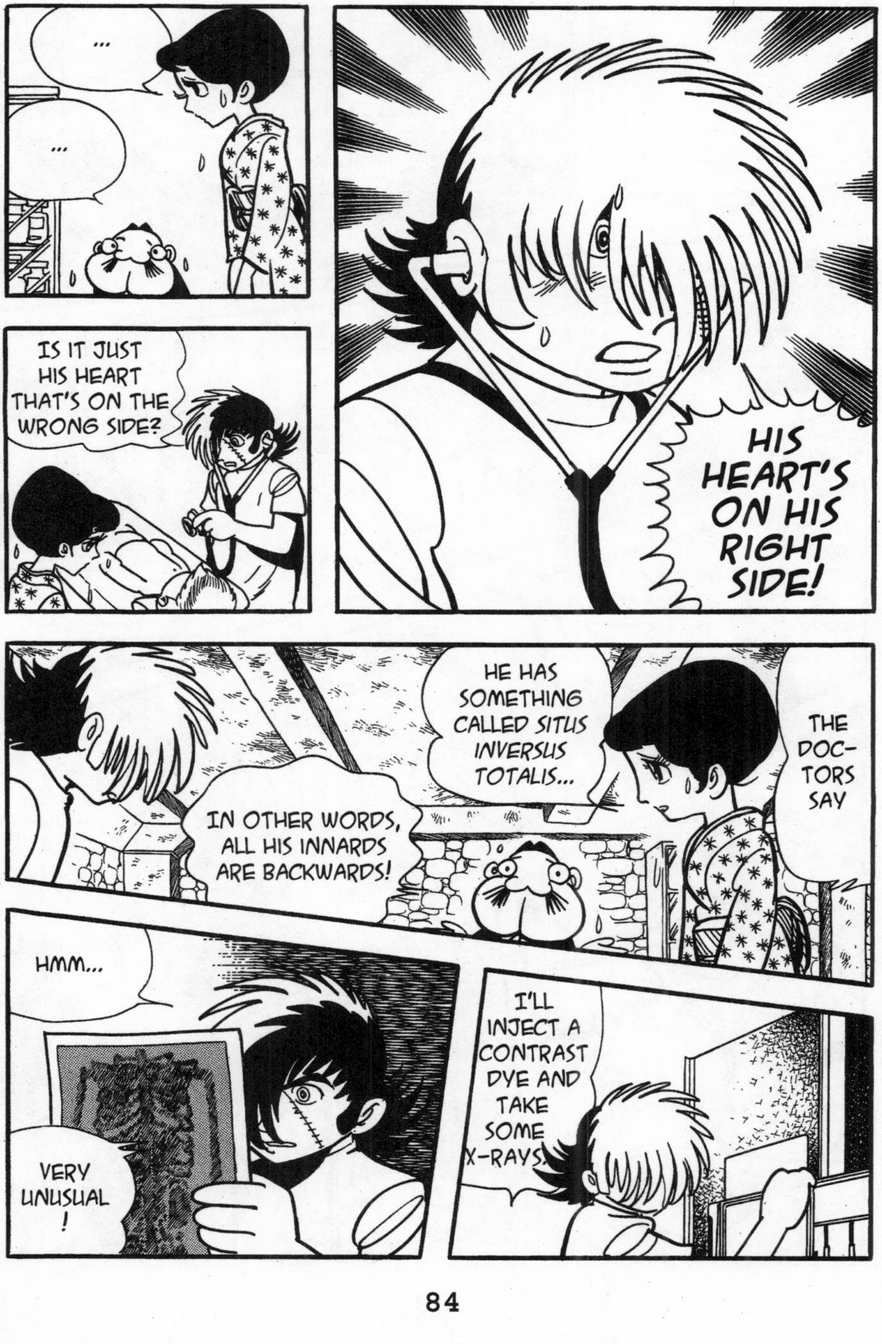

HIS HEART'S ON HIS RIGHT SIDE!
...
...
IS IT JUST HIS HEART THAT'S ON THE WRONG SIDE?
THE DOC-TORS SAY
HE HAS SOMETHING CALLED SITUS INVERSUS TOTALIS...
IN OTHER WORDS, ALL HIS INNARDS ARE BACKWARDS!
I'LL INJECT A CONTRAST DYE AND TAKE SOME X-RAYS.
HMM...
VERY UNUSUAL!

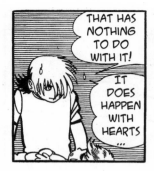

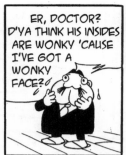

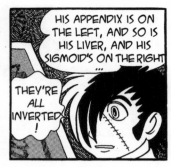

HIS APPENDIX IS ON THE LEFT, AND SO IS HIS LIVER, AND HIS SIGMOID'S ON THE RIGHT ...
THEY'RE ALL INVERTED!
ER, DOCTOR? D'YA THINK HIS INSIDES ARE WONKY 'CAUSE I'VE GOT A WONKY FACE?
THAT HAS NOTHING TO DO WITH IT!
IT DOES HAPPEN WITH HEARTS ...
BUT IT'S EXTREMELY RARE TO SEE SOMEONE WITH EVERYTHING BACKWARDS.
Normal
lungs
heart
stomach
intestines
Backwards
heart
intestines
stomach
INVERSION TENDS TO CAUSE VARIOUS HEALTH PROBLEMS.
OWW...
IT HUUURTS ...
WHERE DOES IT HURT?
SWELLING, LEFT OF THE EPIGASTRIC.
NORMALLY, THAT WOULD BE THE RIGHT SIDE... GALL BLADDER OR BILE DUCT.

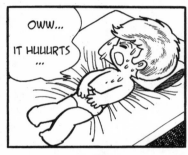

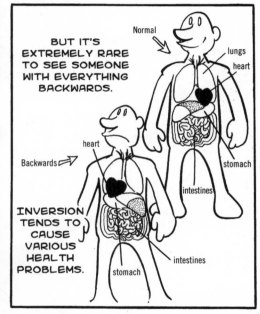

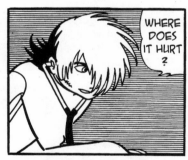

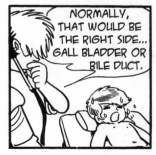

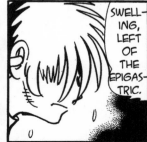

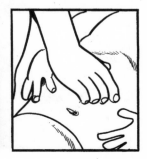

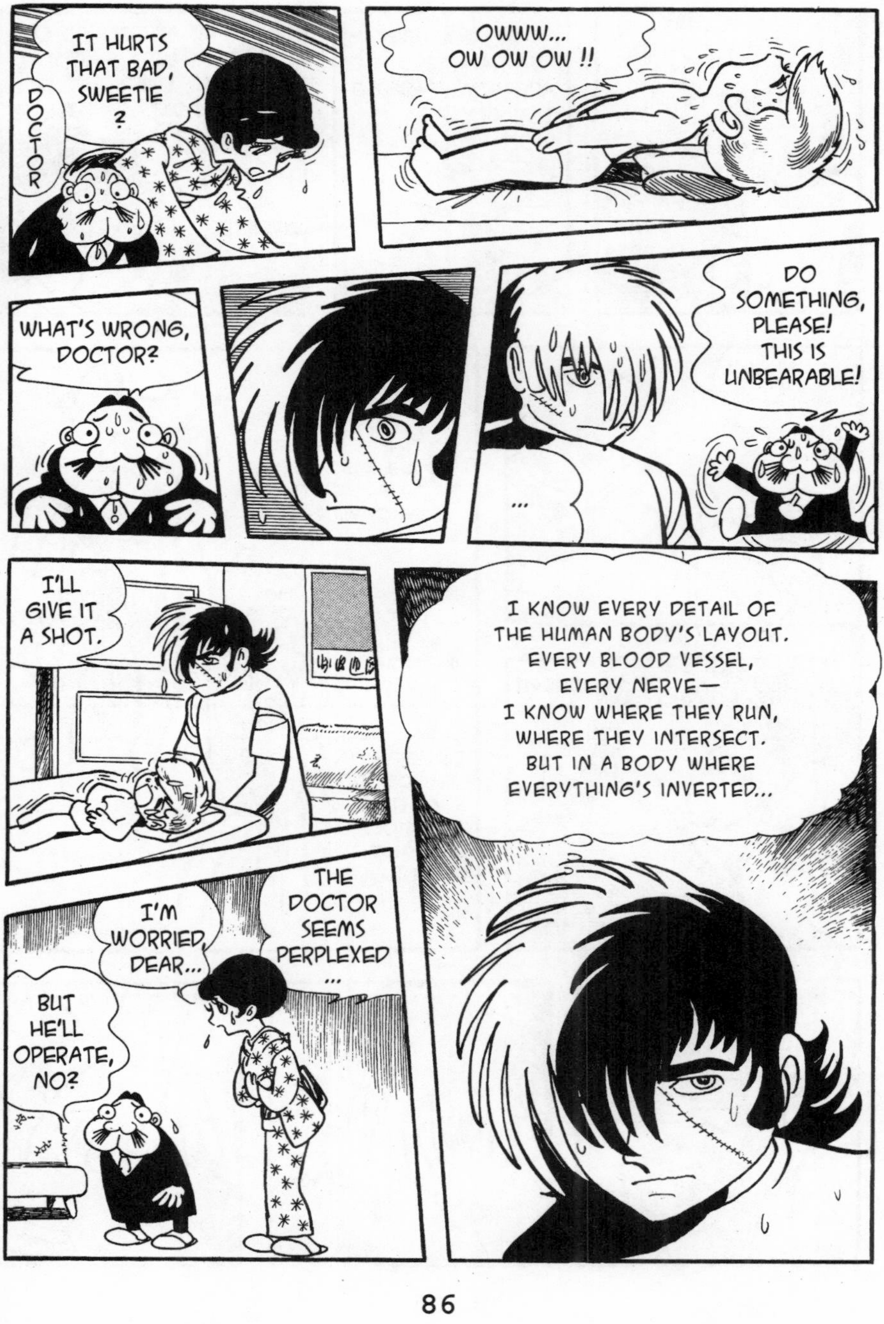

OWWW... OW OW OW !!
IT HURTS THAT BAD, SWEETIE ?
DOCTOR
DO SOMETHING, PLEASE! THIS IS UNBEARABLE!
...
WHAT'S WRONG, DOCTOR?
I KNOW EVERY DETAIL OF THE HUMAN BODY'S LAYOUT. EVERY BLOOD VESSEL, EVERY NERVE— I KNOW WHERE THEY RUN, WHERE THEY INTERSECT. BUT IN A BODY WHERE EVERYTHING'S INVERTED...
I'LL GIVE IT A SHOT.
THE DOCTOR SEEMS PERPLEXED ...
I'M WORRIED, DEAR...
BUT HE'LL OPERATE, NO?

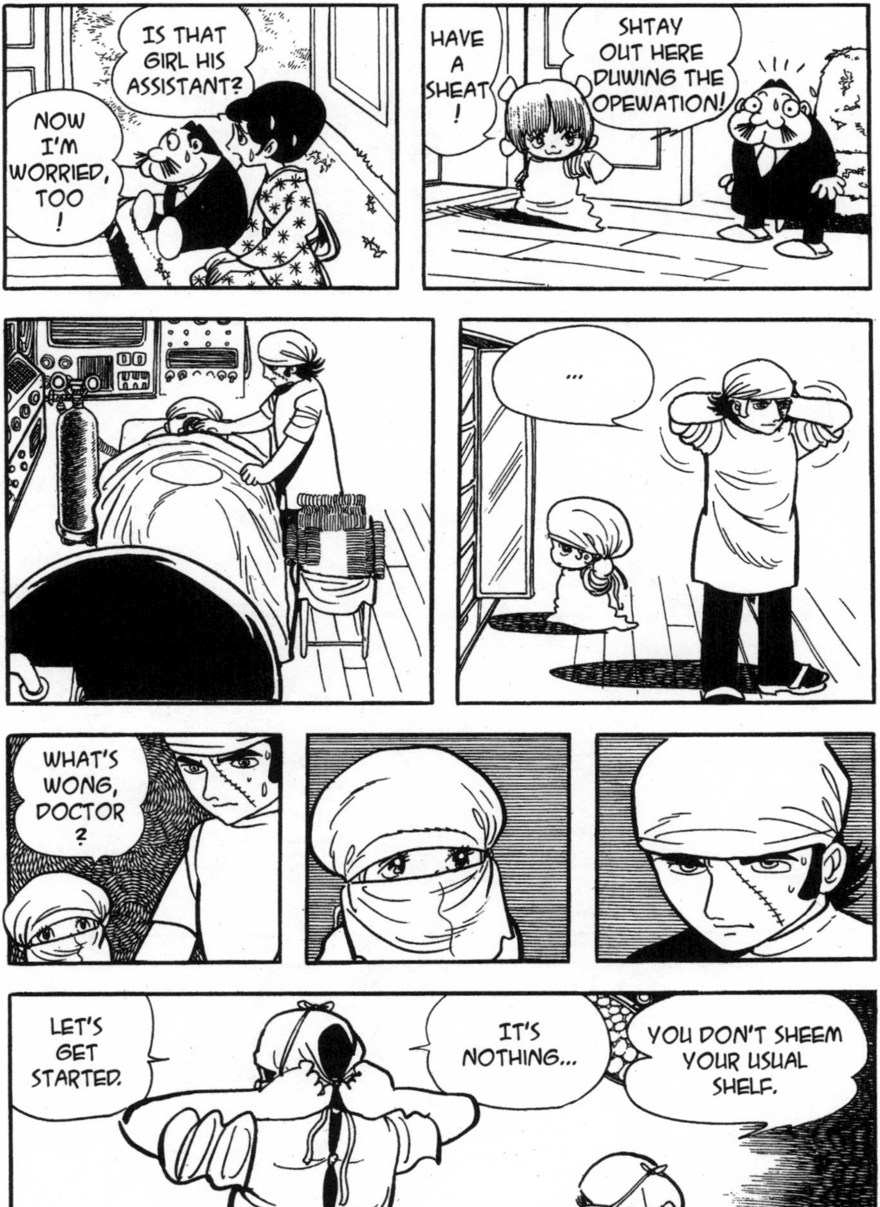

SHTAY OUT HERE DUWING THE OPEWATION!
HAVE A SHEAT!
IS THAT GIRL HIS ASSISTANT?
NOW I'M WORRIED, TOO!
...
WHAT'S WONG, DOCTOR?
YOU DON'T SHEEM YOUR USUAL SHELF.
IT'S NOTHING...
LET'S GET STARTED.

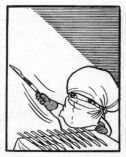

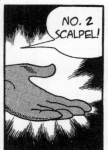

NO. 2
SCALPEL!

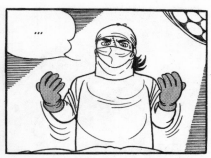

...

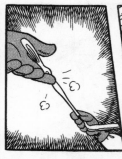

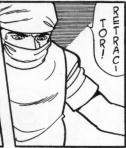

RETRACT! TORI!

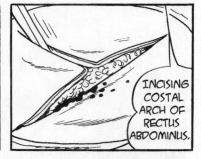

INCISING COSTAL ARCH OF RECTUS ABDOMINUS.

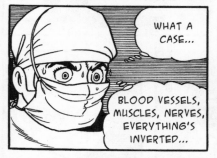

WHAT A CASE...

BLOOD VESSELS, MUSCLES, NERVES, EVERYTHING'S INVERTED...

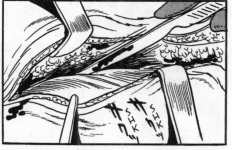

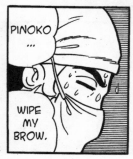

PINOKO ...

WIPE MY BROW.

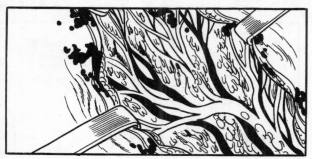

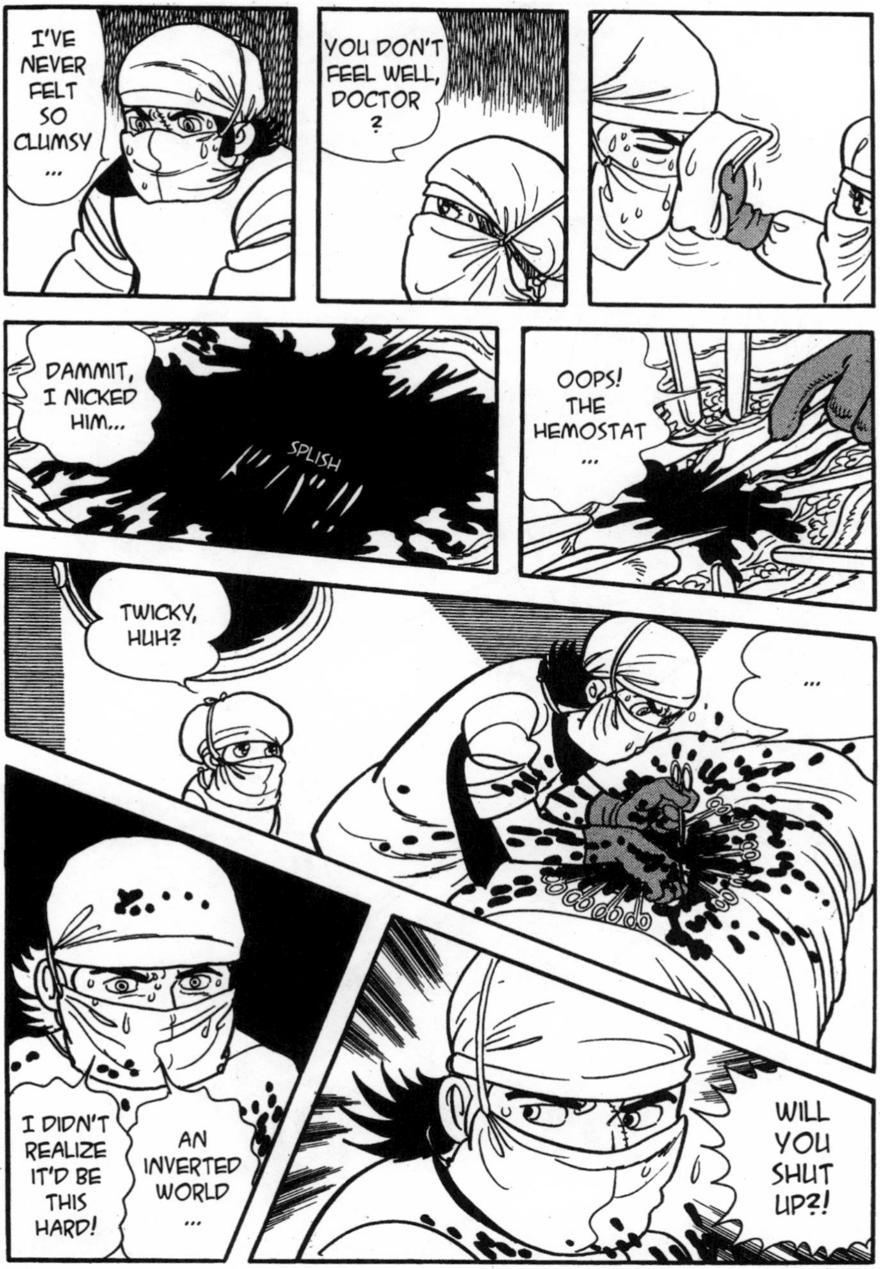
YOU DON'T FEEL WELL, DOCTOR?
I'VE NEVER FELT SO CLUMSY...
OOPS! THE HEMOSTAT...
DAMMIT, I NICKED HIM...
SPLISH
...
TWICKY, HUH?
WILL YOU SHUT UP?!
AN INVERTED WORLD...
I DIDN'T REALIZE IT'D BE THIS HARD!

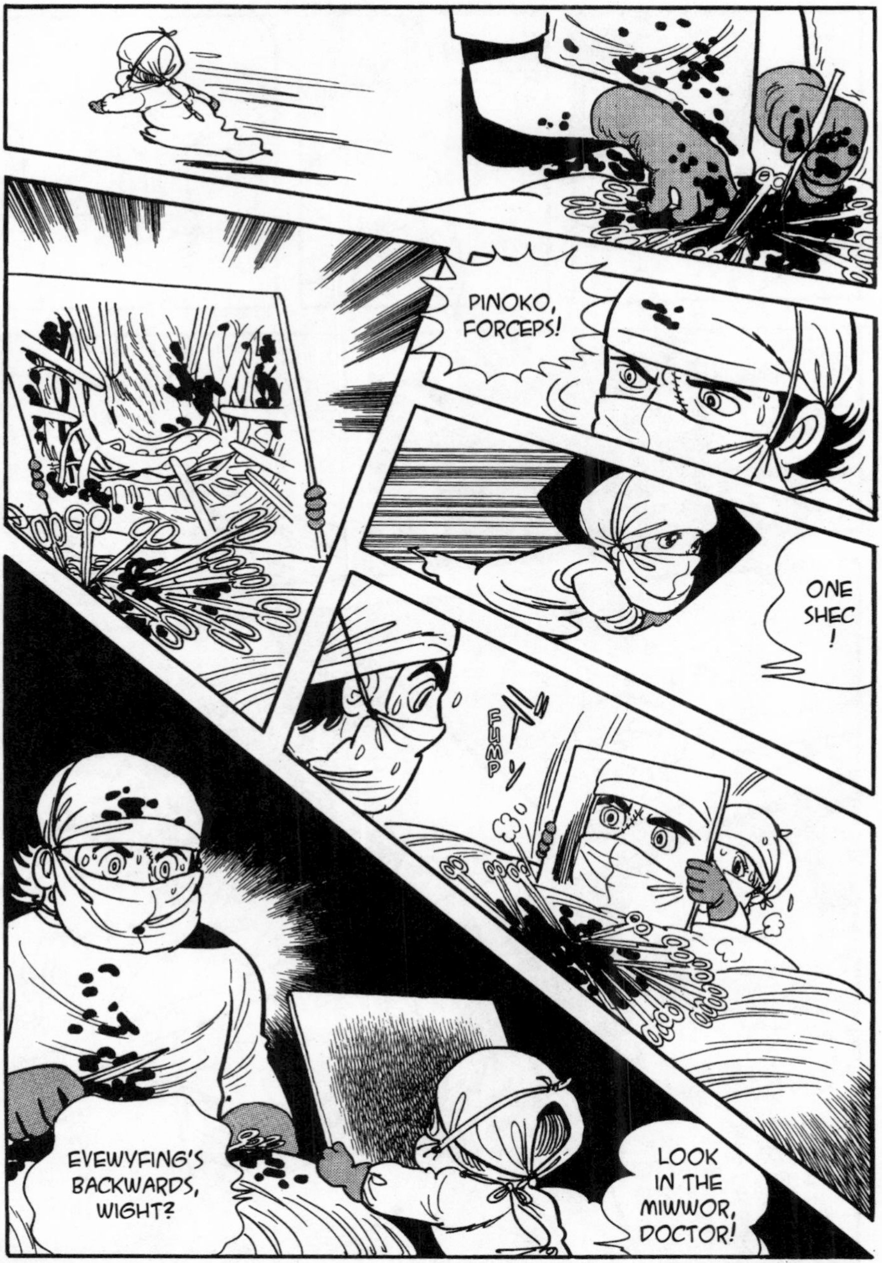
PINOKO, FORCEPS!
ONE SHEC!
FUMP
LOOK IN THE MIWWOR, DOCTOR!
EVEWYFING'S BACKWARDS, WIGHT?

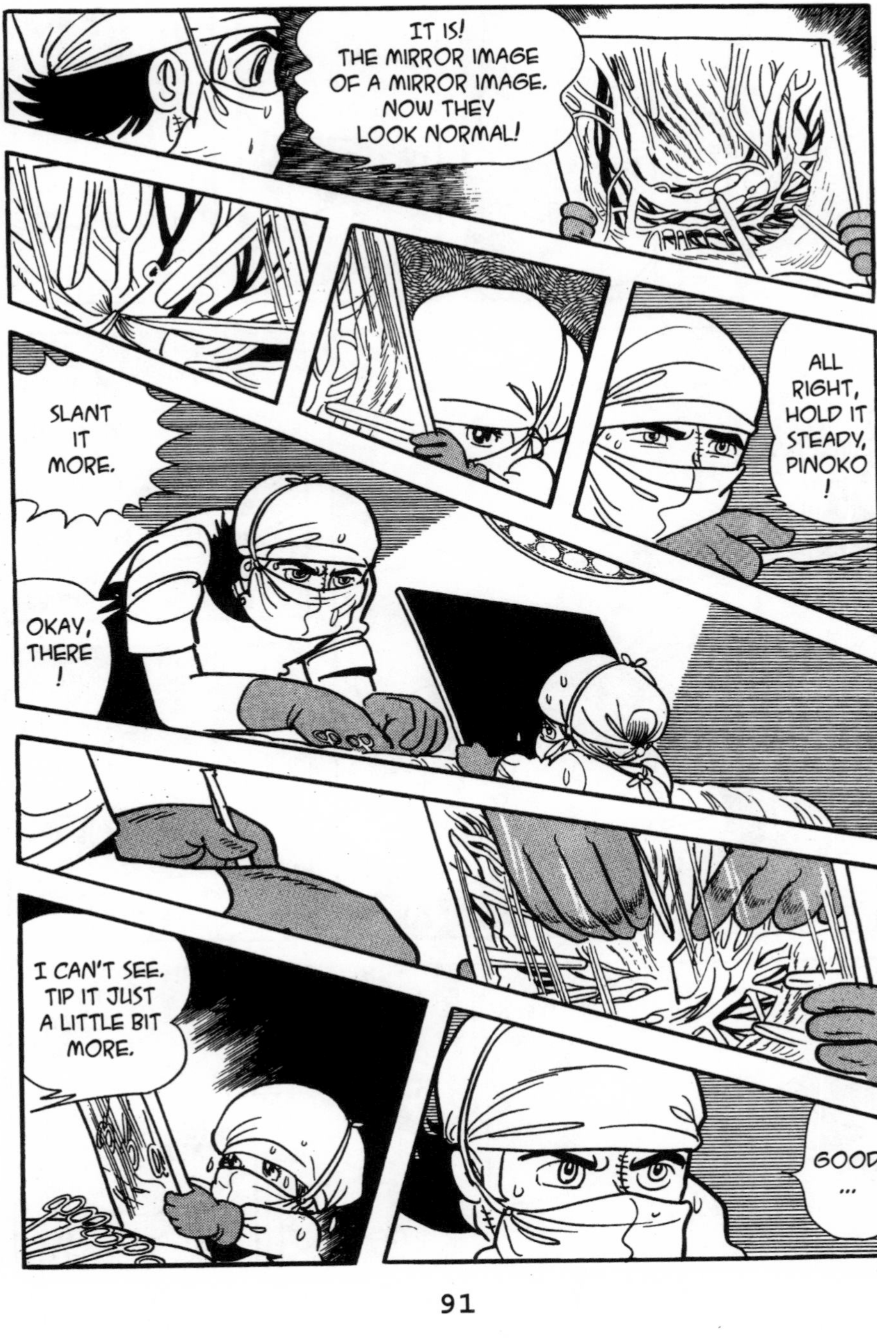
IT IS! THE MIRROR IMAGE OF A MIRROR IMAGE. NOW THEY LOOK NORMAL!
ALL RIGHT, HOLD IT STEADY, PINOKO!
SLANT IT MORE.
OKAY, THERE!
GOOD ...
I CAN'T SEE. TIP IT JUST A LITTLE BIT MORE.

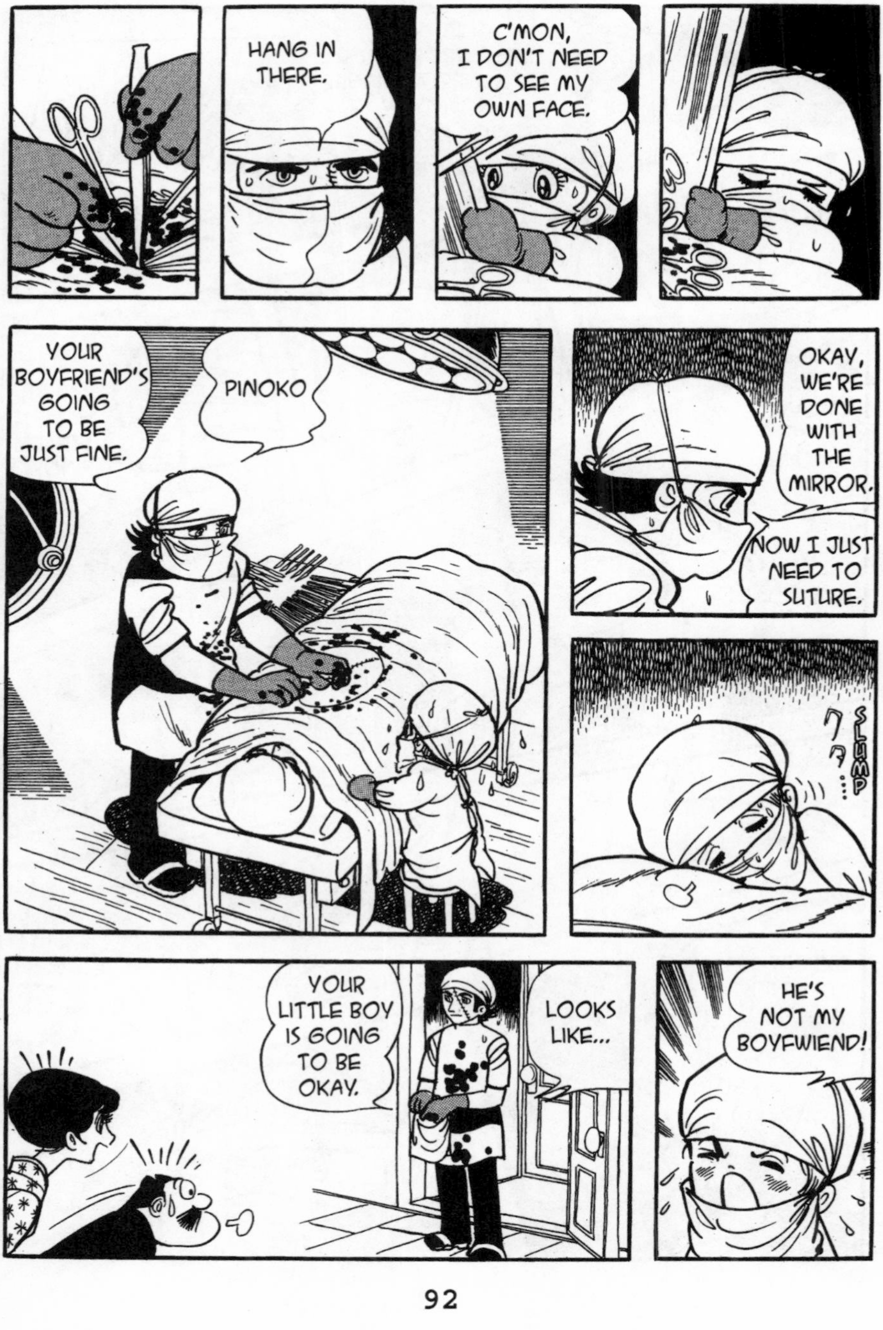
C'MON, I DON'T NEED TO SEE MY OWN FACE.
HANG IN THERE.
OKAY, WE'RE DONE WITH THE MIRROR.
NOW I JUST NEED TO SUTURE.
クタ…
SLUMP
PINOKO
YOUR BOYFRIEND'S GOING TO BE JUST FINE.
HE'S NOT MY BOYFWIEND!
LOOKS LIKE...
YOUR LITTLE BOY IS GOING TO BE OKAY.

YOUR SON WAS ALSO BORN WITH AN ENLARGED BILE DUCT.
TH... THANK YOU SO MUCH.
YOU NEED TO THANK PINOKO ...
WHO?
MY SUPERB ASSISTANT.
MAIL!
THANK YOU.
WHAT'S THIS? PINOKO'S LOVE LETTERS CAME BACK.

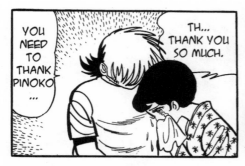

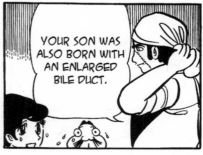

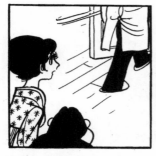

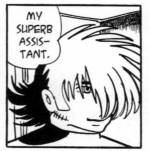

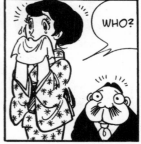

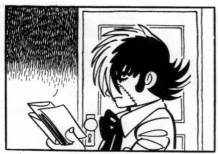

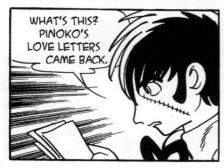

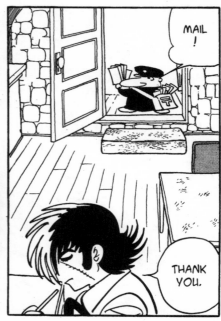

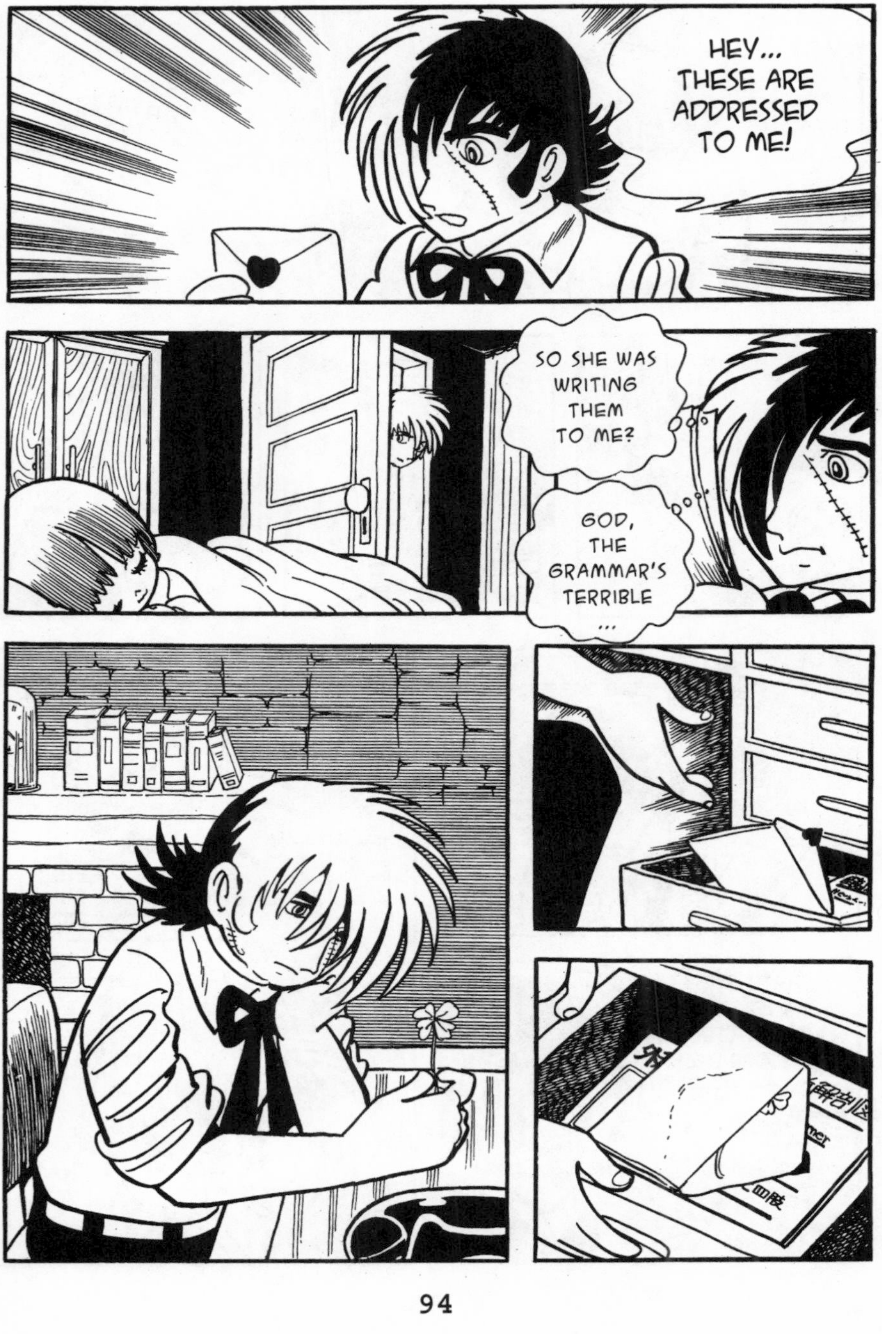
HEY... THESE ARE ADDRESSED TO ME!
SO SHE WAS WRITING THEM TO ME?
GOD, THE GRAMMAR'S TERRIBLE ...

THE SEWER WAY

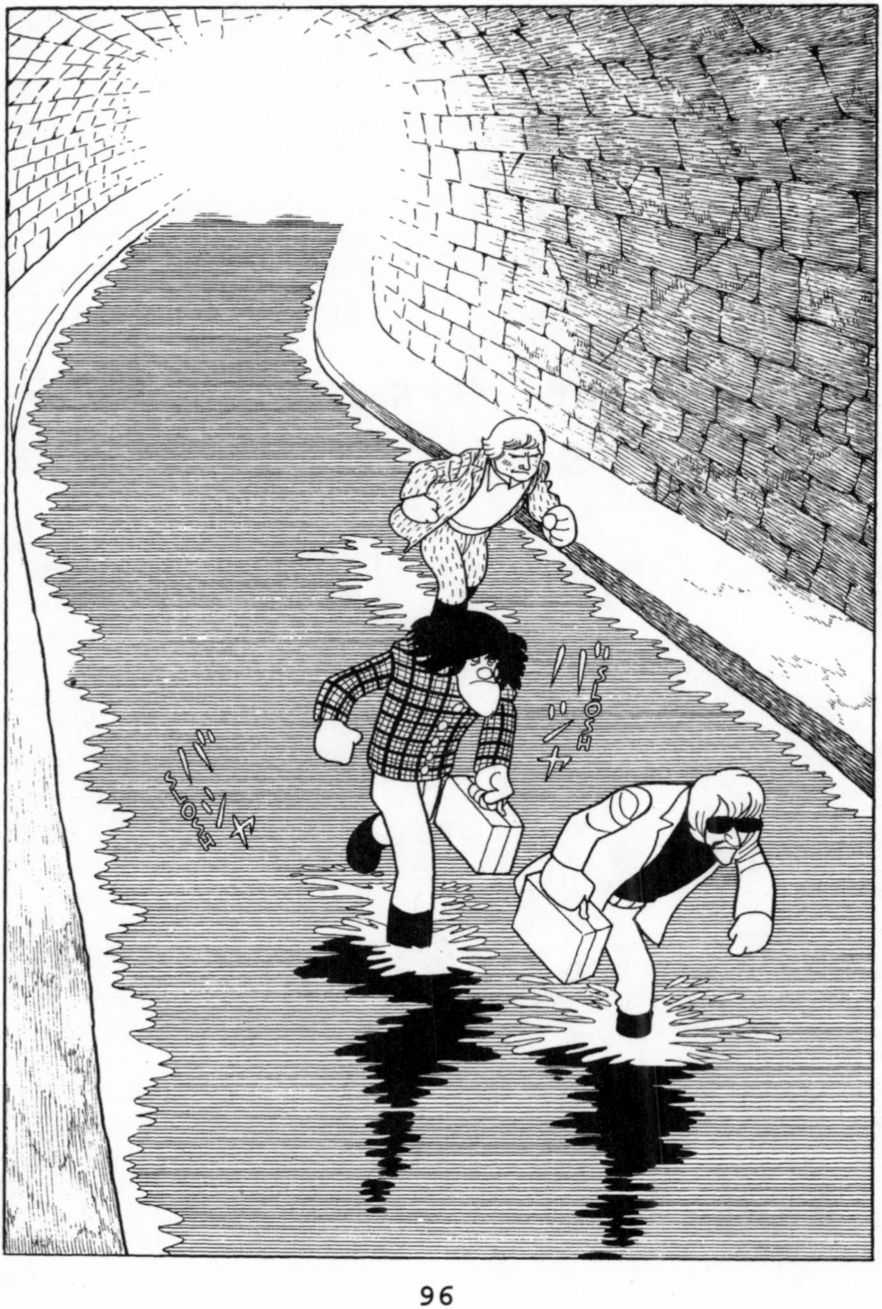
SLOSH
SLOSH

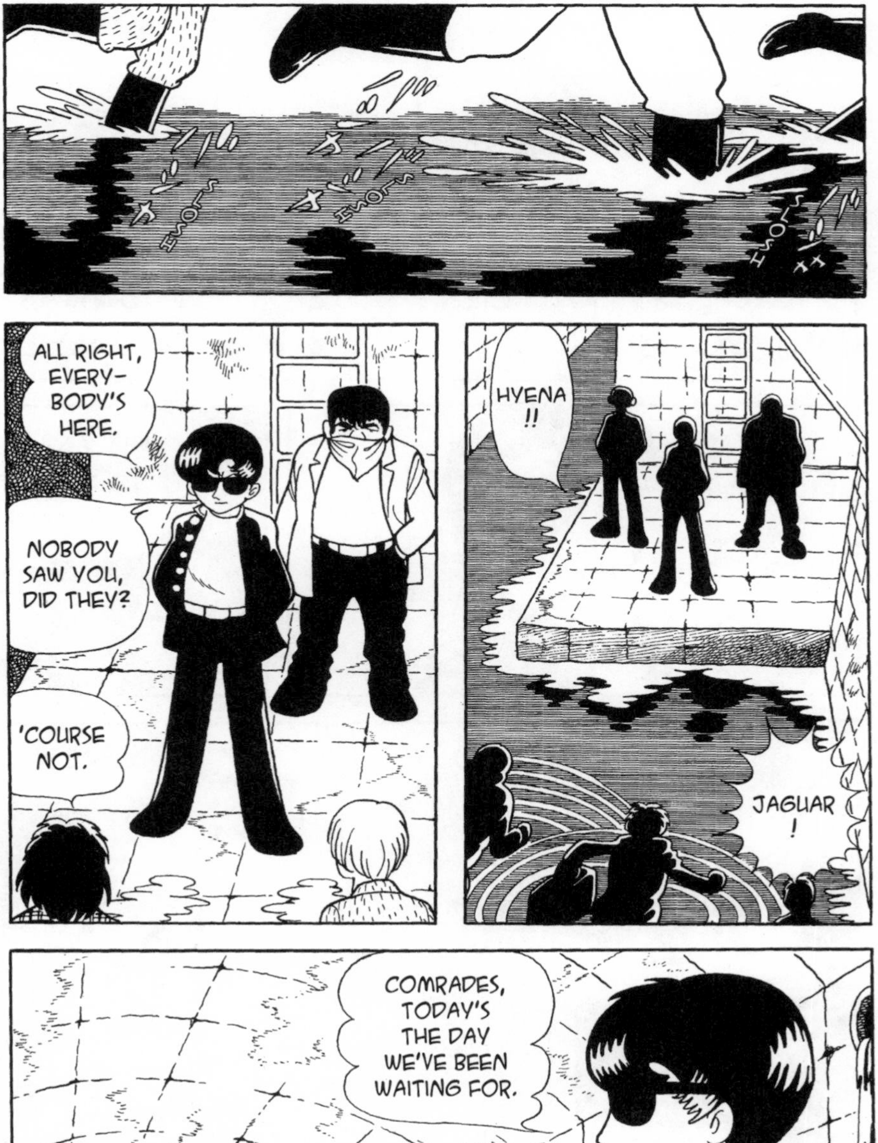
SLOSH
SLOSH
SLOSH
HYENA !!
JAGUAR !
ALL RIGHT, EVERYBODY'S HERE.
NOBODY SAW YOU, DID THEY?
'COURSE NOT.
COMRADES, TODAY'S THE DAY WE'VE BEEN WAITING FOR.

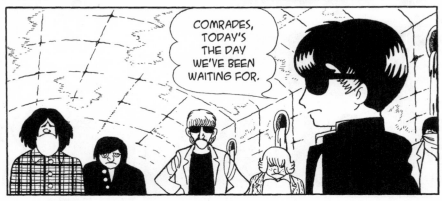

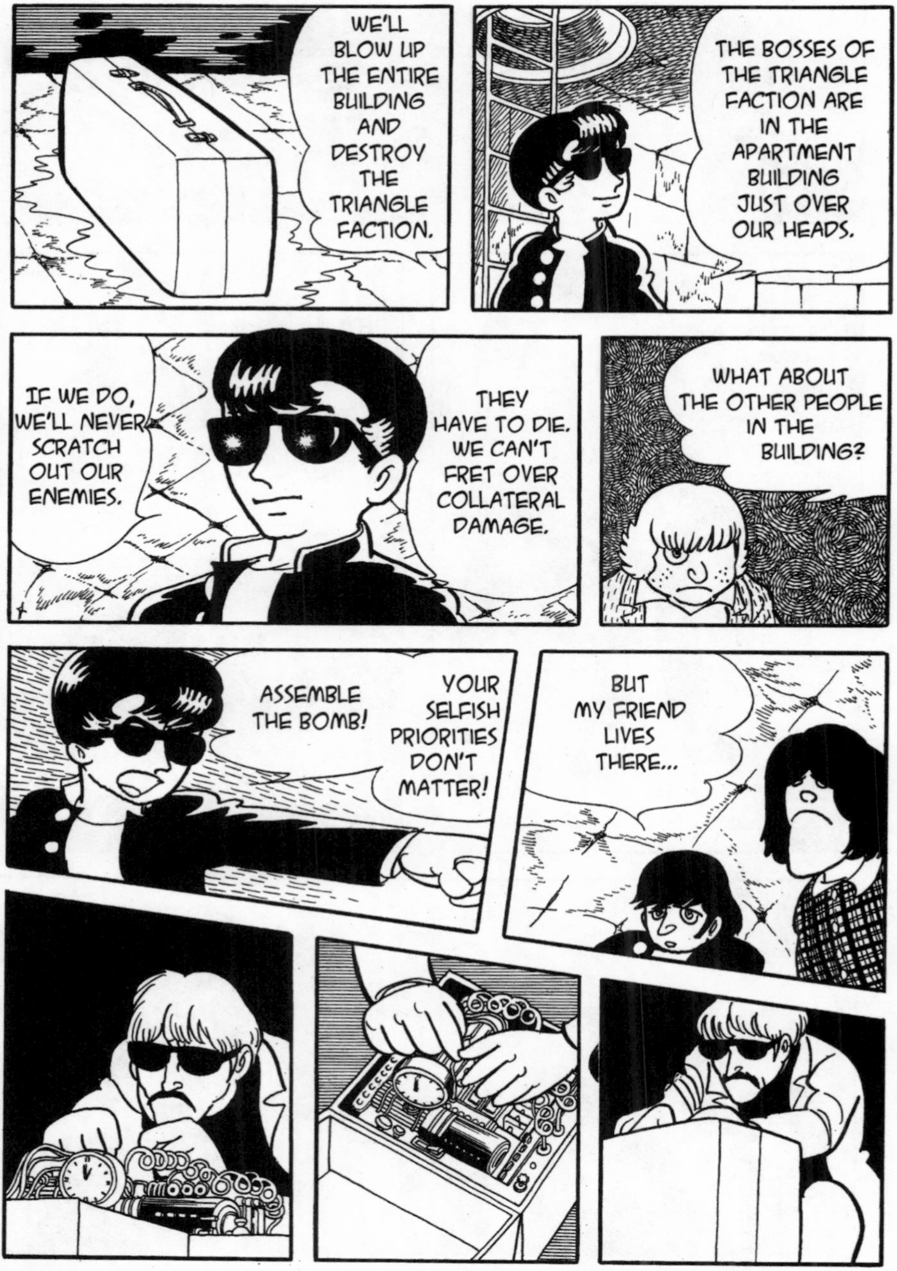
THE BOSSES OF THE TRIANGLE FACTION ARE IN THE APARTMENT BUILDING JUST OVER OUR HEADS.
WE'LL BLOW UP THE ENTIRE BUILDING AND DESTROY THE TRIANGLE FACTION.
WHAT ABOUT THE OTHER PEOPLE IN THE BUILDING?
THEY HAVE TO DIE. WE CAN'T FRET OVER COLLATERAL DAMAGE.
IF WE DO, WE'LL NEVER SCRATCH OUT OUR ENEMIES.
BUT MY FRIEND LIVES THERE...
YOUR SELFISH PRIORITIES DON'T MATTER!
ASSEMBLE THE BOMB!

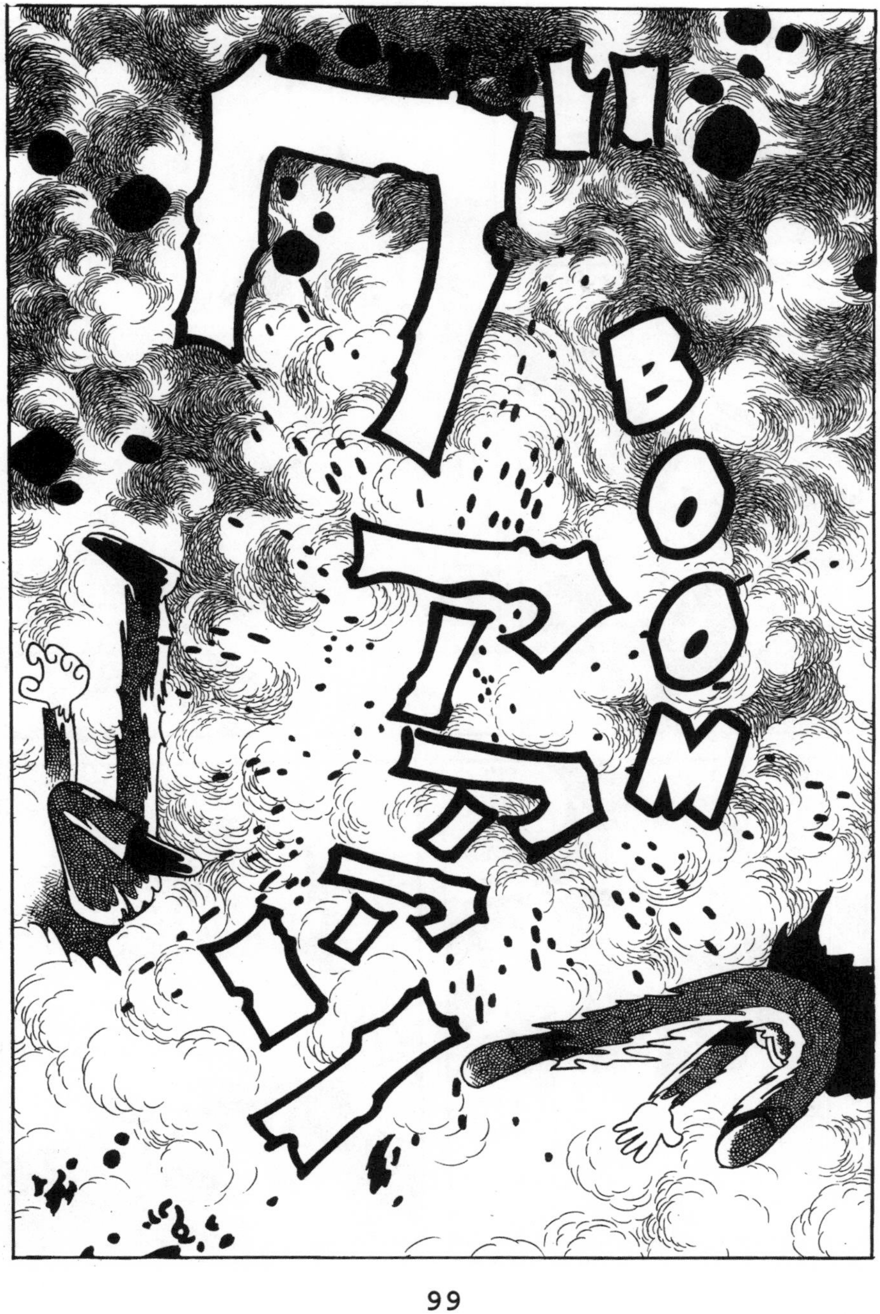
BOOM

NNNG...
UHH...
CHIEF ...
CHIEF !
IT'S FROM A CAR ACCIDENT ...
THE BURNS, TOO ?
YEAH. IT CAUGHT FIRE.

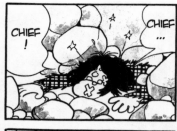

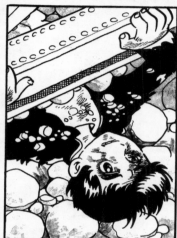

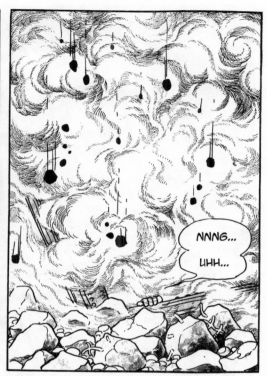

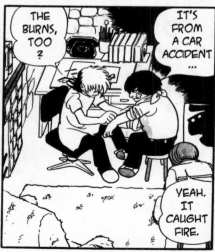

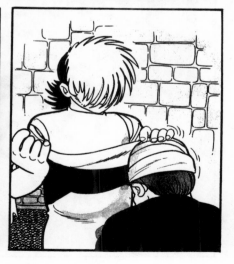

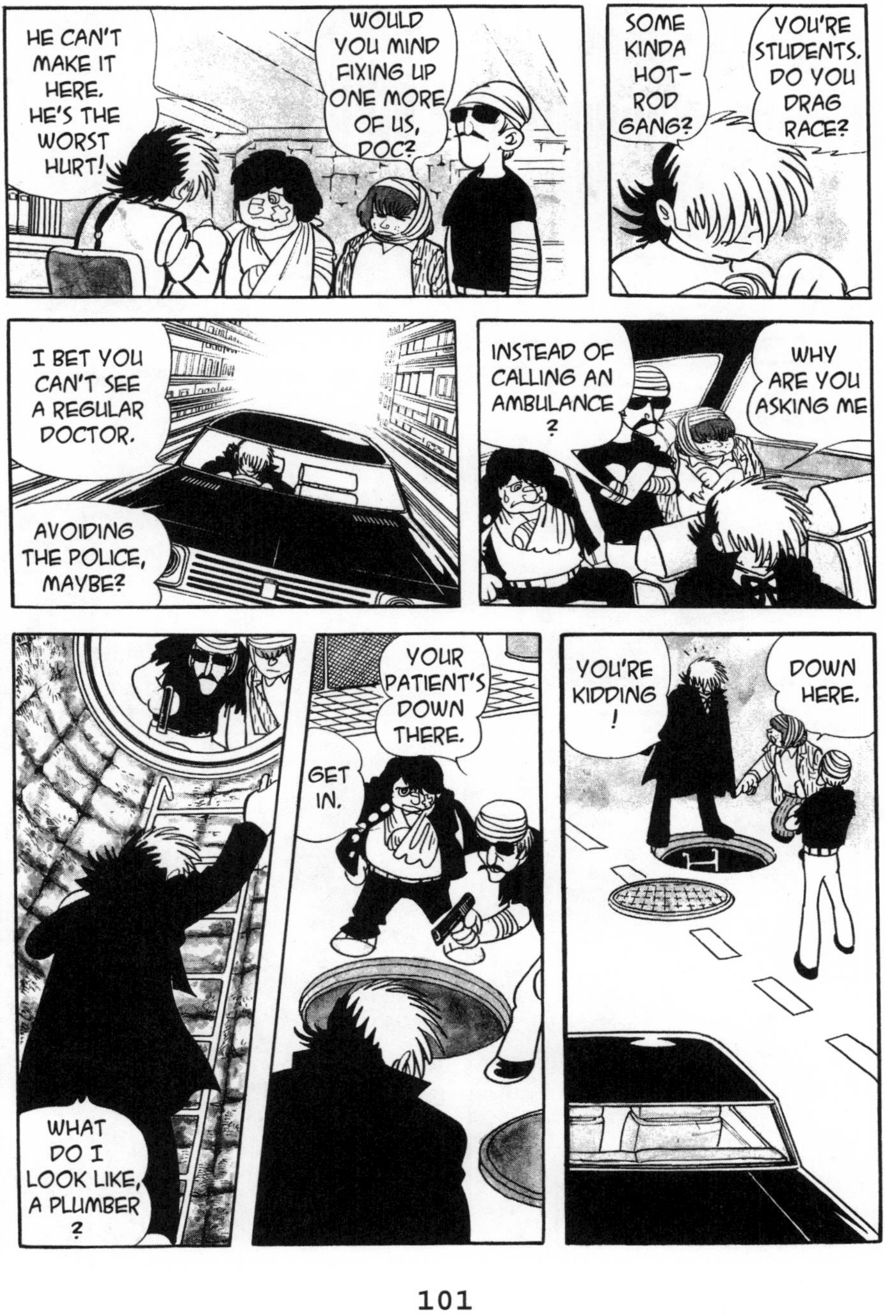
YOU'RE STUDENTS. DO YOU DRAG RACE?
SOME KINDA HOT-ROD GANG?
WOULD YOU MIND FIXING UP ONE MORE OF US, DOC?
HE CAN'T MAKE IT HERE. HE'S THE WORST HURT!
WHY ARE YOU ASKING ME
INSTEAD OF CALLING AN AMBULANCE?
I BET YOU CAN'T SEE A REGULAR DOCTOR.
AVOIDING THE POLICE, MAYBE?
DOWN HERE.
YOU'RE KIDDING!
YOUR PATIENT'S DOWN THERE.
GET IN.
WHAT DO I LOOK LIKE, A PLUMBER?

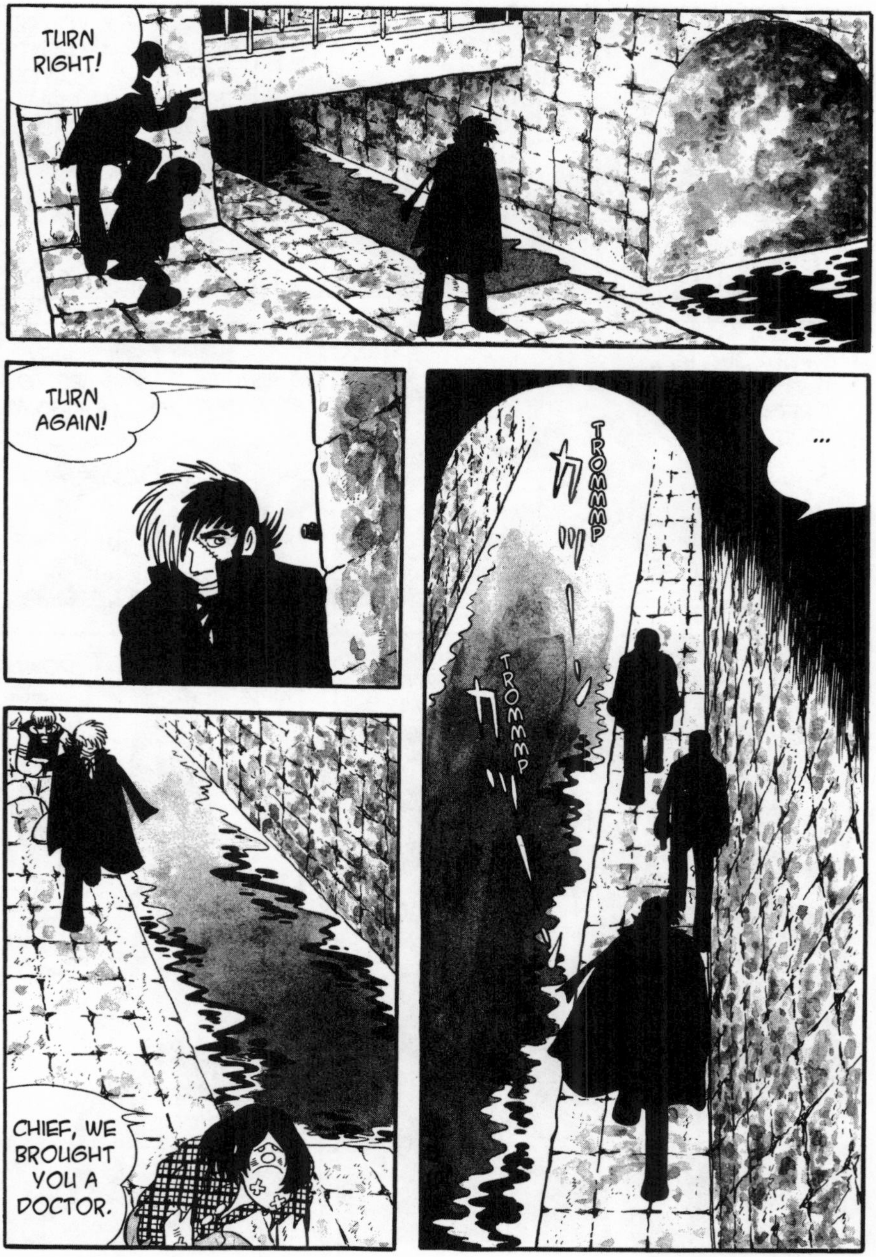
TURN RIGHT!
...
TROMMMP
TROMMMP
TURN AGAIN!
CHIEF, WE BROUGHT YOU A DOCTOR.

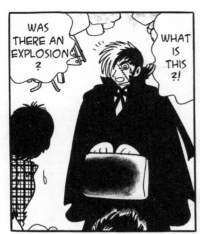

WAS THERE AN EXPLOSION?

WHAT IS THIS?!

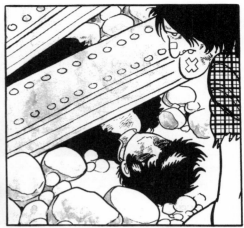

WE TRIED, BUT HE'S TRAPPED UNDER THAT HUGE BEAM.

IN ANY CASE, WE HAVE TO GET HIM OUT OF HERE.

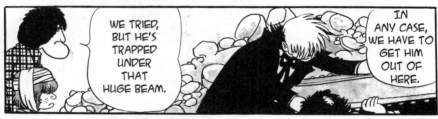

THE HIDEOUT OF AN ENEMY GROUP IS OVERHEAD. WE WERE GONNA WIPE THEM OUT BY SETTING OFF A BOMB, BUT IT WENT OFF ON US INSTEAD.

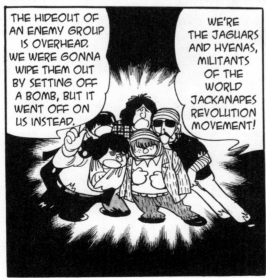

WE'RE THE JAGUARS AND HYENAS, MILITANTS OF THE WORLD JACKANAPES REVOLUTION MOVEMENT!

HE HAS BROKEN BONES AND MAJOR BLEEDING. HE'LL DIE.

THEN CALL THE COPS!

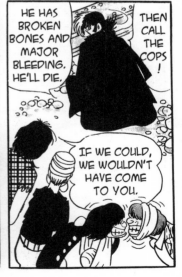

IF WE COULD, WE WOULDN'T HAVE COME TO YOU.

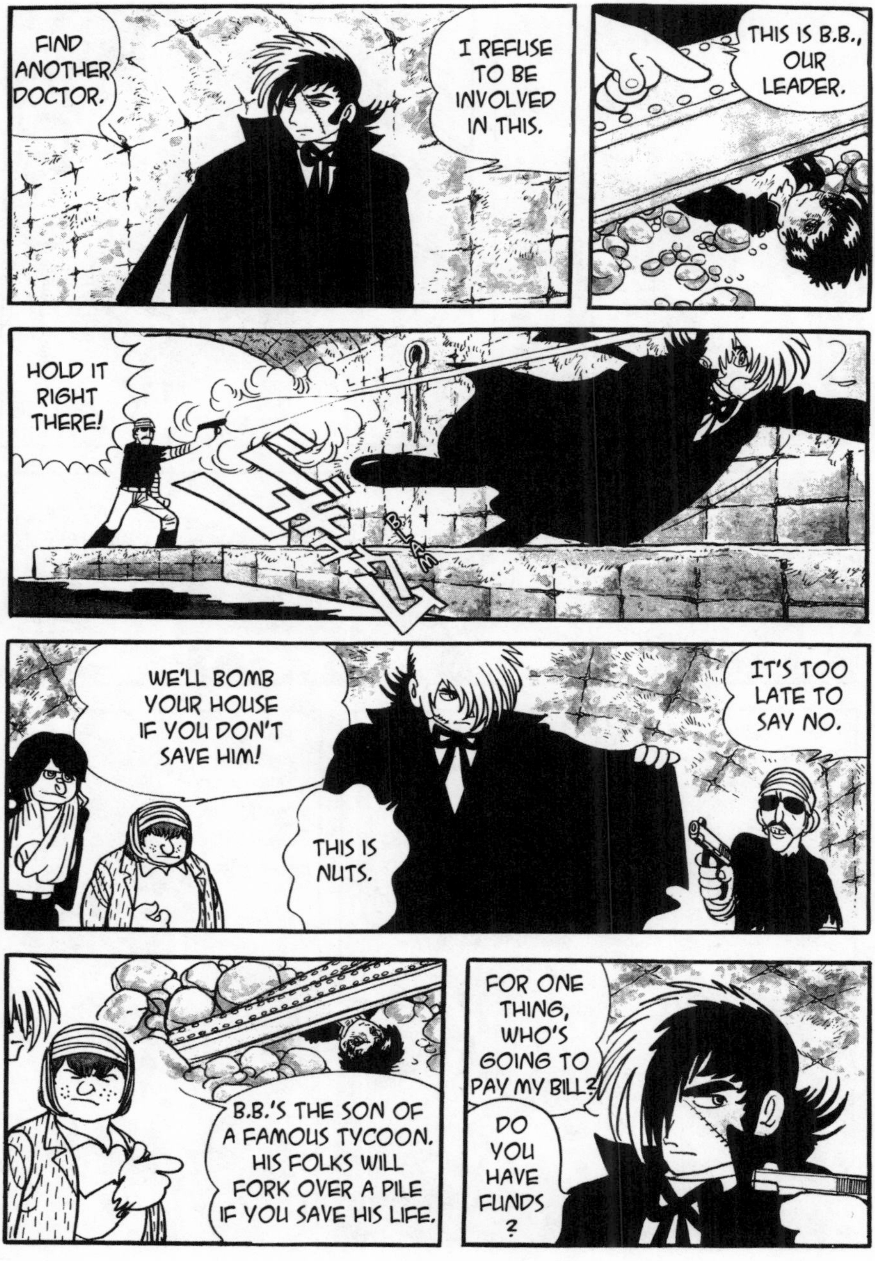
THIS IS B.B., OUR LEADER.
I REFUSE TO BE INVOLVED IN THIS.
FIND ANOTHER DOCTOR.
HOLD IT RIGHT THERE!
BLAM
IT'S TOO LATE TO SAY NO.
WE'LL BOMB YOUR HOUSE IF YOU DON'T SAVE HIM!
THIS IS NUTS.
FOR ONE THING, WHO'S GOING TO PAY MY BILL?
DO YOU HAVE FUNDS?
B.B.'S THE SON OF A FAMOUS TYCOON. HIS FOLKS WILL FORK OVER A PILE IF YOU SAVE HIS LIFE.

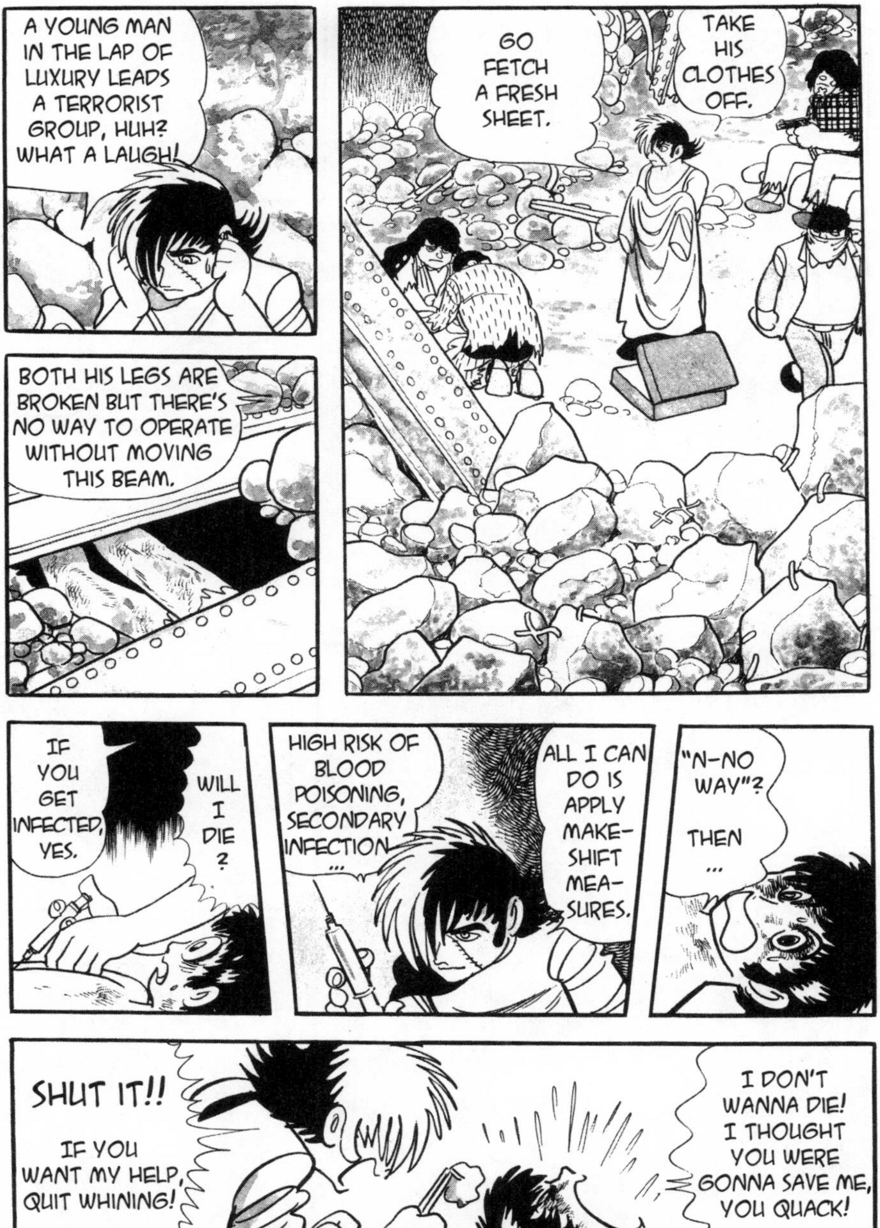
TAKE HIS CLOTHES OFF.
GO FETCH A FRESH SHEET.
A YOUNG MAN IN THE LAP OF LUXURY LEADS A TERRORIST GROUP, HUH? WHAT A LAUGH!
BOTH HIS LEGS ARE BROKEN BUT THERE'S NO WAY TO OPERATE WITHOUT MOVING THIS BEAM.
"N-NO WAY"?
THEN ...
ALL I CAN DO IS APPLY MAKE-SHIFT MEA-SURES.
HIGH RISK OF BLOOD POISONING, SECONDARY INFECTION ...
WILL I DIE ?
IF YOU GET INFECTED, YES.
I DON'T WANNA DIE! I THOUGHT YOU WERE GONNA SAVE ME, YOU QUACK!
SHUT IT!!
IF YOU WANT MY HELP, QUIT WHINING!

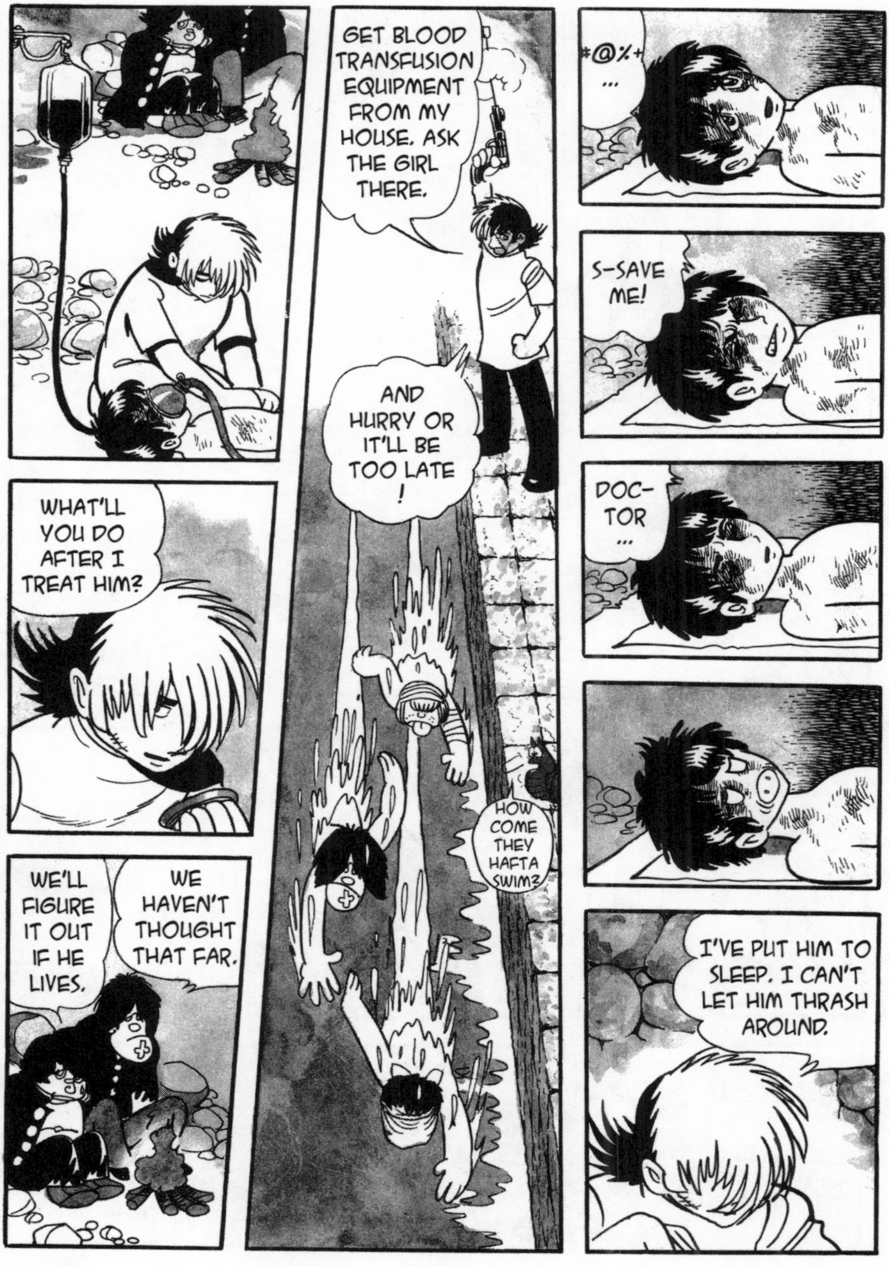
*@%+ ...
S-SAVE ME!
DOC-TOR ...
I'VE PUT HIM TO SLEEP. I CAN'T LET HIM THRASH AROUND.
GET BLOOD TRANSFUSION EQUIPMENT FROM MY HOUSE. ASK THE GIRL THERE.
AND HURRY OR IT'LL BE TOO LATE!
HOW COME THEY HAFTA SWIM?
WHAT'LL YOU DO AFTER I TREAT HIM?
WE HAVEN'T THOUGHT THAT FAR.
WE'LL FIGURE IT OUT IF HE LIVES.

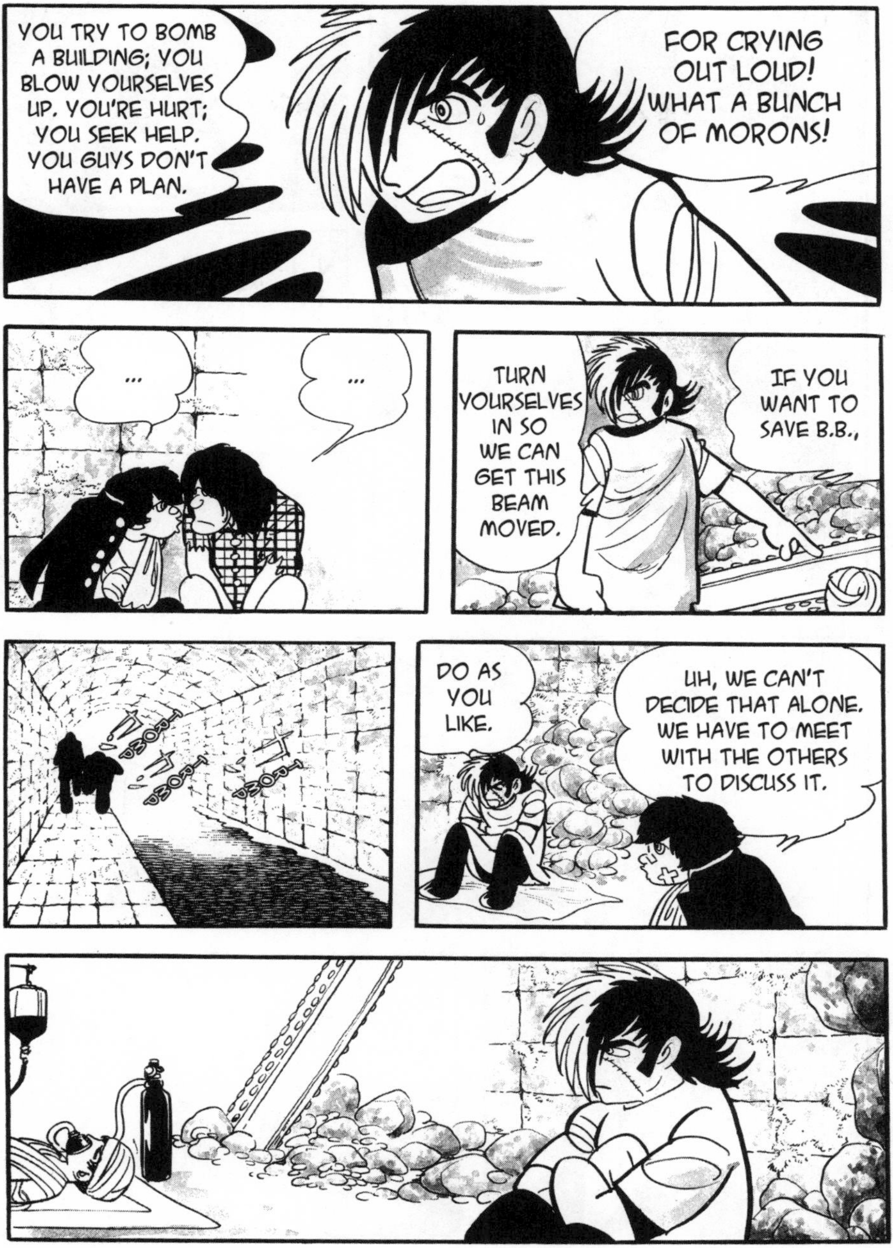
FOR CRYING OUT LOUD! WHAT A BUNCH OF MORONS!
YOU TRY TO BOMB A BUILDING; YOU BLOW YOURSELVES UP. YOU'RE HURT; YOU SEEK HELP. YOU GUYS DON'T HAVE A PLAN.
IF YOU WANT TO SAVE B.B.,
TURN YOURSELVES IN SO WE CAN GET THIS BEAM MOVED.
...
...
UH, WE CAN'T DECIDE THAT ALONE. WE HAVE TO MEET WITH THE OTHERS TO DISCUSS IT.
DO AS YOU LIKE.
TROMP
TROMP
TROMP

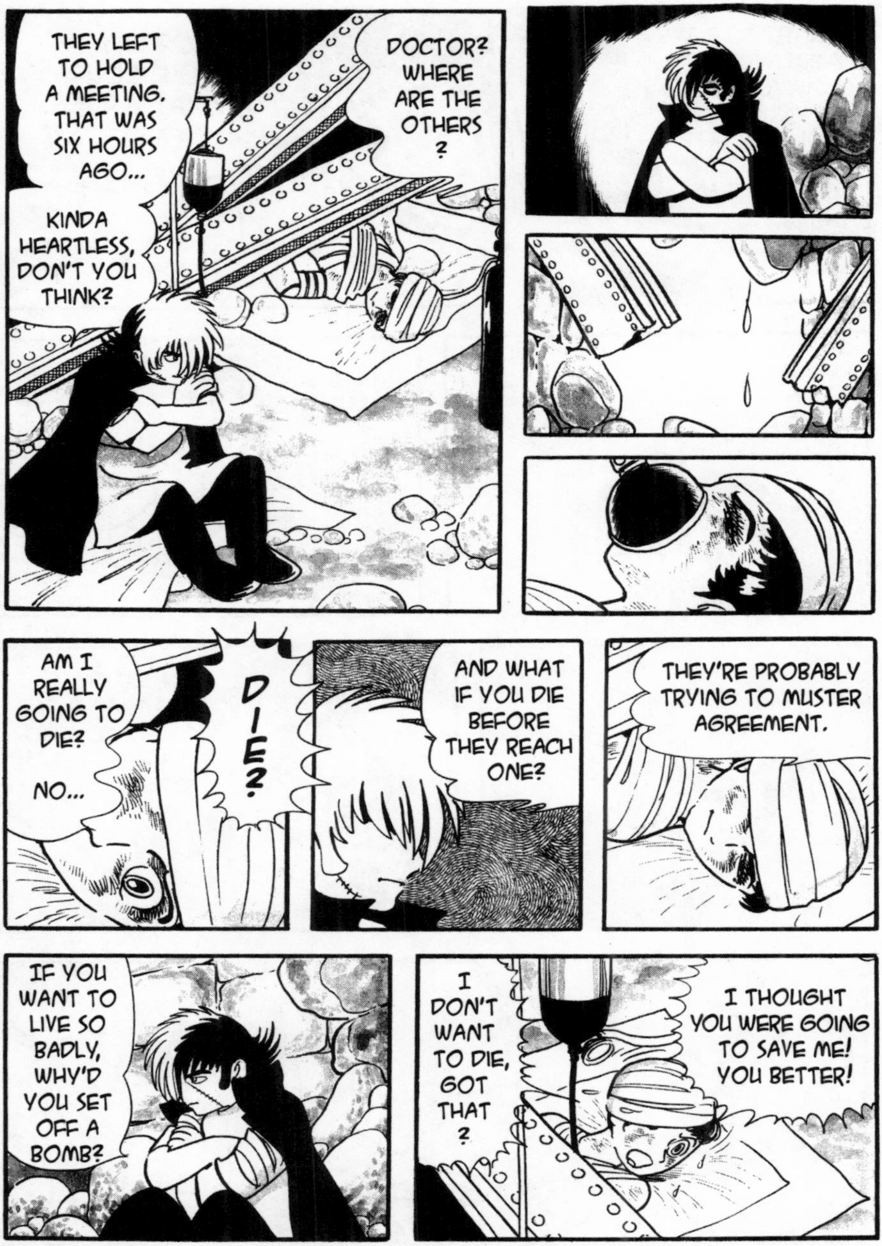
DOCTOR? WHERE ARE THE OTHERS?
THEY LEFT TO HOLD A MEETING. THAT WAS SIX HOURS AGO...
KINDA HEARTLESS, DON'T YOU THINK?
THEY'RE PROBABLY TRYING TO MUSTER AGREEMENT.
AND WHAT IF YOU DIE BEFORE THEY REACH ONE?
DIE?
AM I REALLY GOING TO DIE?
NO...
I THOUGHT YOU WERE GOING TO SAVE ME! YOU BETTER!
I DON'T WANT TO DIE, GOT THAT?
IF YOU WANT TO LIVE SO BADLY, WHY'D YOU SET OFF A BOMB?

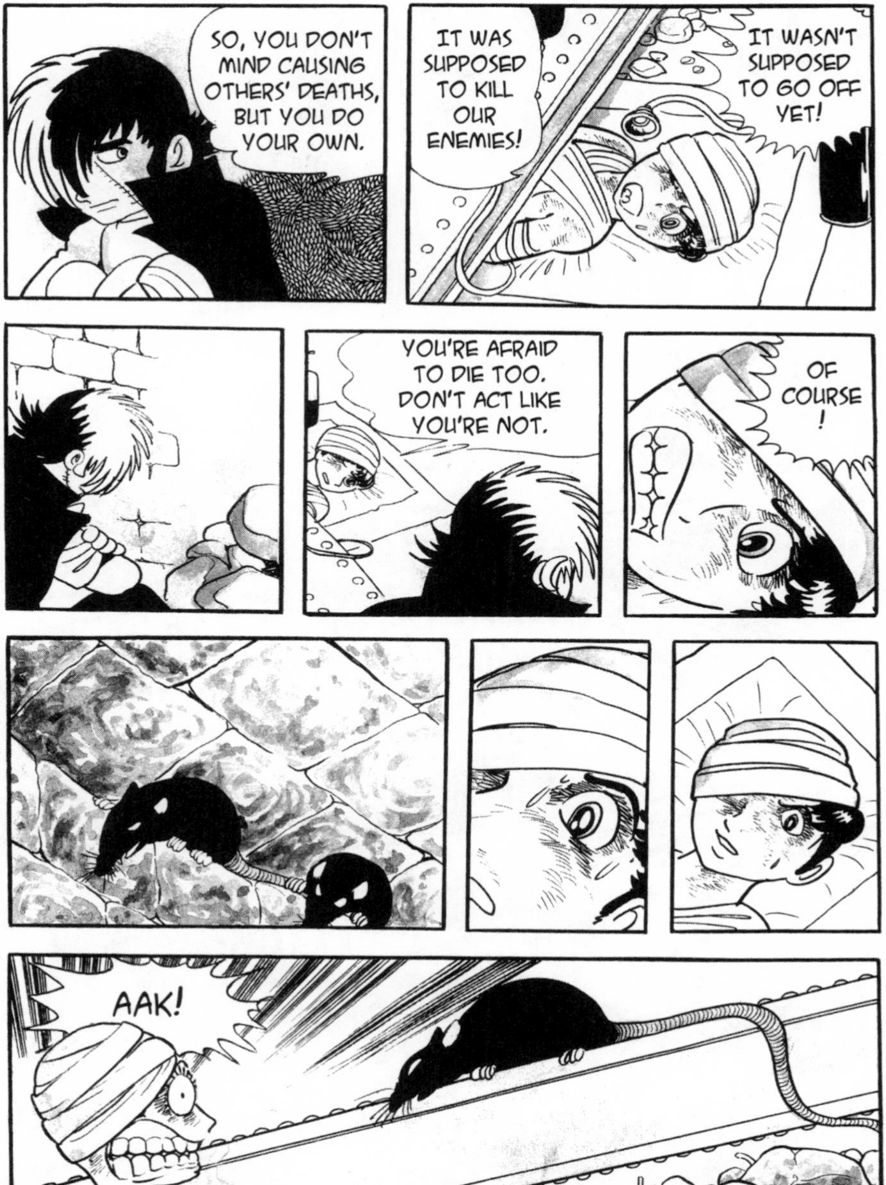
IT WASN'T SUPPOSED TO GO OFF YET!
IT WAS SUPPOSED TO KILL OUR ENEMIES!
SO, YOU DON'T MIND CAUSING OTHERS' DEATHS, BUT YOU DO YOUR OWN.
OF COURSE!
YOU'RE AFRAID TO DIE TOO. DON'T ACT LIKE YOU'RE NOT.
AAK!

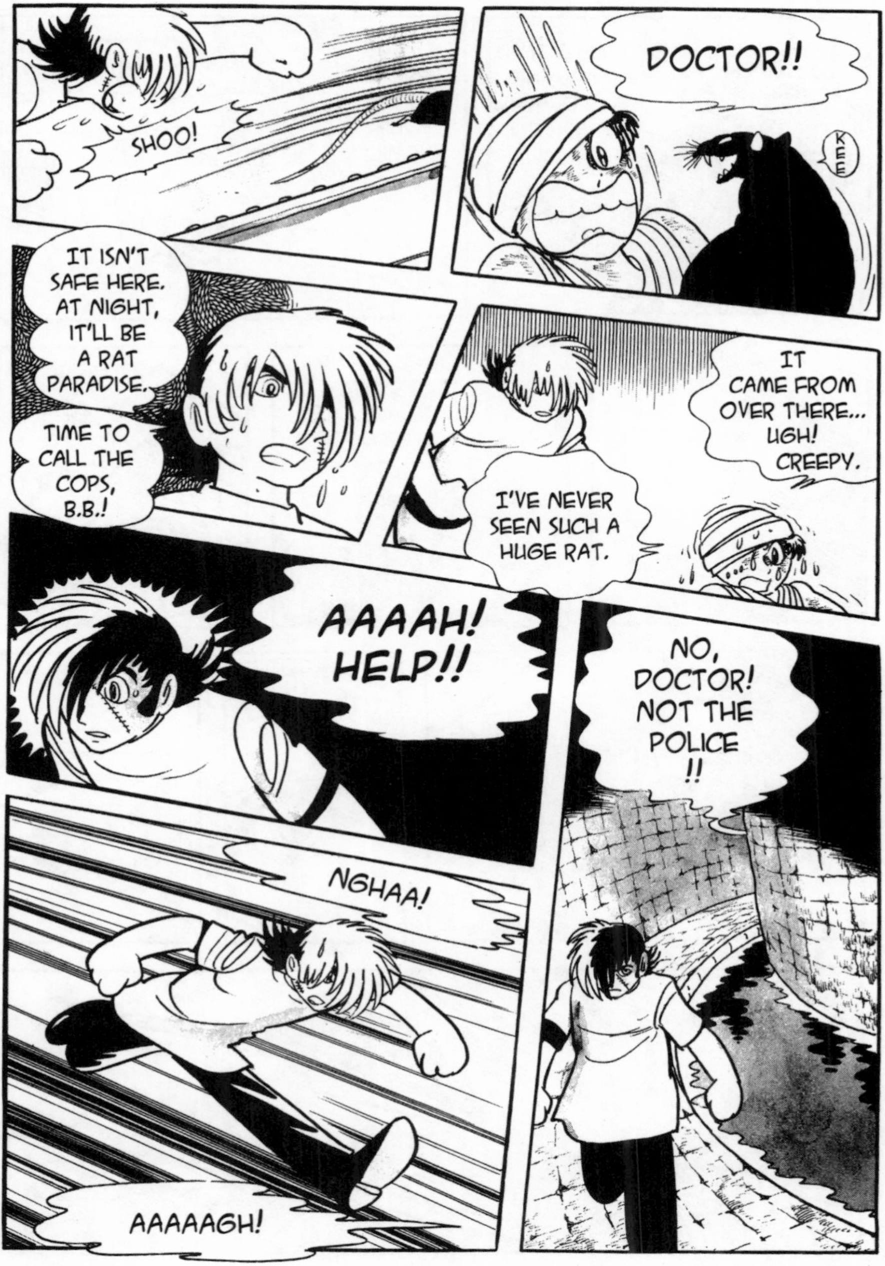
DOCTOR!!
KEEE
SHOO!
IT CAME FROM OVER THERE... UGH! CREEPY.
I'VE NEVER SEEN SUCH A HUGE RAT.
IT ISN'T SAFE HERE. AT NIGHT, IT'LL BE A RAT PARADISE.
TIME TO CALL THE COPS, B.B.!
NO, DOCTOR! NOT THE POLICE !!
AAAAH! HELP!!
NGHAA!
AAAAAGH!

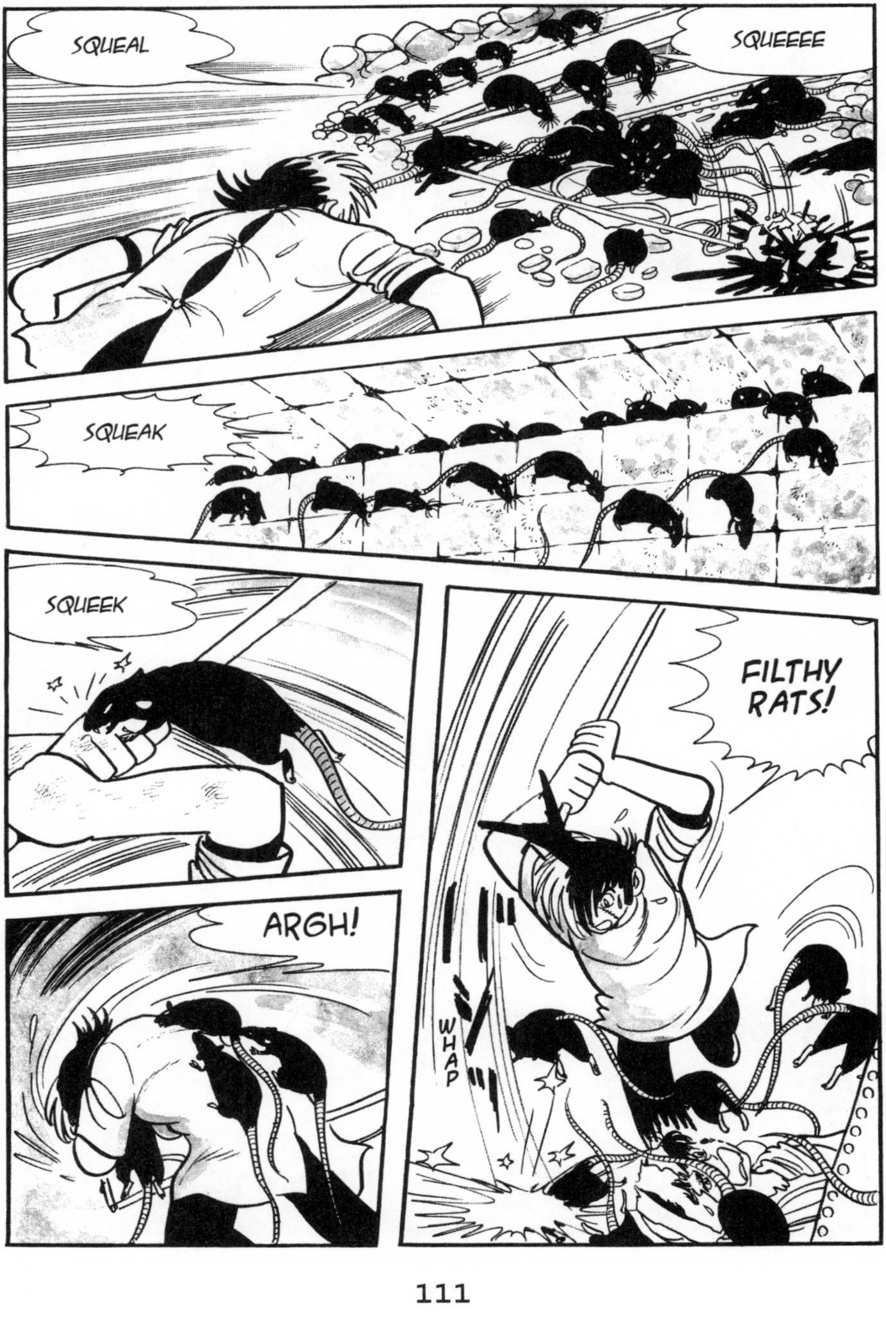
SQUEEEE
SQUEAL
SQUEAK
FILTHY RATS!
WHAP
SQUEEK
ARGH!

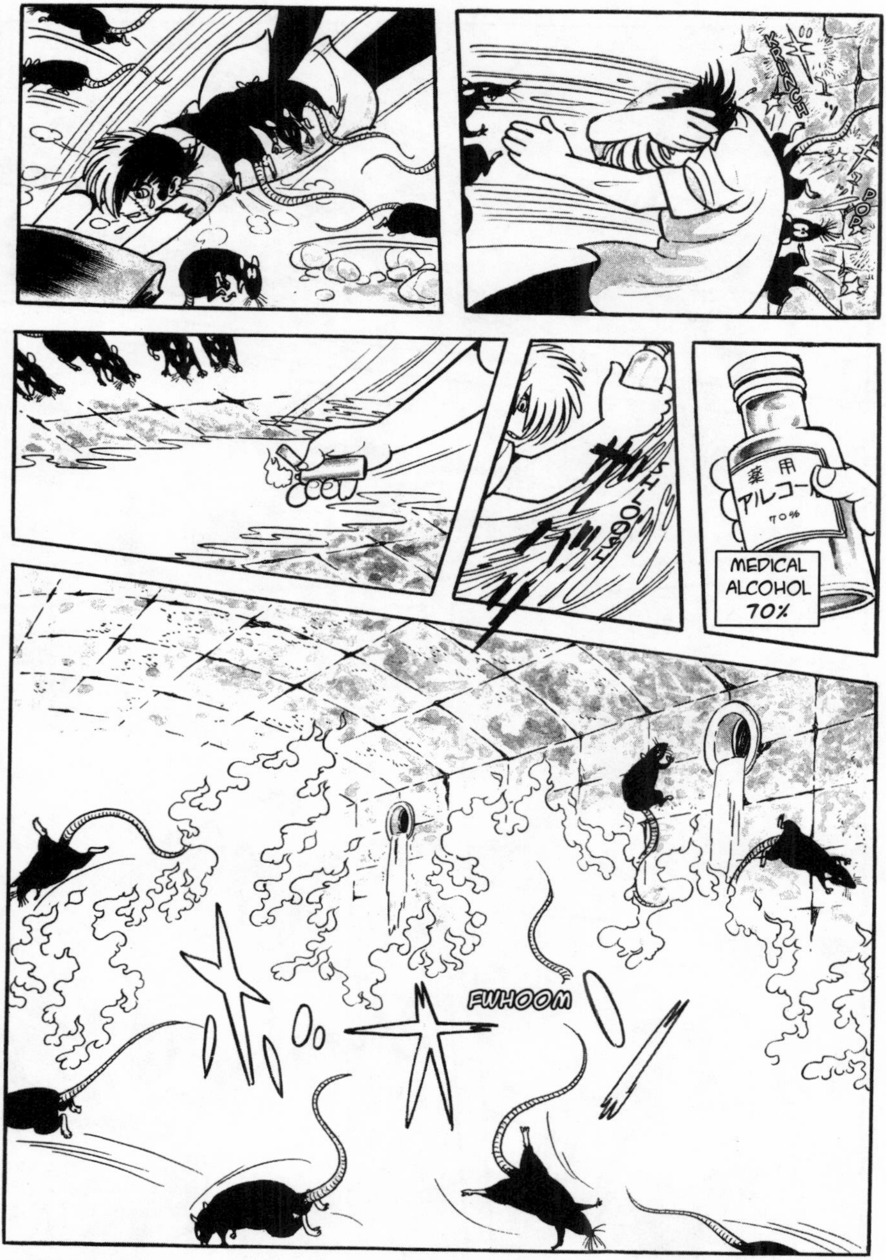
KRUNCH
POP POP
薬用
アルコール
70%
MEDICAL ALCOHOL 70%
SHLOOSH
FWHOOM

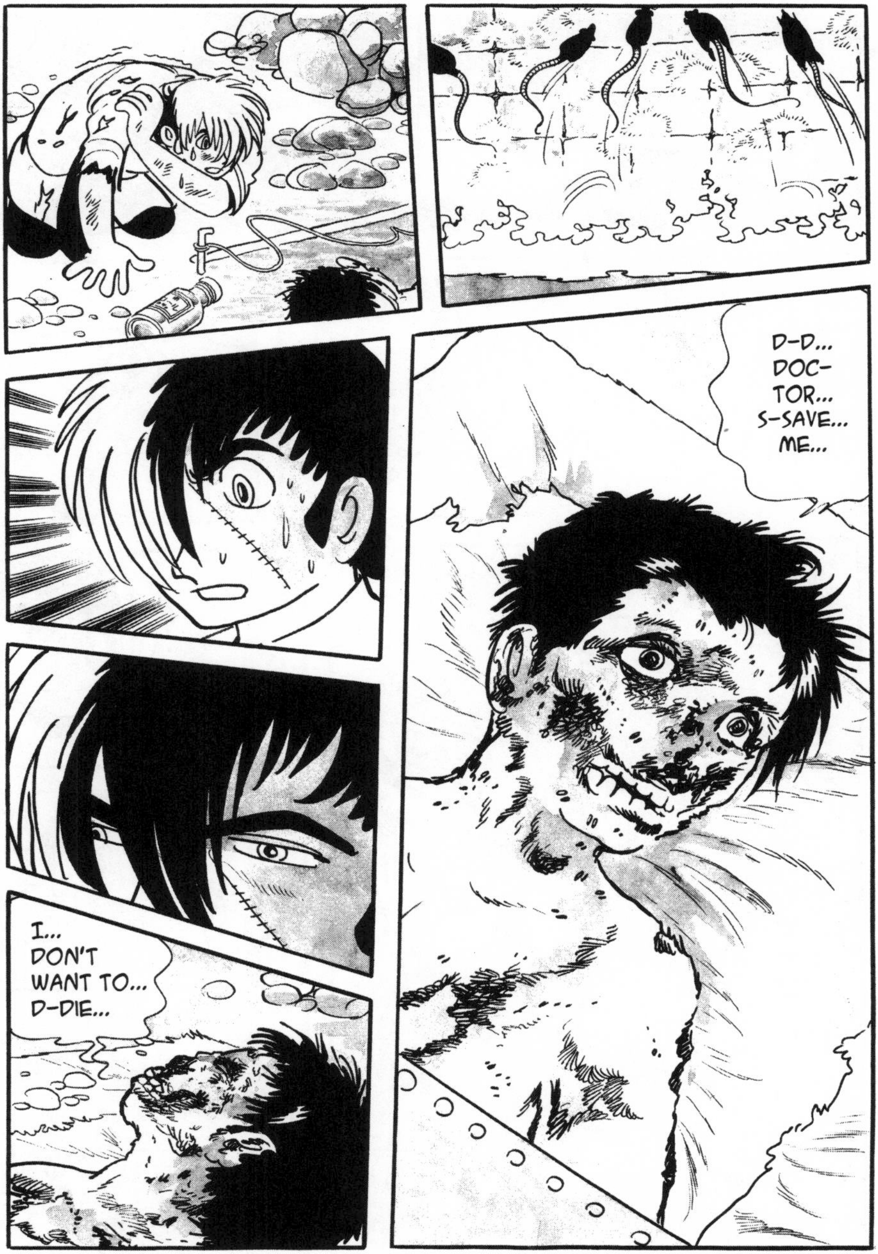
D-D... DOCTOR... S-SAVE... ME...
I... DON'T WANT TO... D-DIE...

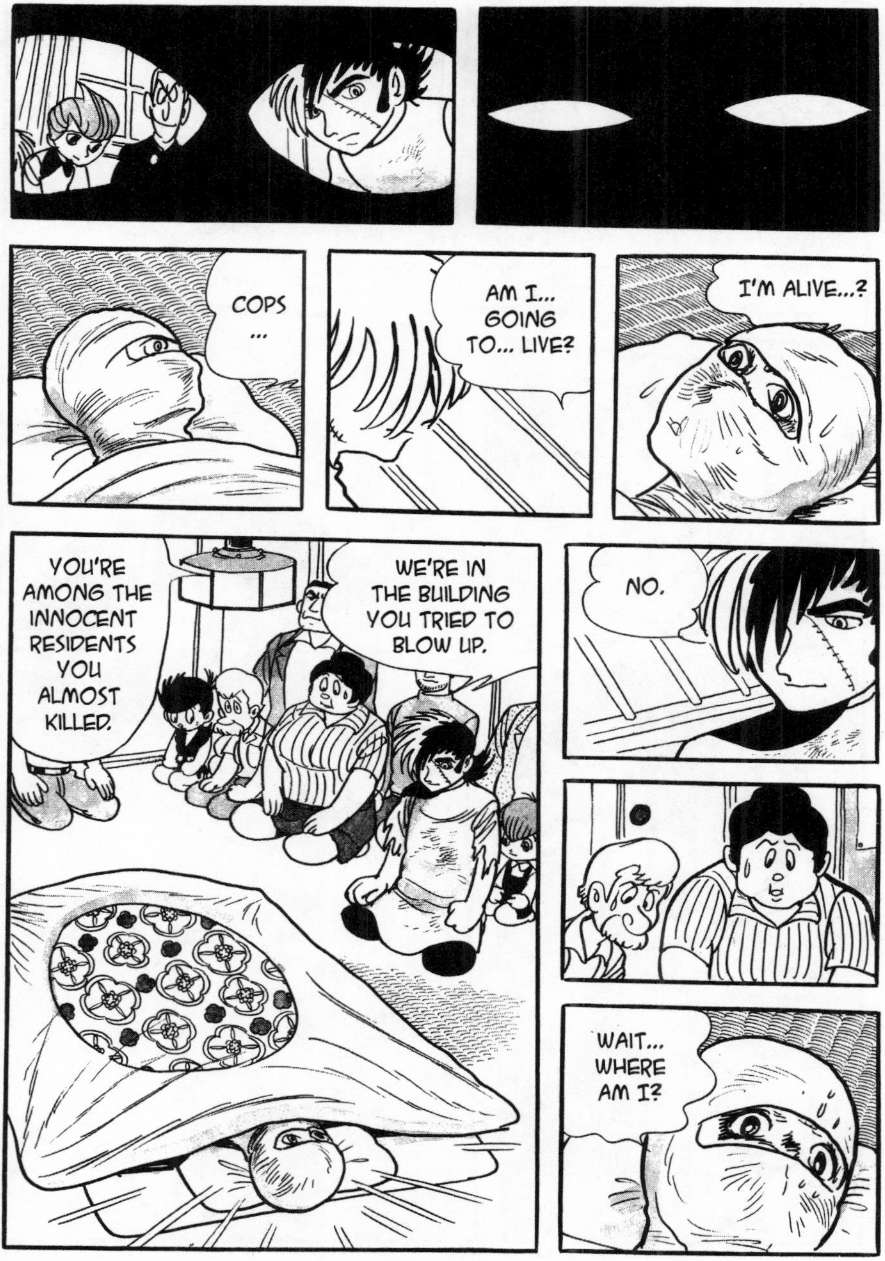
I'M ALIVE...?
AM I... GOING TO... LIVE?
COPS ...
NO.
WAIT... WHERE AM I?
WE'RE IN THE BUILDING YOU TRIED TO BLOW UP.
YOU'RE AMONG THE INNOCENT RESIDENTS YOU ALMOST KILLED.

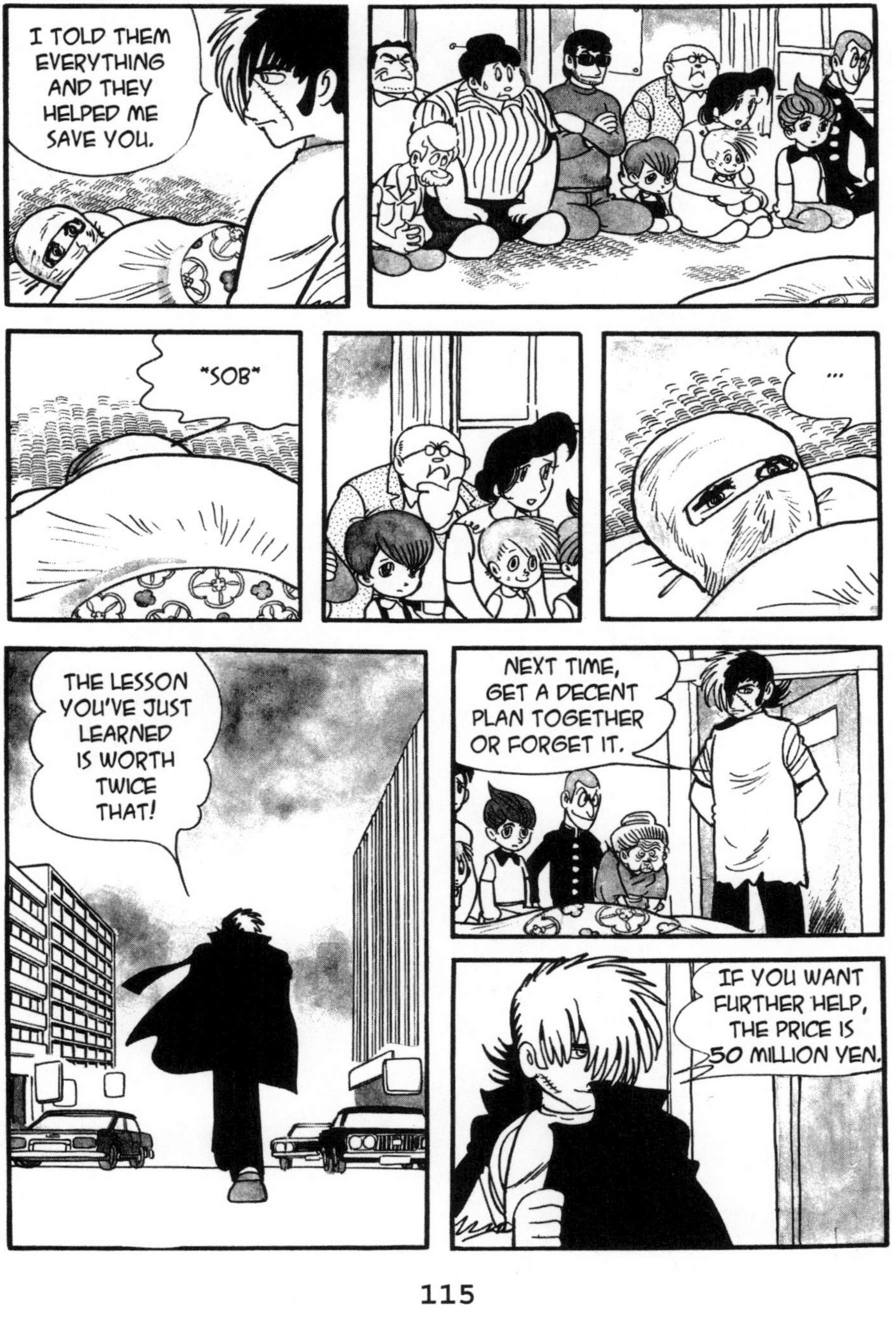
I TOLD THEM EVERYTHING AND THEY HELPED ME SAVE YOU.
...
SOB
NEXT TIME, GET A DECENT PLAN TOGETHER OR FORGET IT.
IF YOU WANT FURTHER HELP, THE PRICE IS 50 MILLION YEN.
THE LESSON YOU'VE JUST LEARNED IS WORTH TWICE THAT!

THE SEA SMELLS OF ROMANCE

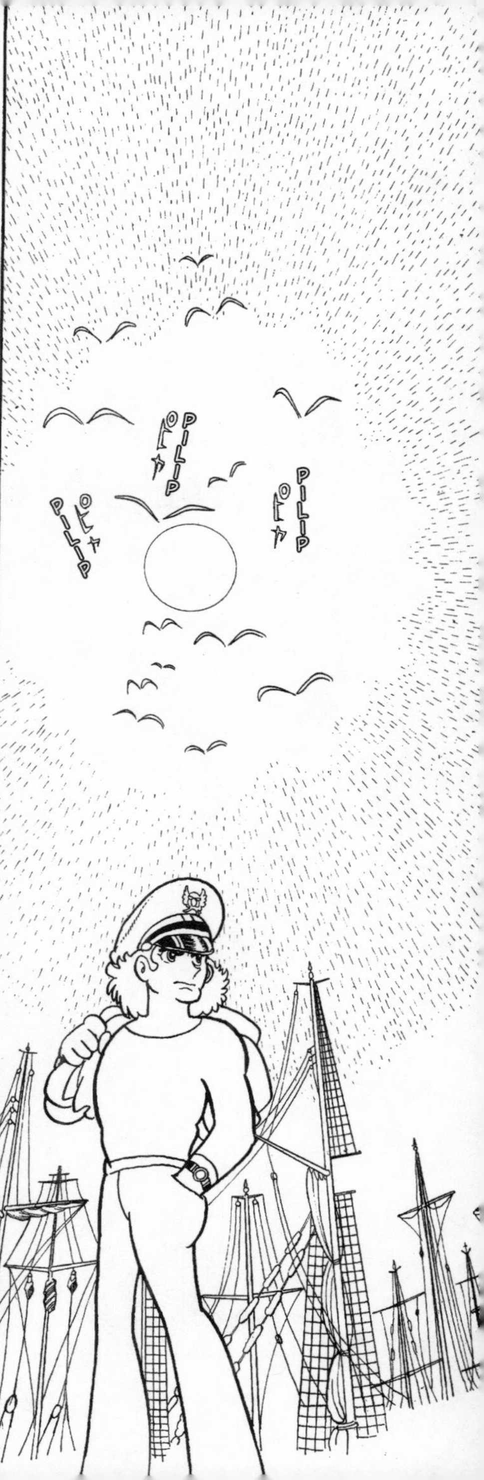
PILIP
PILIP
PILIP

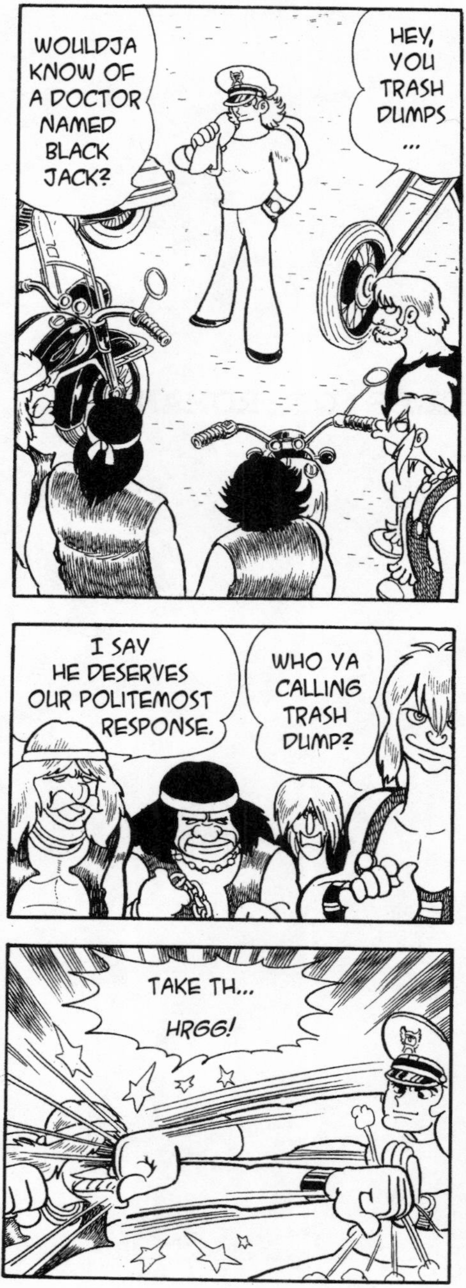
HEY, YOU TRASH DUMPS ...
WOULDJA KNOW OF A DOCTOR NAMED BLACK JACK?
WHO YA CALLING TRASH DUMP?
I SAY HE DESERVES OUR POLITEMOST RESPONSE.
TAKE TH...
HRGG!

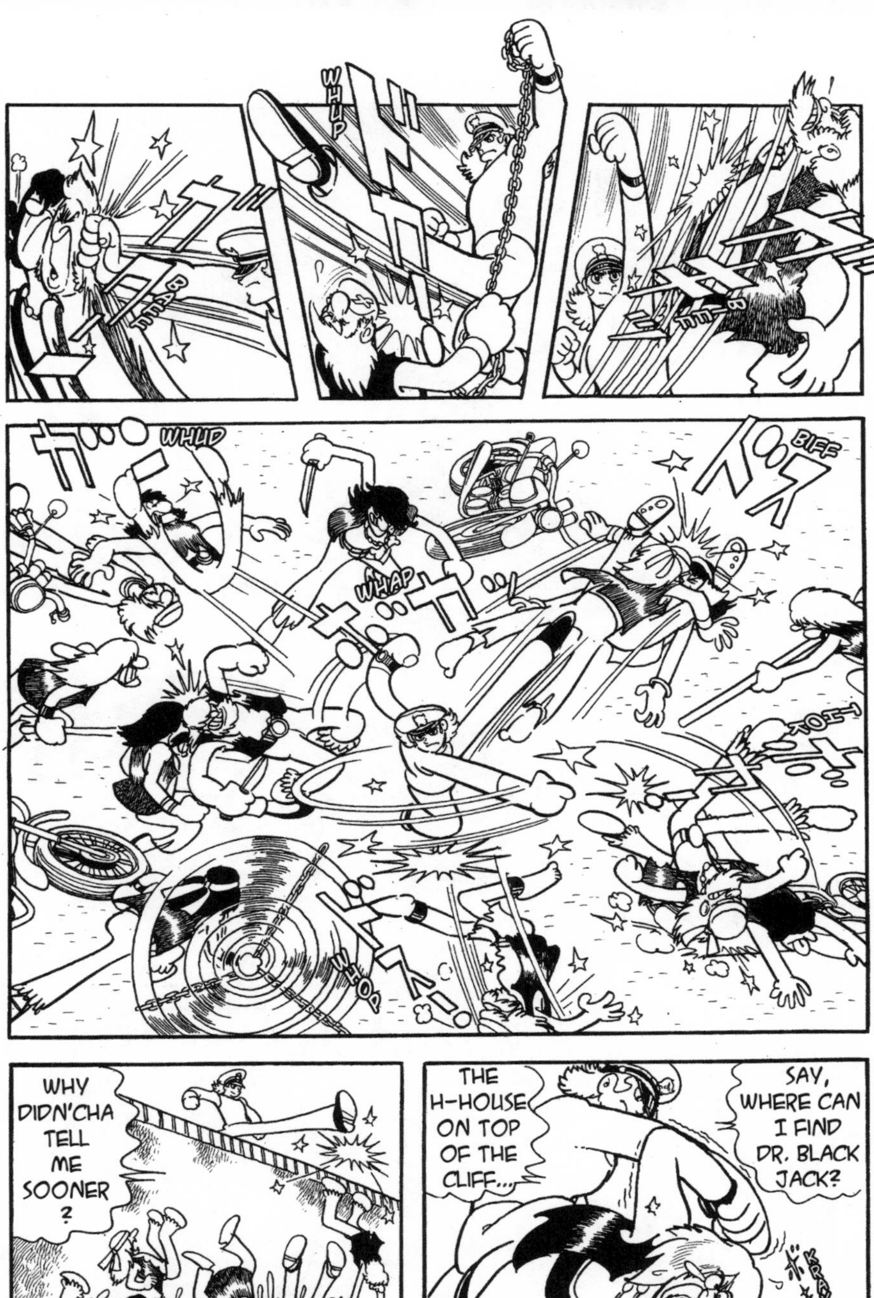
WHUP
BIFF
WHAP
WHUD
WHOP
SAY, WHERE CAN I FIND DR. BLACK JACK?
THE H-HOUSE ON TOP OF THE CLIFF...
KRAK
WHY DIDN'CHA TELL ME SOONER?

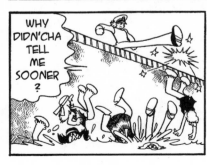

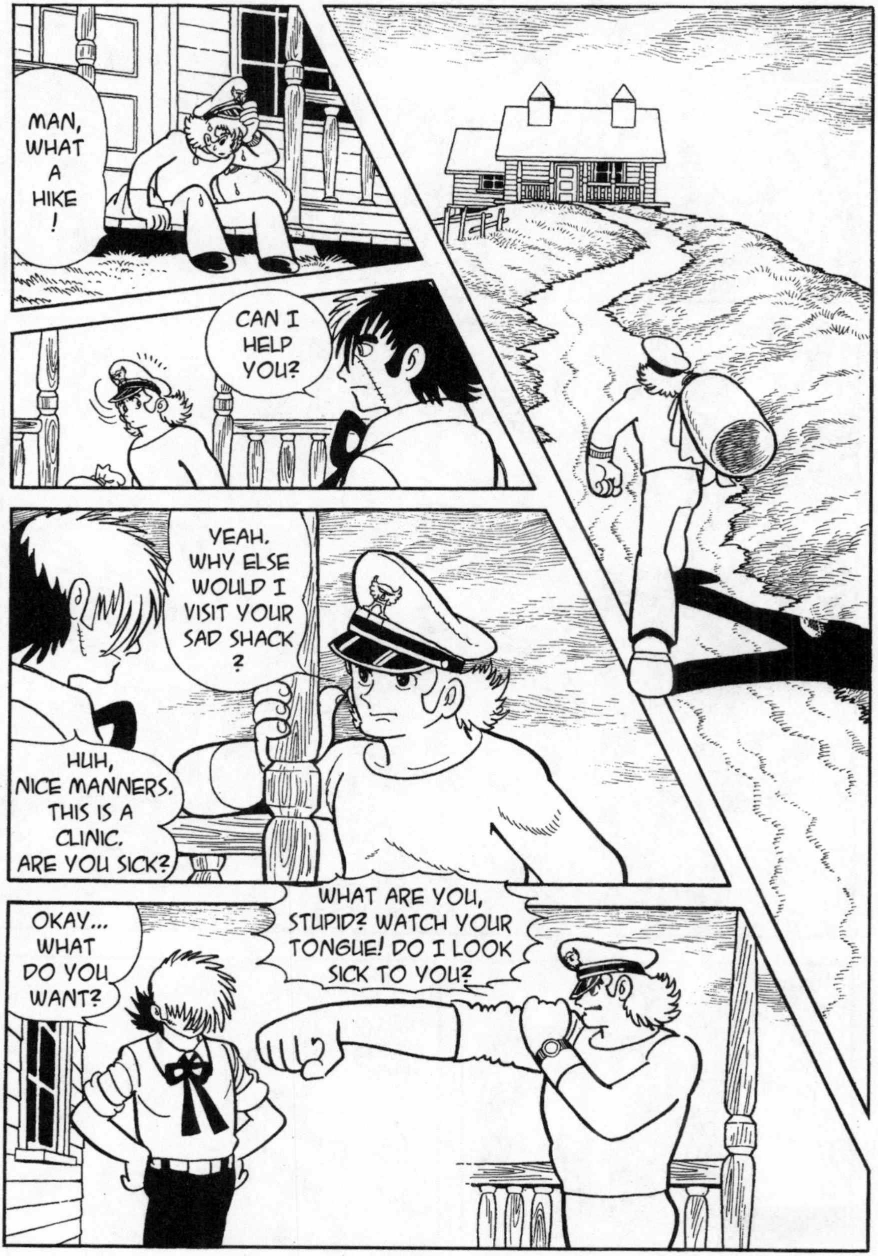
MAN, WHAT A HIKE!
CAN I HELP YOU?
YEAH. WHY ELSE WOULD I VISIT YOUR SAD SHACK?
HUH, NICE MANNERS. THIS IS A CLINIC. ARE YOU SICK?
WHAT ARE YOU, STUPID? WATCH YOUR TONGUE! DO I LOOK SICK TO YOU?
OKAY... WHAT DO YOU WANT?

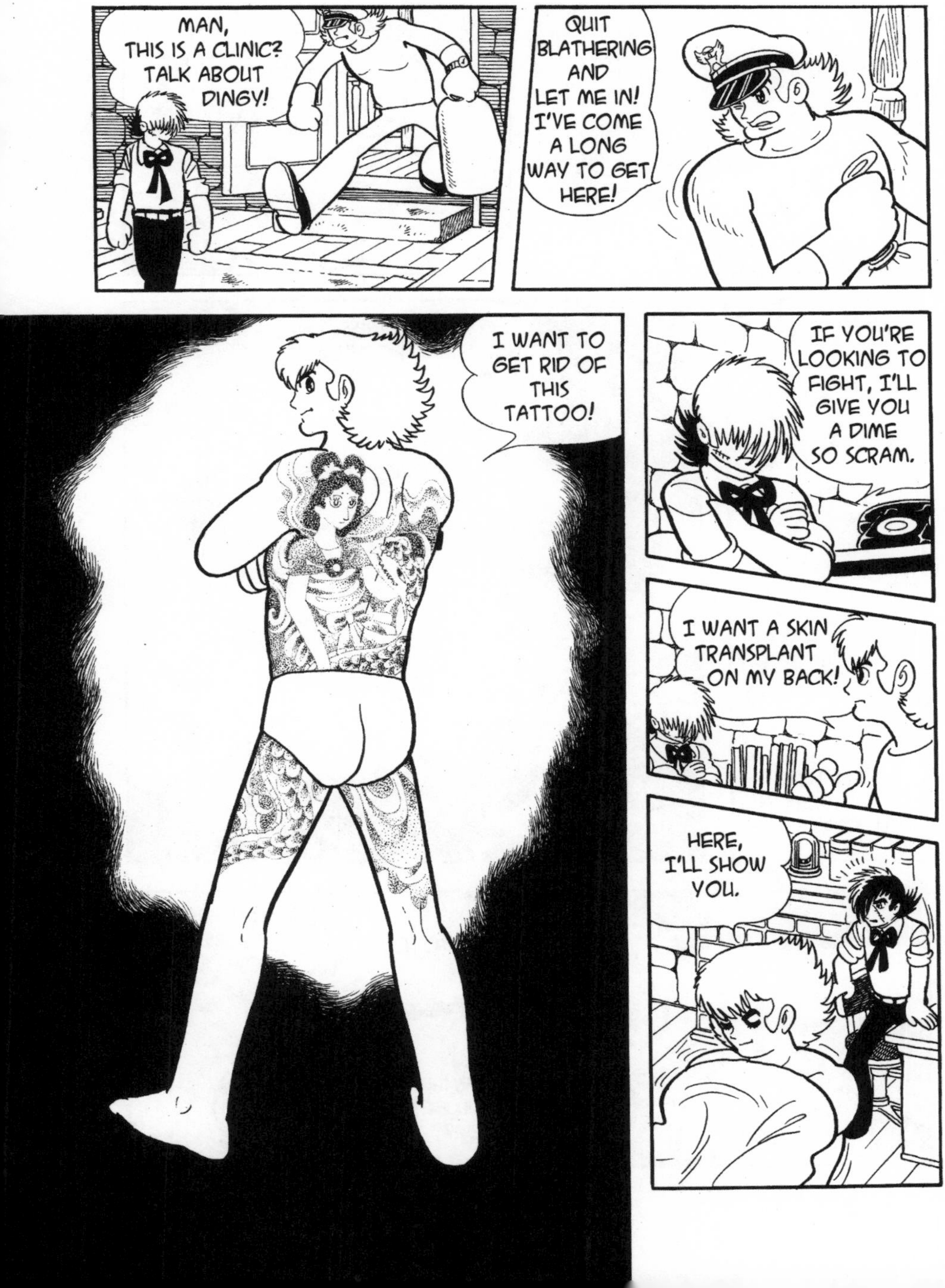
QUIT BLATHERING AND LET ME IN! I'VE COME A LONG WAY TO GET HERE!
MAN, THIS IS A CLINIC? TALK ABOUT DINGY!
IF YOU'RE LOOKING TO FIGHT, I'LL GIVE YOU A DIME SO SCRAM.
I WANT A SKIN TRANSPLANT ON MY BACK!
HERE, I'LL SHOW YOU.
I WANT TO GET RID OF THIS TATTOO!

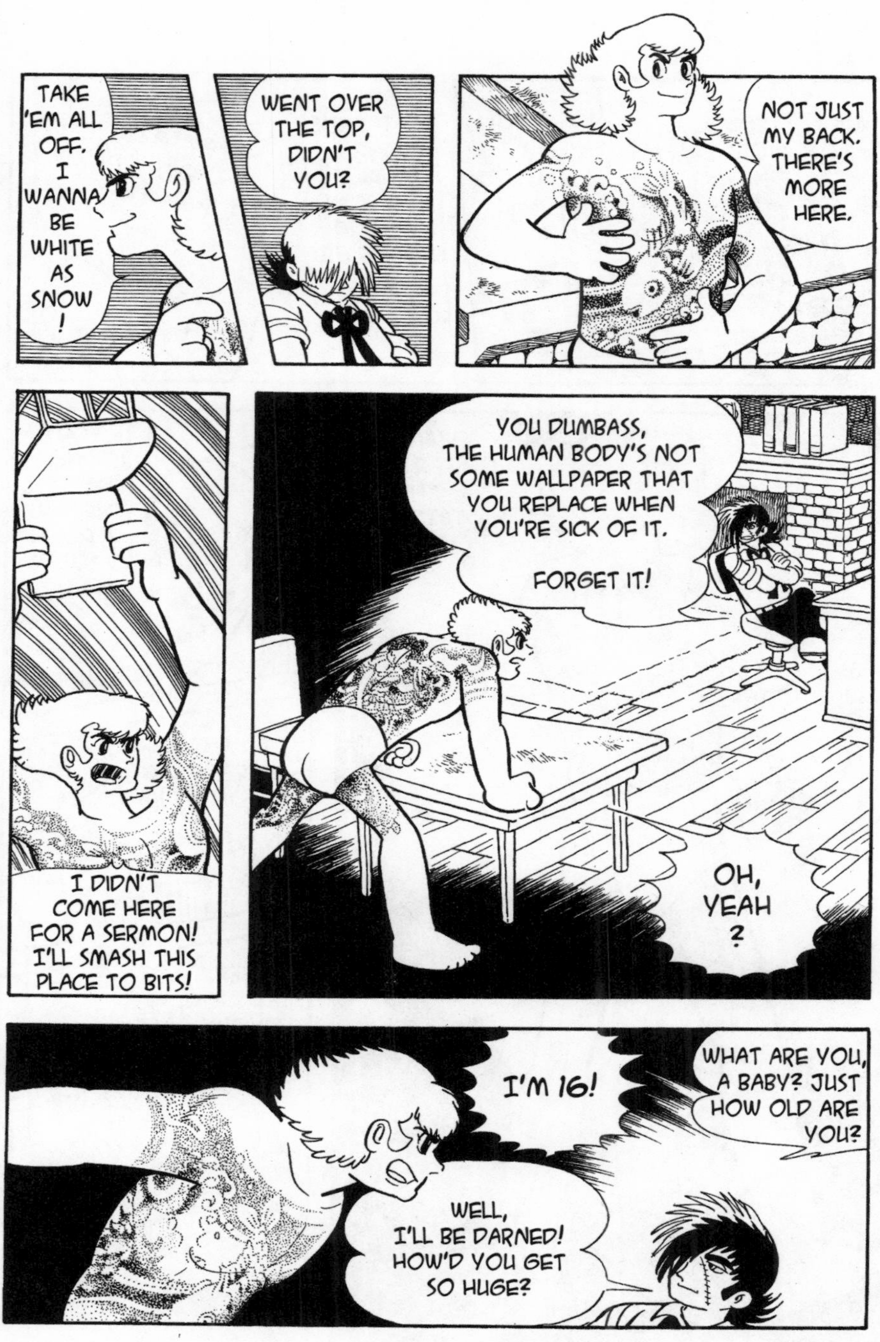
NOT JUST MY BACK. THERE'S MORE HERE.
WENT OVER THE TOP, DIDN'T YOU?
TAKE 'EM ALL OFF. I WANNA BE WHITE AS SNOW!
YOU DUMBASS, THE HUMAN BODY'S NOT SOME WALLPAPER THAT YOU REPLACE WHEN YOU'RE SICK OF IT.
FORGET IT!
OH, YEAH?
I DIDN'T COME HERE FOR A SERMON! I'LL SMASH THIS PLACE TO BITS!
WHAT ARE YOU, A BABY? JUST HOW OLD ARE YOU?
I'M 16!
WELL, I'LL BE DARNED! HOW'D YOU GET SO HUGE?

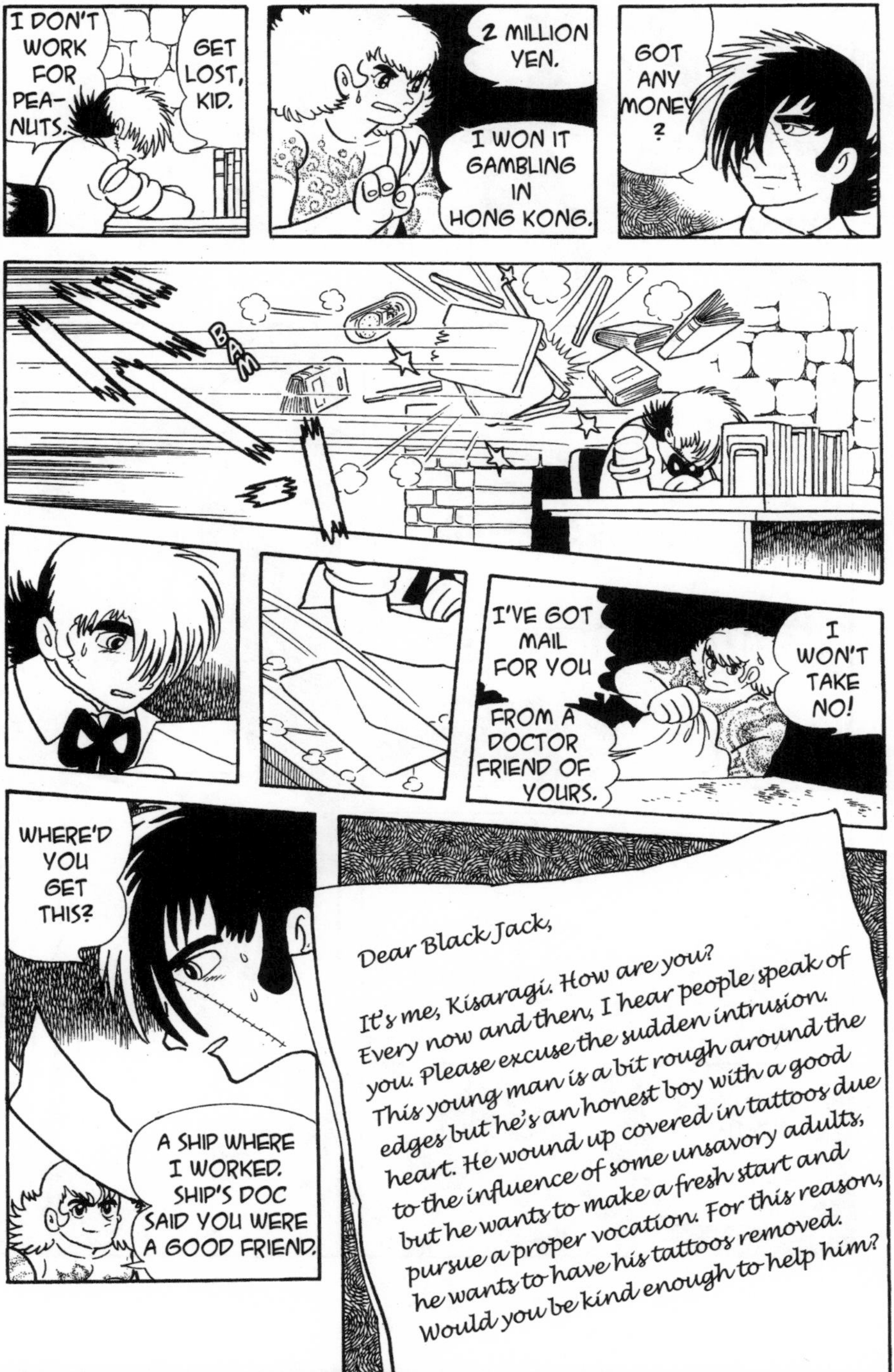
GOT ANY MONEY?
2 MILLION YEN.
I WON IT GAMBLING IN HONG KONG.
GET LOST, KID.
I DON'T WORK FOR PEA-NUTS.
BAM
I WON'T TAKE NO!
I'VE GOT MAIL FOR YOU
FROM A DOCTOR FRIEND OF YOURS.
Dear Black Jack,
It's me, Kisaragi. How are you? Every now and then, I hear people speak of you. Please excuse the sudden intrusion. This young man is a bit rough around the edges but he's an honest boy with a good heart. He wound up covered in tattoos due to the influence of some unsavory adults, but he wants to make a fresh start and pursue a proper vocation. For this reason, he wants to have his tattoos removed. Would you be kind enough to help him?
WHERE'D YOU GET THIS?
A SHIP WHERE I WORKED. SHIP'S DOC SAID YOU WERE A GOOD FRIEND.

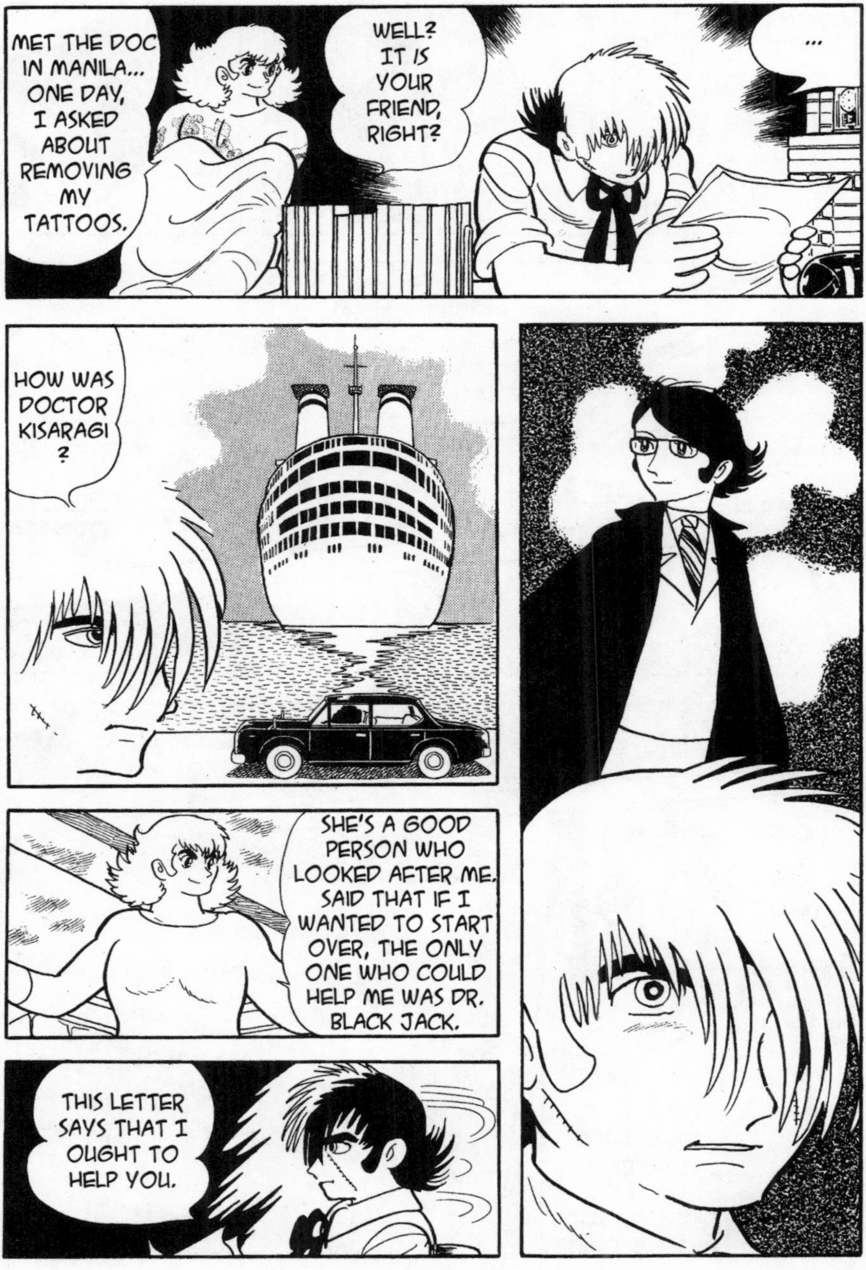
...
WELL? IT IS YOUR FRIEND, RIGHT?
MET THE DOC IN MANILA... ONE DAY, I ASKED ABOUT REMOVING MY TATTOOS.
HOW WAS DOCTOR KISARAGI?
SHE'S A GOOD PERSON WHO LOOKED AFTER ME. SAID THAT IF I WANTED TO START OVER, THE ONLY ONE WHO COULD HELP ME WAS DR. BLACK JACK.
THIS LETTER SAYS THAT I OUGHT TO HELP YOU.

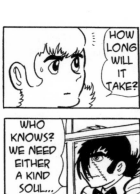

SEE?
SO HURRY AND DO IT!
HOW LONG WILL IT TAKE?
WHO KNOWS? WE NEED EITHER A KIND SOUL...
LISTEN UP.
GETTING RID OF YOUR TATTOO WILL BE A MAJOR OPERATION.
YOU NEED SOMEONE ELSE'S SKIN. UNDERSTAND?
NOT JUST THE EPIDERMIS, EITHER. WE NEED SUBCUTANEOUS TISSUE AS WELL. IT'S CUMBERSOME. IT TAKES A LOT OF TIME AND FIRST WE NEED TO FIND A SKIN DONOR.
OR A CORPSE. GO HOME AND WAIT FOR ME TO SEND WORD.
I FIGURED. I BROUGHT A TENT. I CAN LIVE OUT HERE FOR DAYS.
BESIDES, THESE EPISODES ARE ONLY 20 PAGES LONG, RIGHT?
YOU'LL HAVE TO COME UP WITH SOMETHING PRETTY SOON.
SHUT UP!

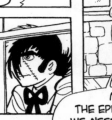

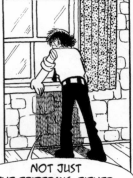

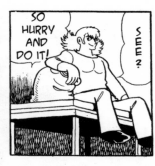

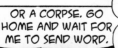

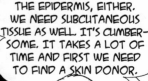

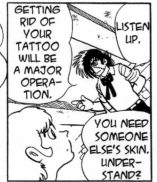

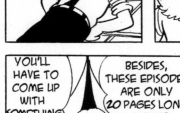

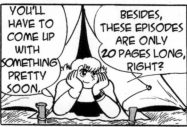

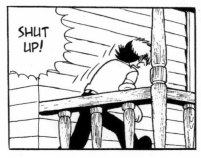

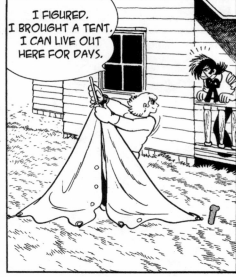

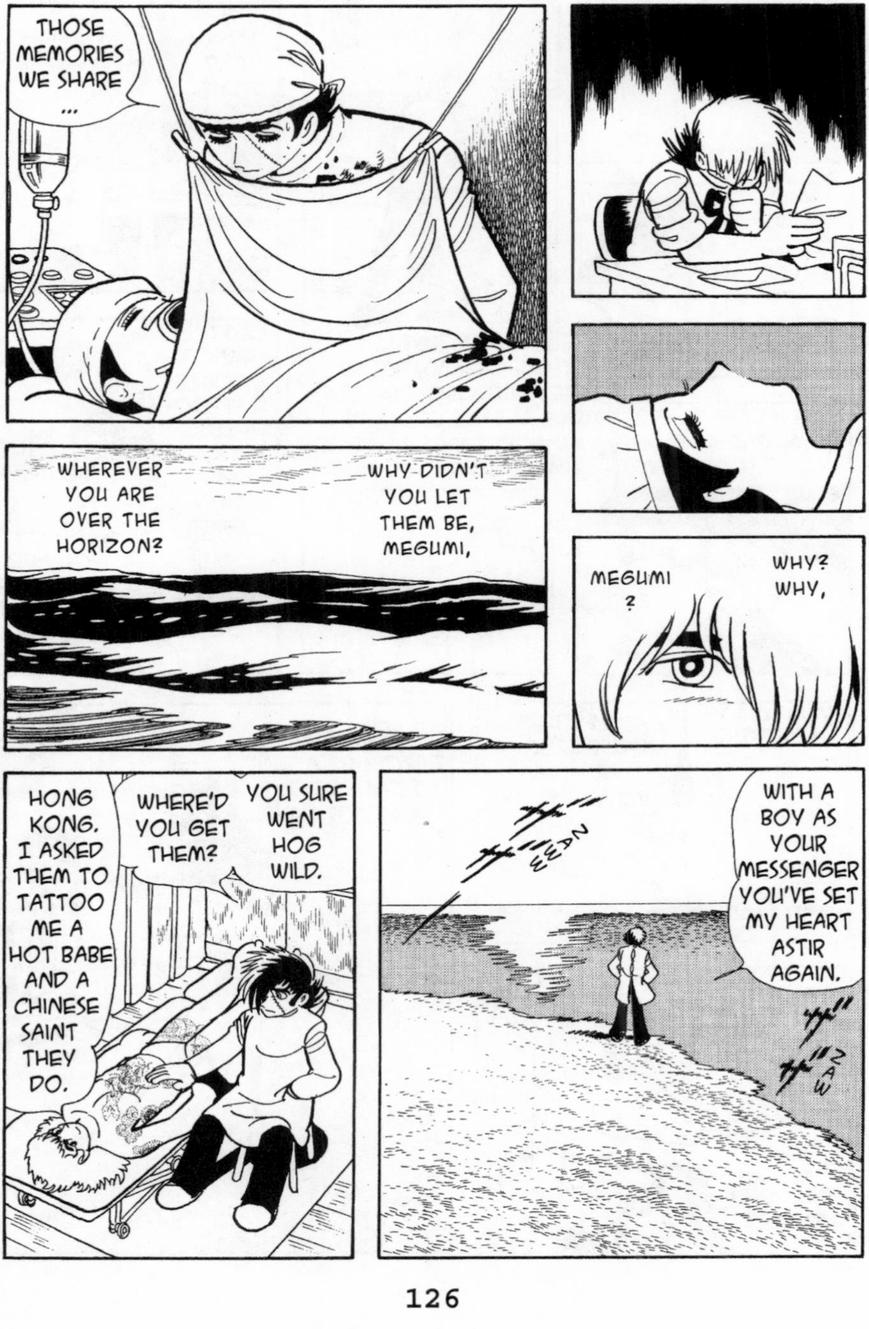
THOSE MEMORIES WE SHARE ...
WHY? WHY,
MEGUMI ?
WHY DIDN'T YOU LET THEM BE, MEGUMI,
WHEREVER YOU ARE OVER THE HORIZON?
ZAW
WITH A BOY AS YOUR MESSENGER YOU'VE SET MY HEART ASTIR AGAIN.
ZAW
YOU SURE WENT HOG WILD.
WHERE'D YOU GET THEM?
HONG KONG. I ASKED THEM TO TATTOO ME A HOT BABE AND A CHINESE SAINT THEY DO.

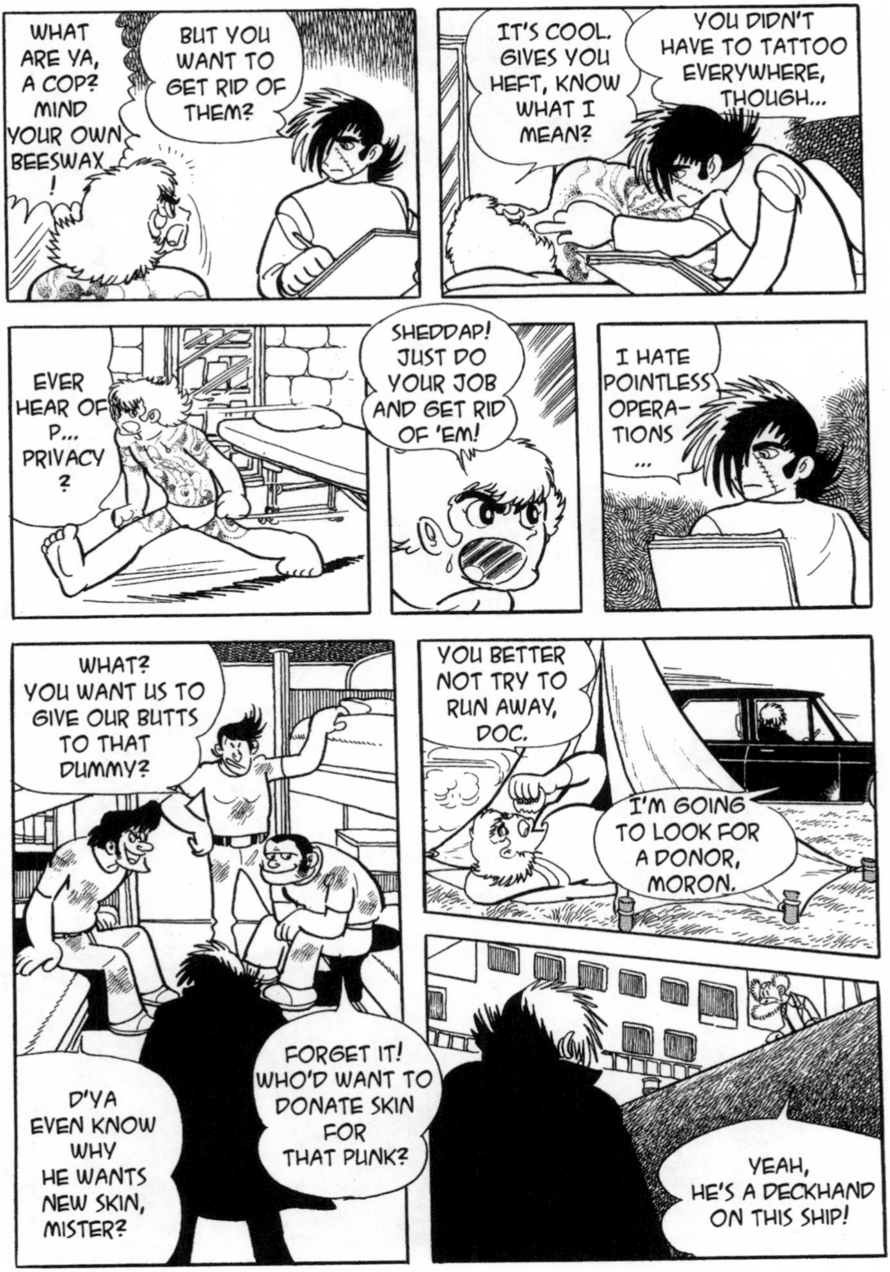
YOU DIDN'T HAVE TO TATTOO EVERYWHERE, THOUGH...
IT'S COOL. GIVES YOU HEFT, KNOW WHAT I MEAN?
BUT YOU WANT TO GET RID OF THEM?
WHAT ARE YA, A COP? MIND YOUR OWN BEESWAX!
I HATE POINTLESS OPERATIONS...
SHEDDAP! JUST DO YOUR JOB AND GET RID OF 'EM!
EVER HEAR OF P... PRIVACY?
YOU BETTER NOT TRY TO RUN AWAY, DOC.
I'M GOING TO LOOK FOR A DONOR, MORON.
YEAH, HE'S A DECKHAND ON THIS SHIP!
WHAT? YOU WANT US TO GIVE OUR BUTTS TO THAT DUMMY?
FORGET IT! WHO'D WANT TO DONATE SKIN FOR THAT PUNK?
D'YA EVEN KNOW WHY HE WANTS NEW SKIN, MISTER?

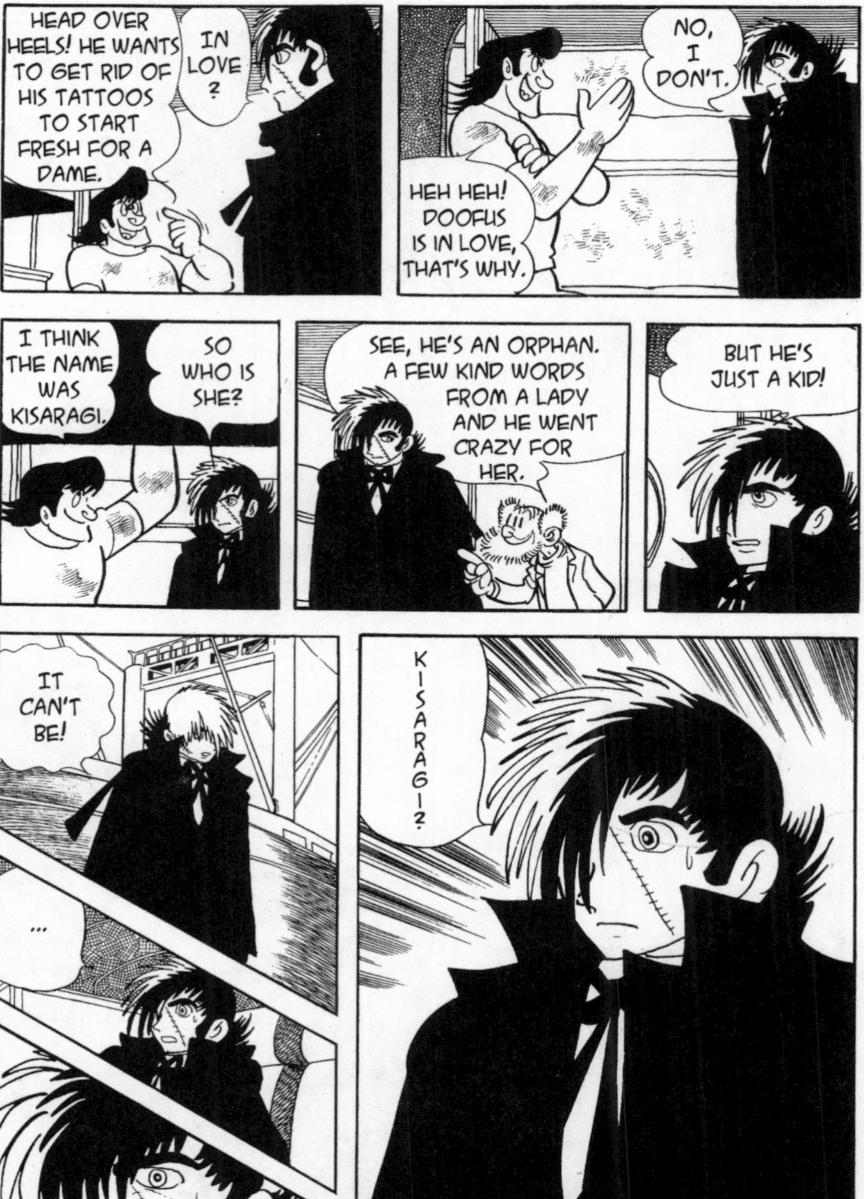
NO, I DON'T.
HEH HEH! DOOFUS IS IN LOVE, THAT'S WHY.
IN LOVE?
HEAD OVER HEELS! HE WANTS TO GET RID OF HIS TATTOOS TO START FRESH FOR A DAME.
BUT HE'S JUST A KID!
SEE, HE'S AN ORPHAN. A FEW KIND WORDS FROM A LADY AND HE WENT CRAZY FOR HER.
SO WHO IS SHE?
I THINK THE NAME WAS KISARAGI.
KISARAGI?
IT CAN'T BE!
...

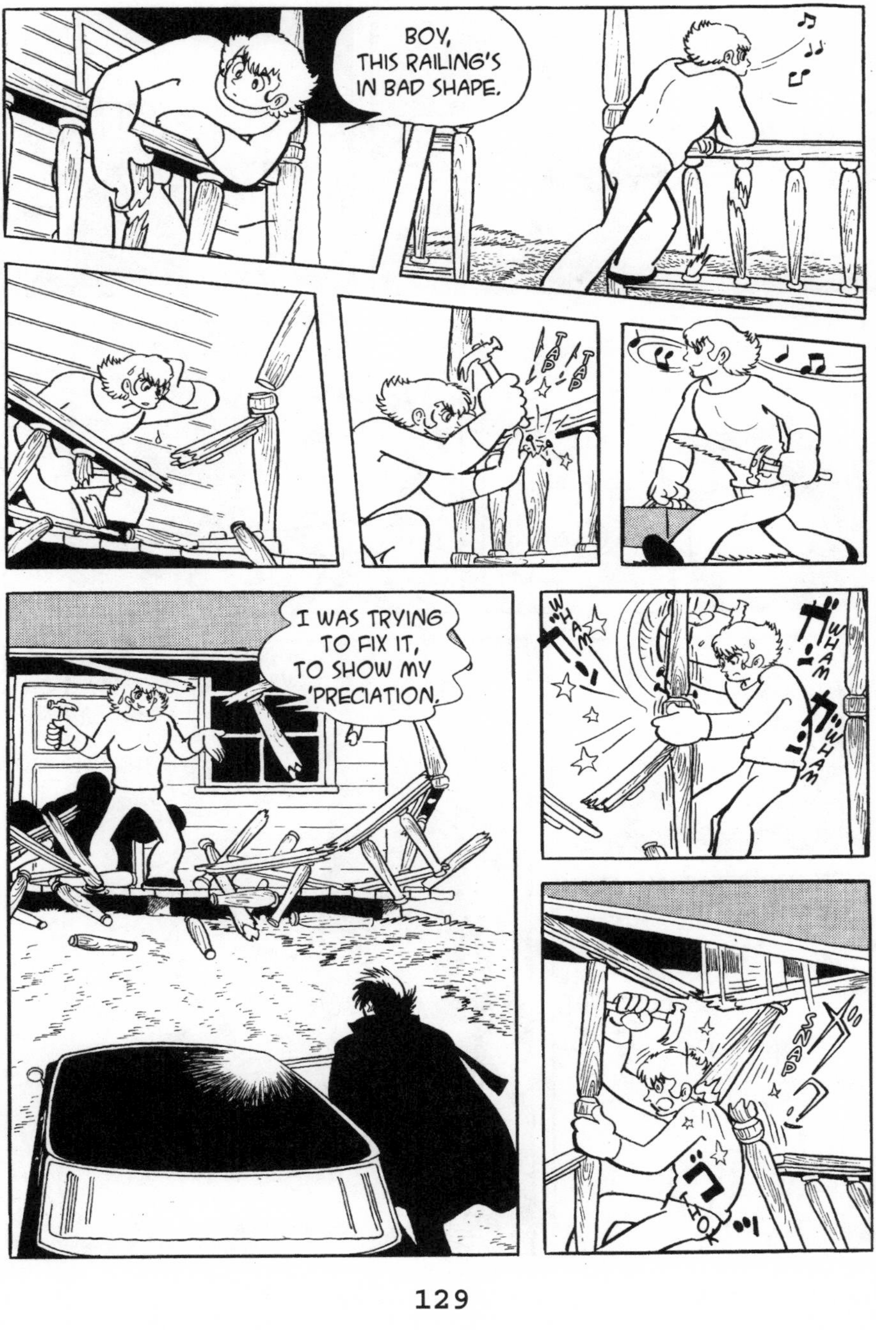
BOY, THIS RAILING'S IN BAD SHAPE.
TAP TAP
WHAM
WHAM
WHAM
SNAP
HOK
I WAS TRYING TO FIX IT, TO SHOW MY 'PRECIATION.

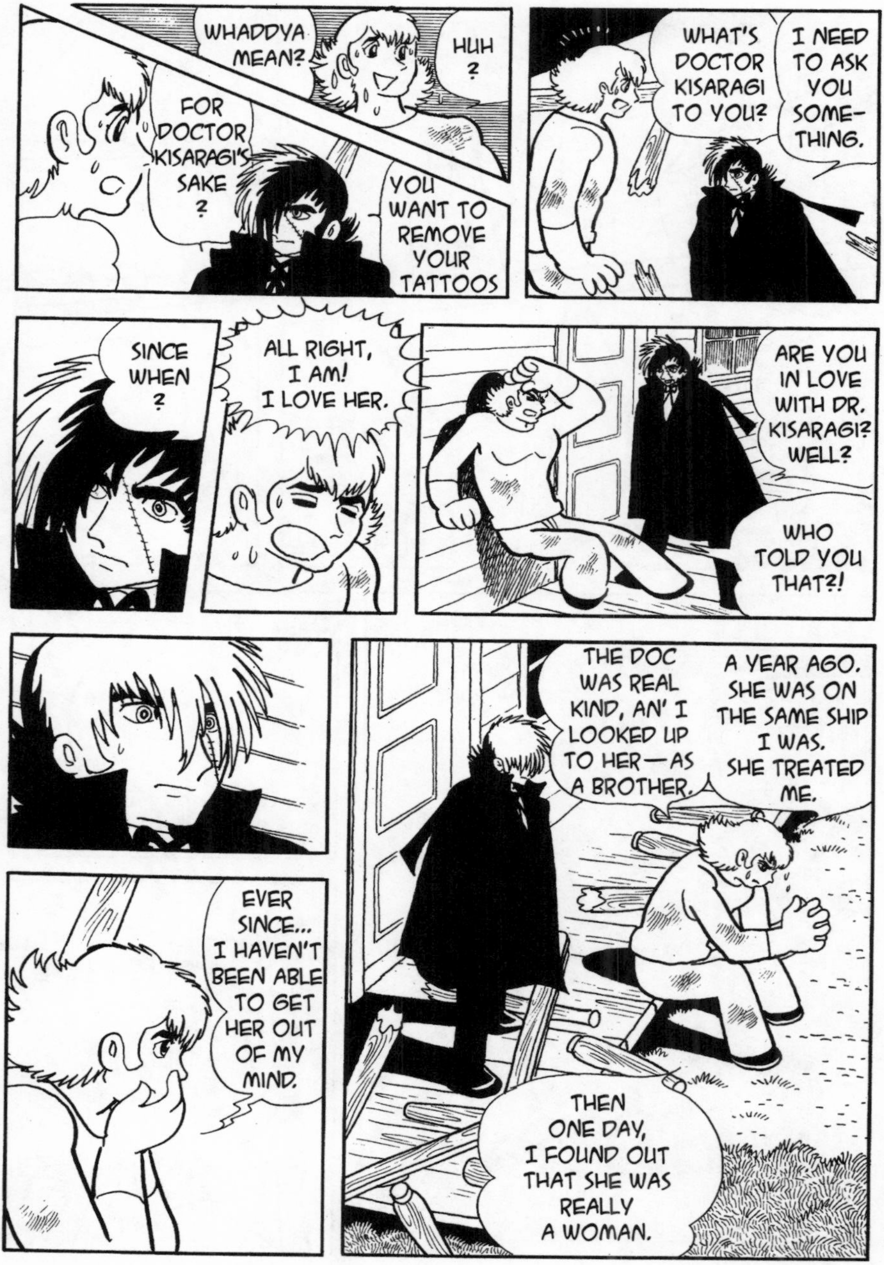
I NEED TO ASK YOU SOMETHING.
WHAT'S DOCTOR KISARAGI TO YOU?
YOU WANT TO REMOVE YOUR TATTOOS
FOR DOCTOR KISARAGI'S SAKE?
HUH?
WHADDYA MEAN?
ARE YOU IN LOVE WITH DR. KISARAGI? WELL?
WHO TOLD YOU THAT?!
ALL RIGHT, I AM! I LOVE HER.
SINCE WHEN?
A YEAR AGO. SHE WAS ON THE SAME SHIP I WAS. SHE TREATED ME.
THE DOC WAS REAL KIND, AN' I LOOKED UP TO HER—AS A BROTHER.
THEN ONE DAY, I FOUND OUT THAT SHE WAS REALLY A WOMAN.
EVER SINCE... I HAVEN'T BEEN ABLE TO GET HER OUT OF MY MIND.

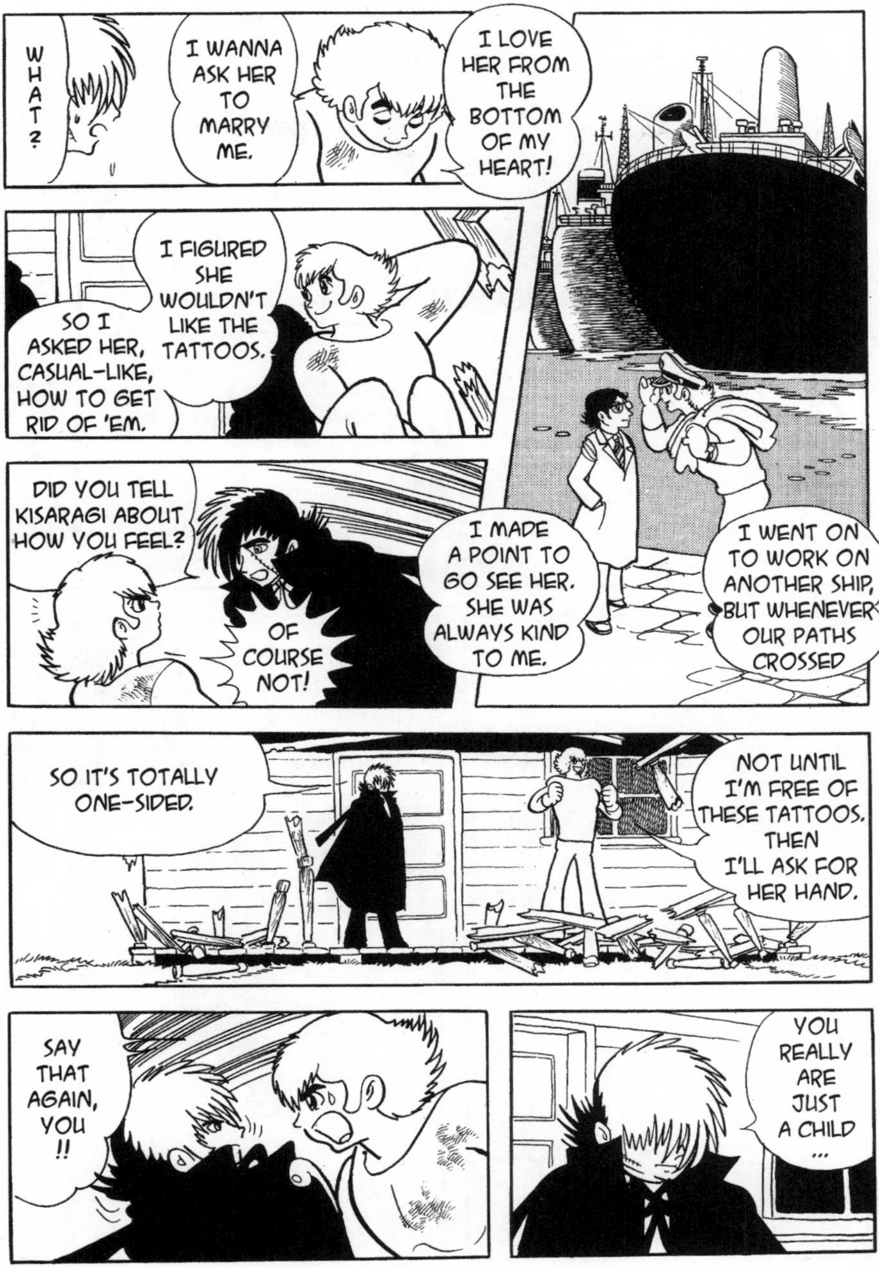

I WENT ON TO WORK ON ANOTHER SHIP, BUT WHENEVER OUR PATHS CROSSED
I MADE A POINT TO GO SEE HER. SHE WAS ALWAYS KIND TO ME.
I LOVE HER FROM THE BOTTOM OF MY HEART!
I WANNA ASK HER TO MARRY ME.
WHAT?
I FIGURED SHE WOULDN'T LIKE THE TATTOOS.
SO I ASKED HER, CASUAL-LIKE, HOW TO GET RID OF 'EM.
DID YOU TELL KISARAGI ABOUT HOW YOU FEEL?
OF COURSE NOT!
SO IT'S TOTALLY ONE-SIDED.
NOT UNTIL I'M FREE OF THESE TATTOOS. THEN I'LL ASK FOR HER HAND.
YOU REALLY ARE JUST A CHILD ...
SAY THAT AGAIN, YOU !!

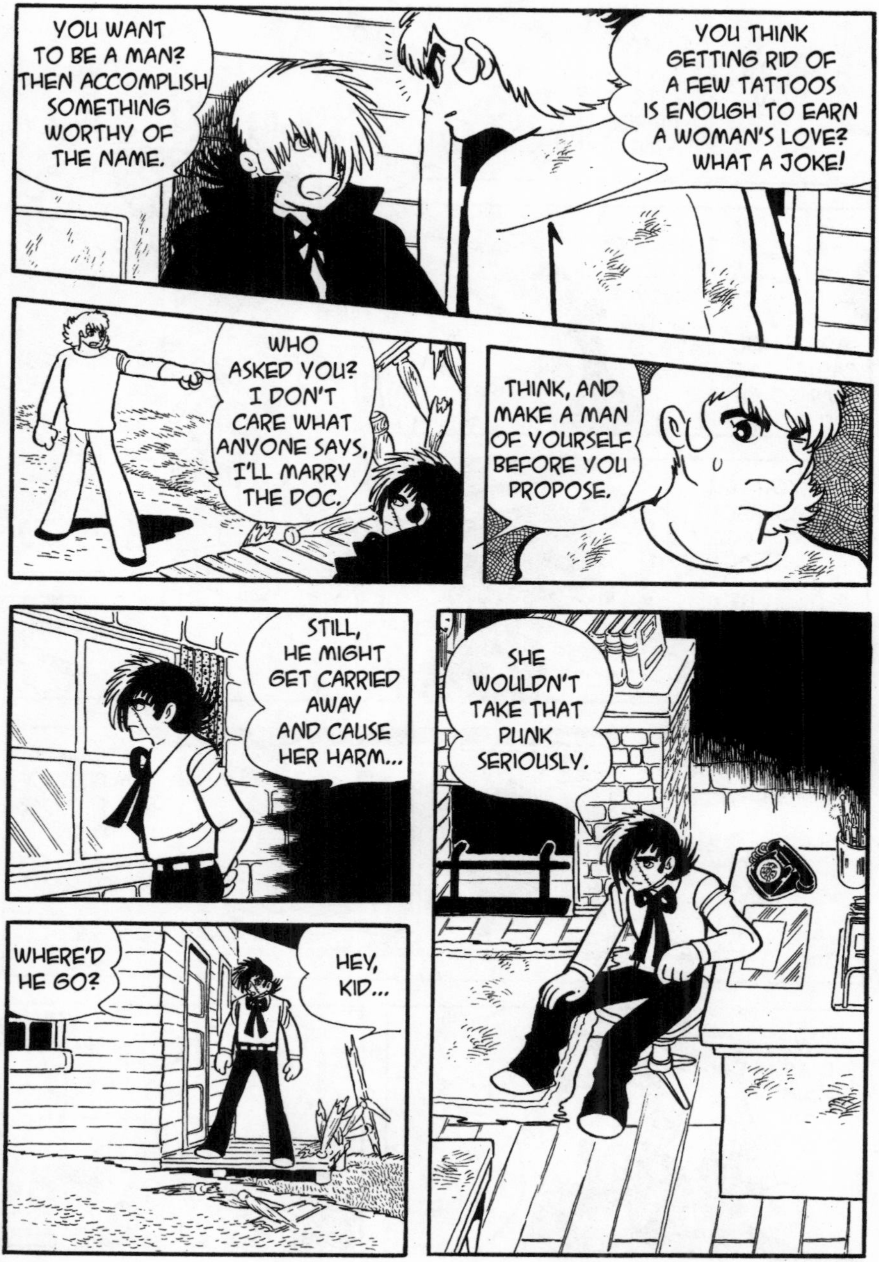
YOU THINK GETTING RID OF A FEW TATTOOS IS ENOUGH TO EARN A WOMAN'S LOVE? WHAT A JOKE!
YOU WANT TO BE A MAN? THEN ACCOMPLISH SOMETHING WORTHY OF THE NAME.
THINK, AND MAKE A MAN OF YOURSELF BEFORE YOU PROPOSE.
WHO ASKED YOU? I DON'T CARE WHAT ANYONE SAYS, I'LL MARRY THE DOC.
SHE WOULDN'T TAKE THAT PUNK SERIOUSLY.
STILL, HE MIGHT GET CARRIED AWAY AND CAUSE HER HARM...
HEY, KID...
WHERE'D HE GO?

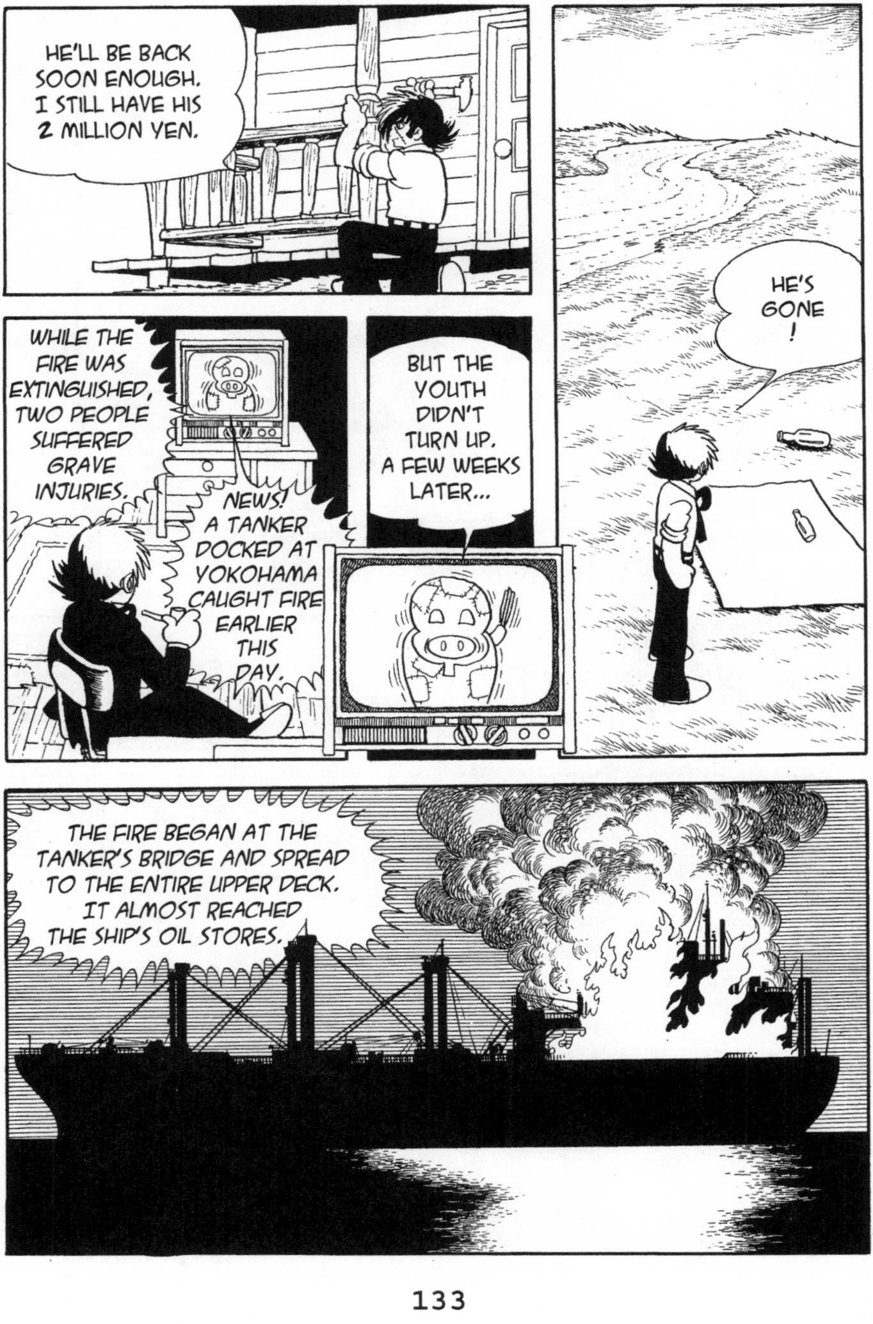
HE'S GONE!
HE'LL BE BACK SOON ENOUGH. I STILL HAVE HIS 2 MILLION YEN.
BUT THE YOUTH DIDN'T TURN UP. A FEW WEEKS LATER...
NEWS! A TANKER DOCKED AT YOKOHAMA CAUGHT FIRE EARLIER THIS DAY.
WHILE THE FIRE WAS EXTINGUISHED, TWO PEOPLE SUFFERED GRAVE INJURIES.
THE FIRE BEGAN AT THE TANKER'S BRIDGE AND SPREAD TO THE ENTIRE UPPER DECK. IT ALMOST REACHED THE SHIP'S OIL STORES.

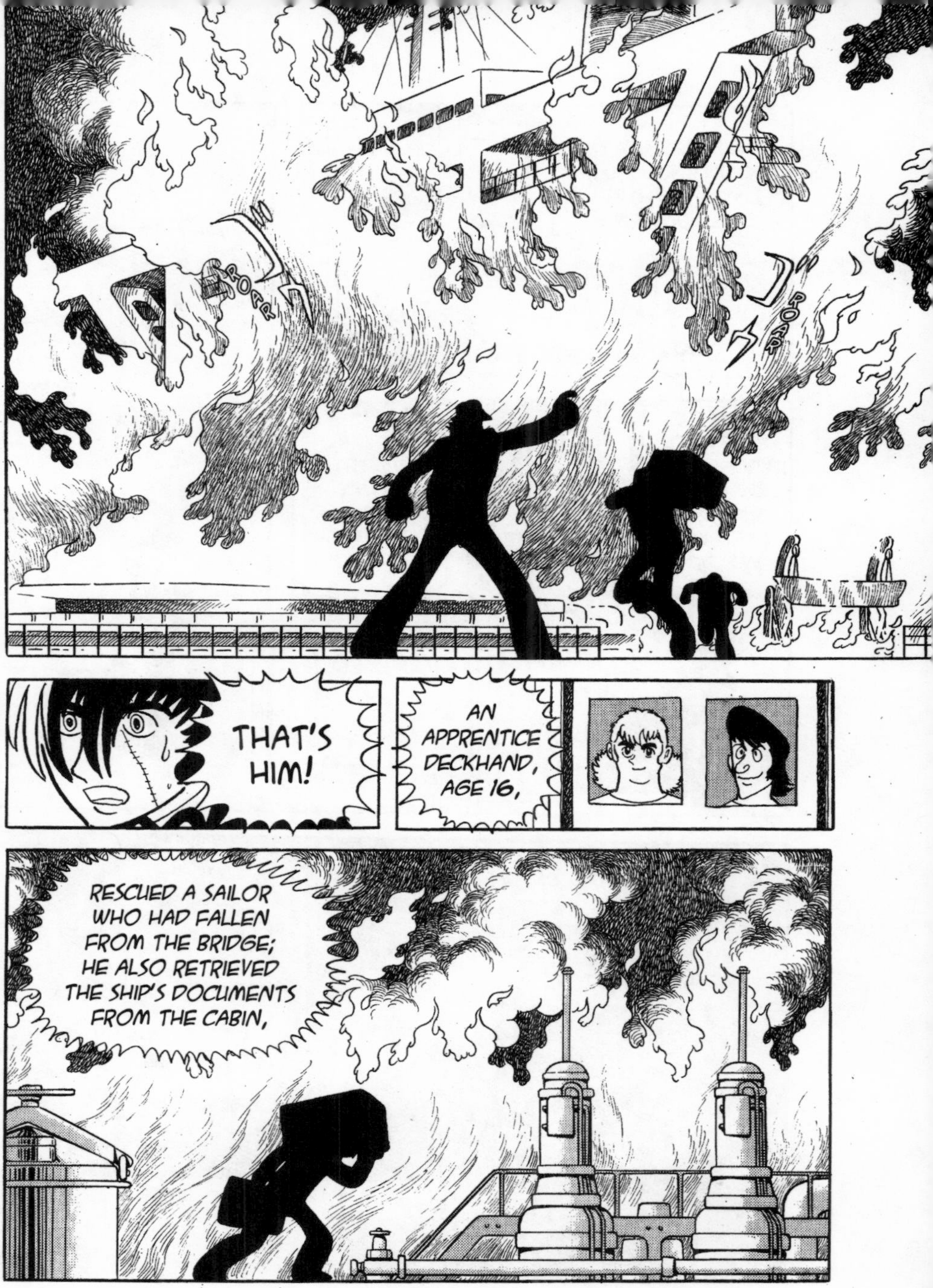
ROAR
ROAR
AN APPRENTICE DECKHAND, AGE 16,
THAT'S HIM!
RESCUED A SAILOR WHO HAD FALLEN FROM THE BRIDGE; HE ALSO RETRIEVED THE SHIP'S DOCUMENTS FROM THE CABIN,

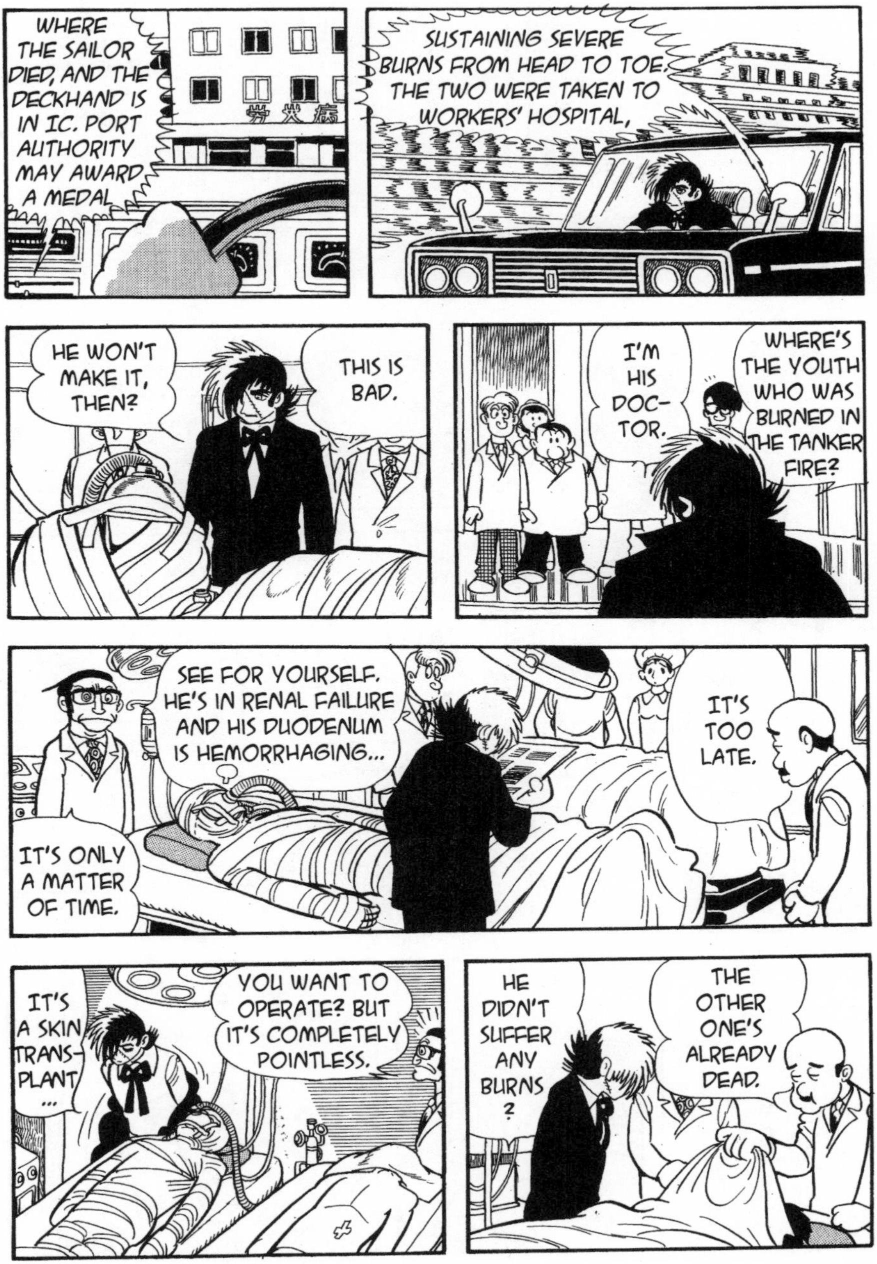
SUSTAINING SEVERE BURNS FROM HEAD TO TOE, THE TWO WERE TAKEN TO WORKERS' HOSPITAL,
WHERE THE SAILOR DIED, AND THE DECKHAND IS IN IC. PORT AUTHORITY MAY AWARD A MEDAL
WHERE'S THE YOUTH WHO WAS BURNED IN THE TANKER FIRE?
I'M HIS DOC-TOR.
THIS IS BAD.
HE WON'T MAKE IT, THEN?
IT'S TOO LATE.
SEE FOR YOURSELF. HE'S IN RENAL FAILURE AND HIS DUODENUM IS HEMORRHAGING...
IT'S ONLY A MATTER OF TIME.
THE OTHER ONE'S ALREADY DEAD.
HE DIDN'T SUFFER ANY BURNS?
YOU WANT TO OPERATE? BUT IT'S COMPLETELY POINTLESS.
IT'S A SKIN TRANS-PLANT...

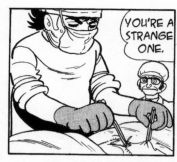

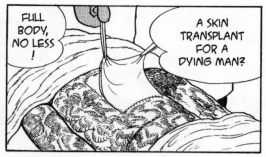

A SKIN TRANSPLANT FOR A DYING MAN?
FULL BODY, NO LESS!
YOU'RE A STRANGE ONE.
HE REGAINED CONSCIOUSNESS. THAT'S SOME WILLPOWER!
HEYA, DOC...
DID YOU OPERATE?
YES.
THEY'RE REALLY GONE?
THANKS... CAN I SEE?
HERE. LOOK IN THE MIRROR.
I CAN SEE, SORT OF...
THE STITCHES WILL COME OUT.
HEY! I'M LIKE A PATCHWORK QUILT!
HEH HEH
NOW I CAN MARRY HER...
GOOD WORK OUT THERE. YOU'RE A MAN NOW.
HE'S DEAD.

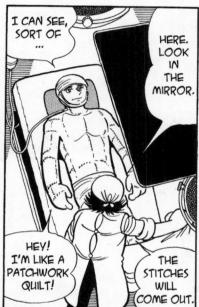

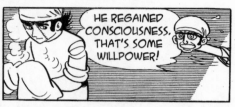

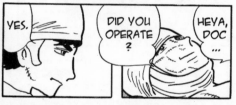

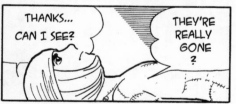

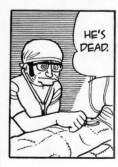

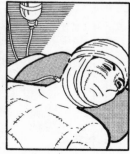

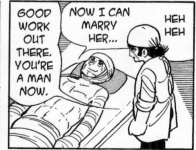

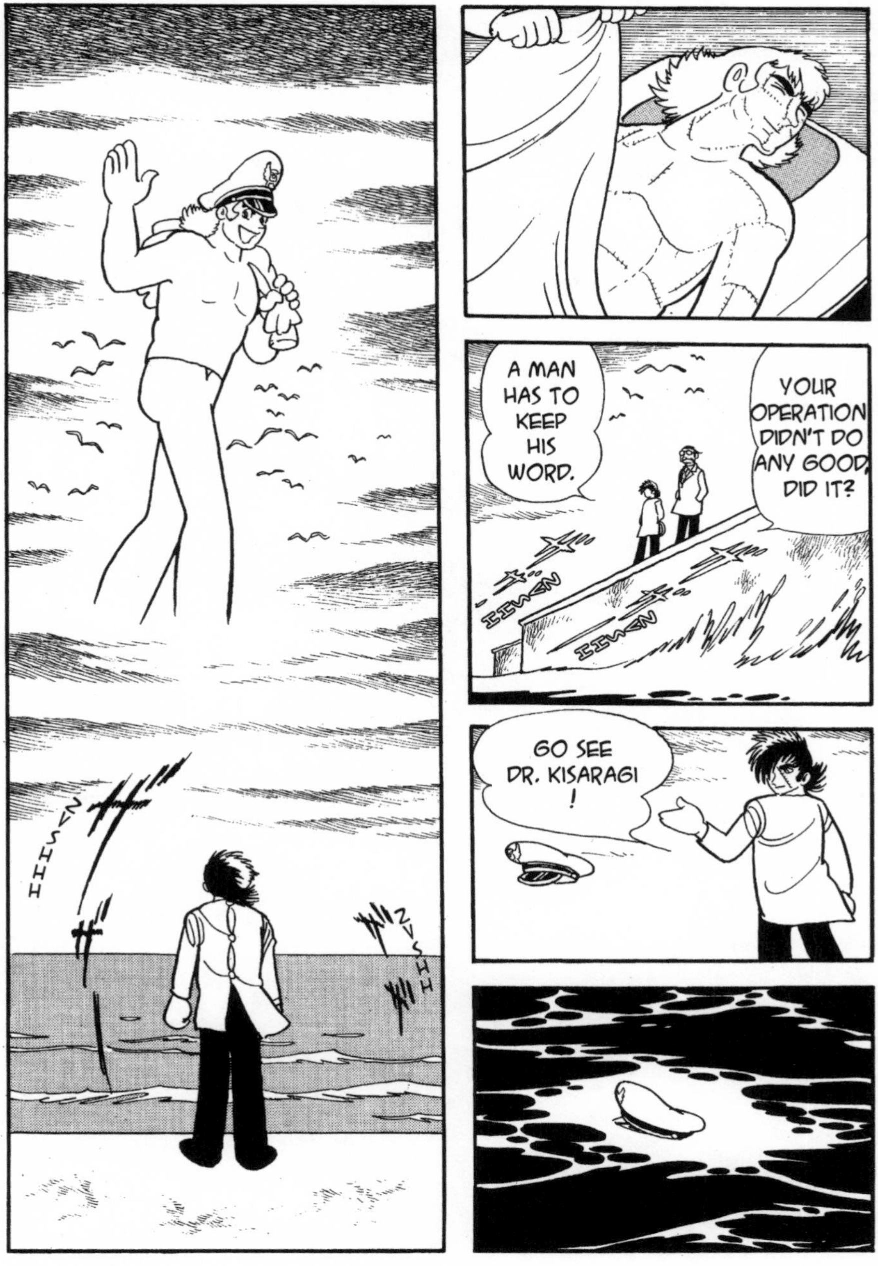
YOUR OPERATION DIDN'T DO ANY GOOD, DID IT?
A MAN HAS TO KEEP HIS WORD.
GO SEE DR. KISARAGI!
ZVSHH
ZVSHHH

TETSU OF THE YAMANOTE LINE

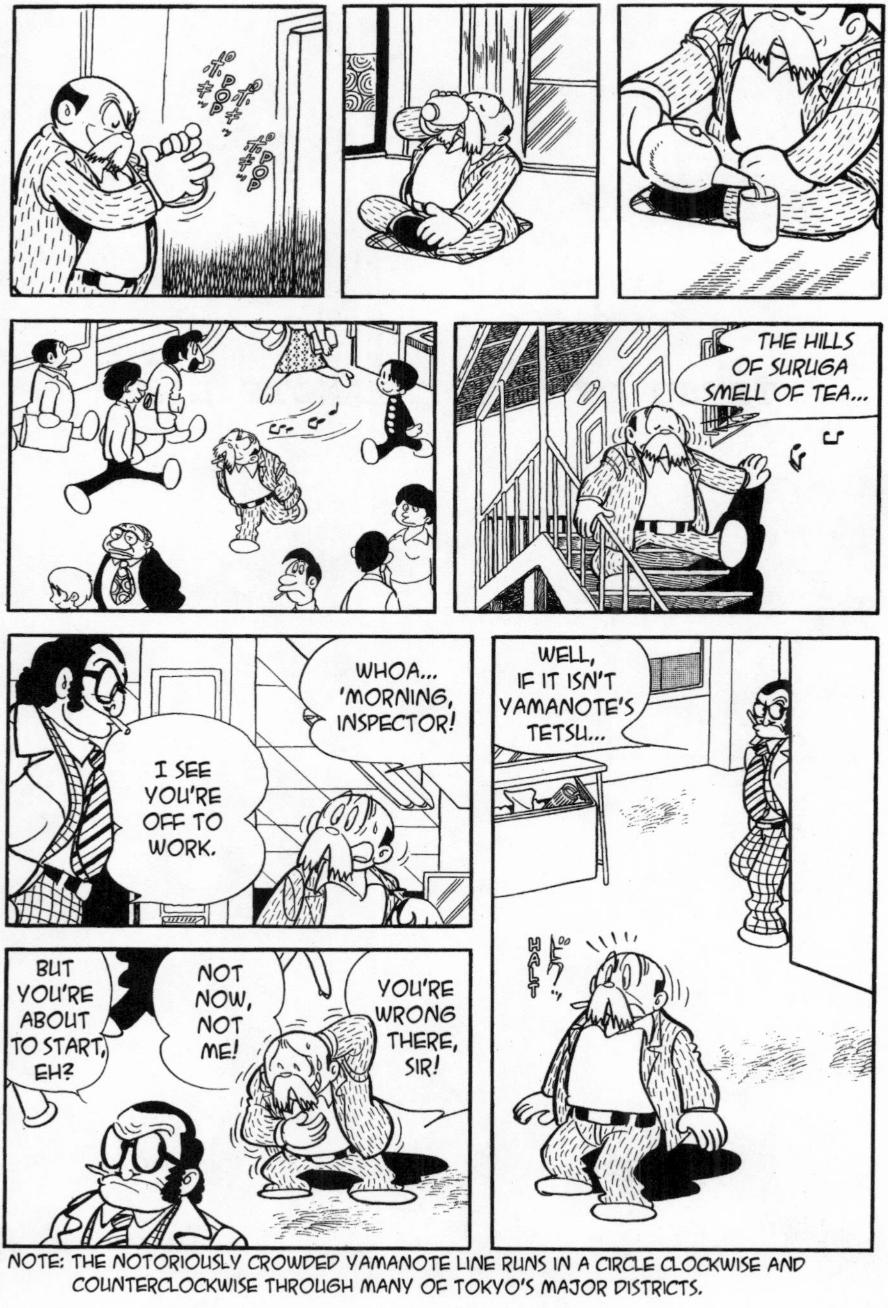
ポキッ POP
ポキッ POP
ポキッ POP
THE HILLS OF SURUGA SMELL OF TEA...
WELL, IF IT ISN'T YAMANOTE'S TETSU...
HALT ドキッ
WHOA... 'MORNING, INSPECTOR!
I SEE YOU'RE OFF TO WORK.
YOU'RE WRONG THERE, SIR!
NOT NOW, NOT ME!
BUT YOU'RE ABOUT TO START, EH?

NOTE: THE NOTORIOUSLY CROWDED YAMANOTE LINE RUNS IN A CIRCLE CLOCKWISE AND COUNTERCLOCKWISE THROUGH MANY OF TOKYO'S MAJOR DISTRICTS.

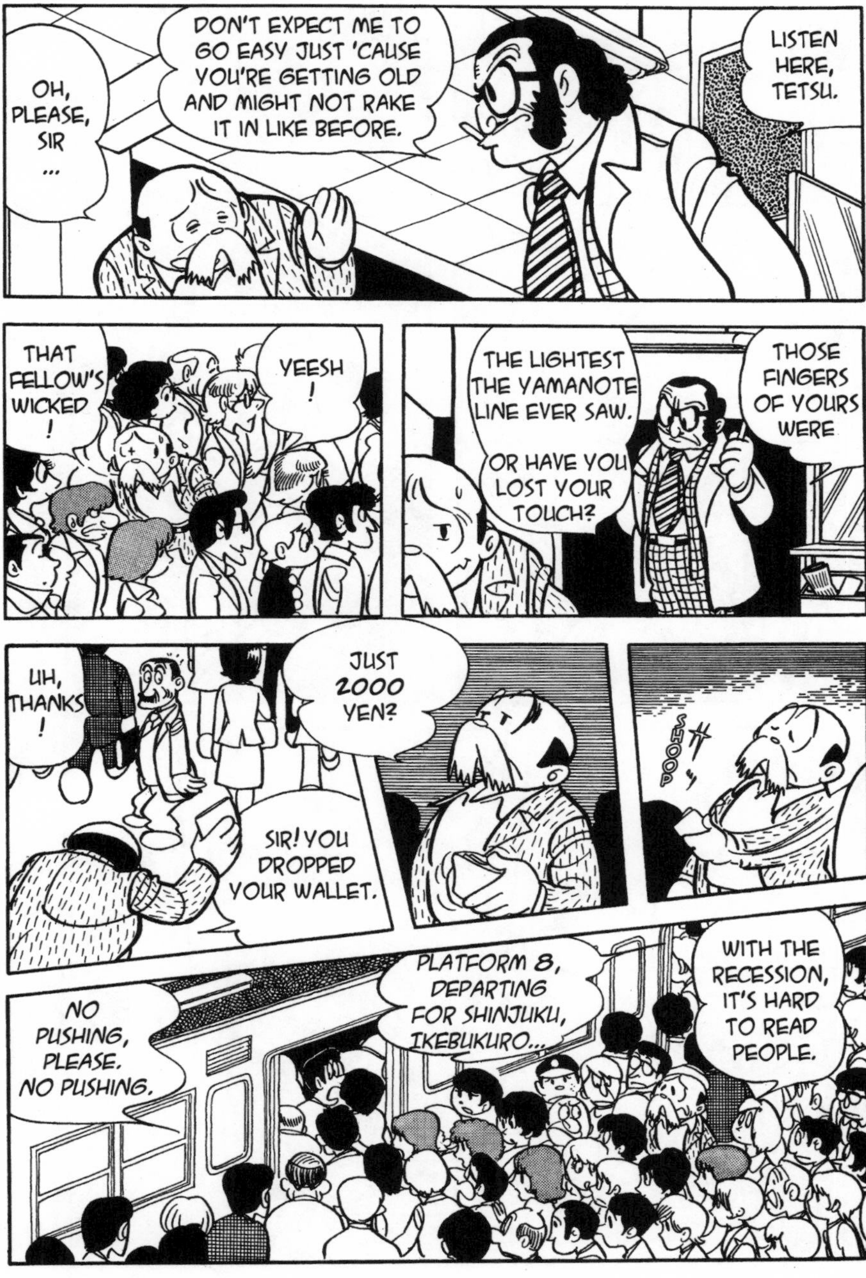
LISTEN HERE, TETSU.
DON'T EXPECT ME TO GO EASY JUST 'CAUSE YOU'RE GETTING OLD AND MIGHT NOT RAKE IT IN LIKE BEFORE.
OH, PLEASE, SIR ...
THOSE FINGERS OF YOURS WERE
THE LIGHTEST THE YAMANOTE LINE EVER SAW.
OR HAVE YOU LOST YOUR TOUCH?
YEESH!
THAT FELLOW'S WICKED!
SHOOP
JUST 2000 YEN?
SIR! YOU DROPPED YOUR WALLET.
UH, THANKS!
WITH THE RECESSION, IT'S HARD TO READ PEOPLE.
PLATFORM 8, DEPARTING FOR SHINJUKU, IKEBUKURO...
NO PUSHING, PLEASE. NO PUSHING.

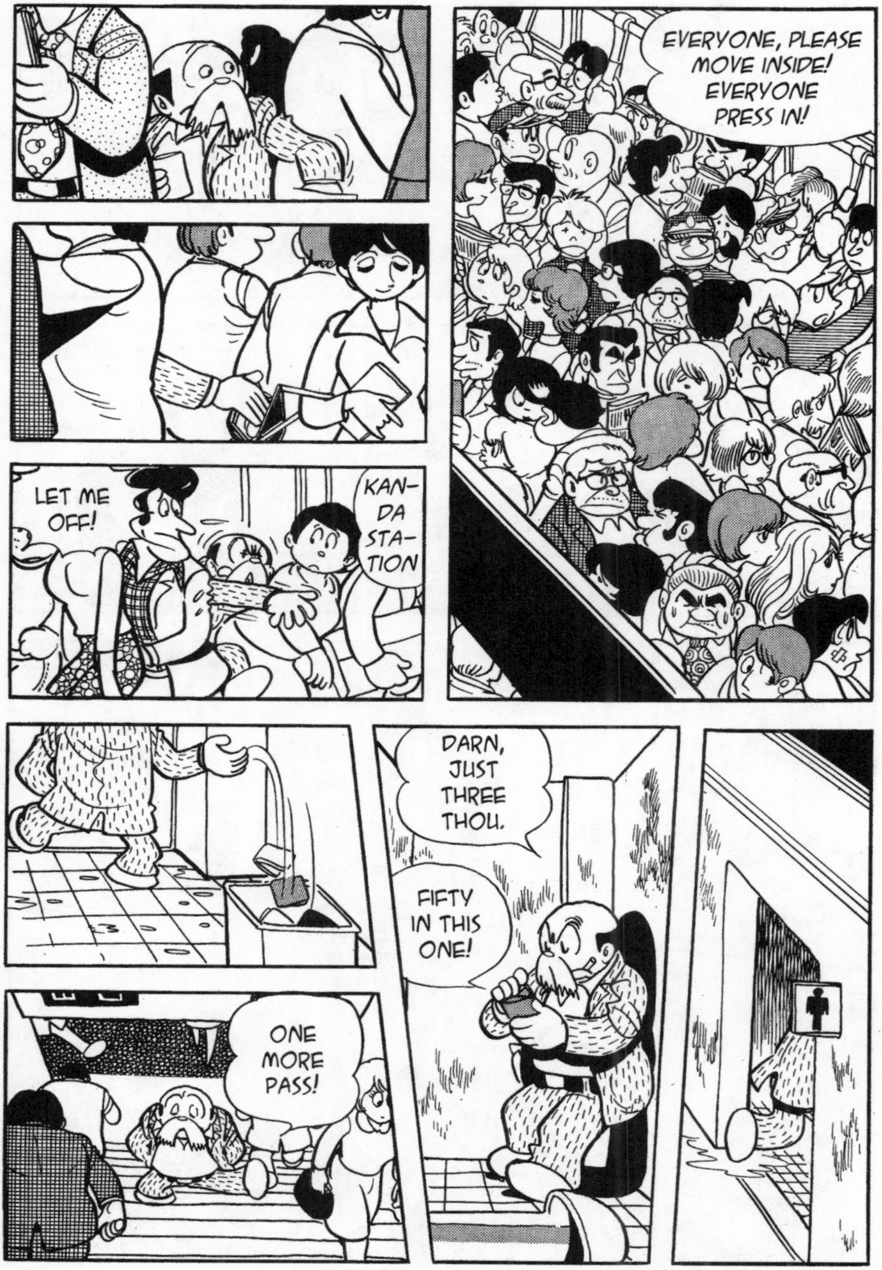
EVERYONE, PLEASE MOVE INSIDE! EVERYONE PRESS IN!
KAN-DA STA-TION
LET ME OFF!
DARN, JUST THREE THOU.
FIFTY IN THIS ONE!
ONE MORE PASS!

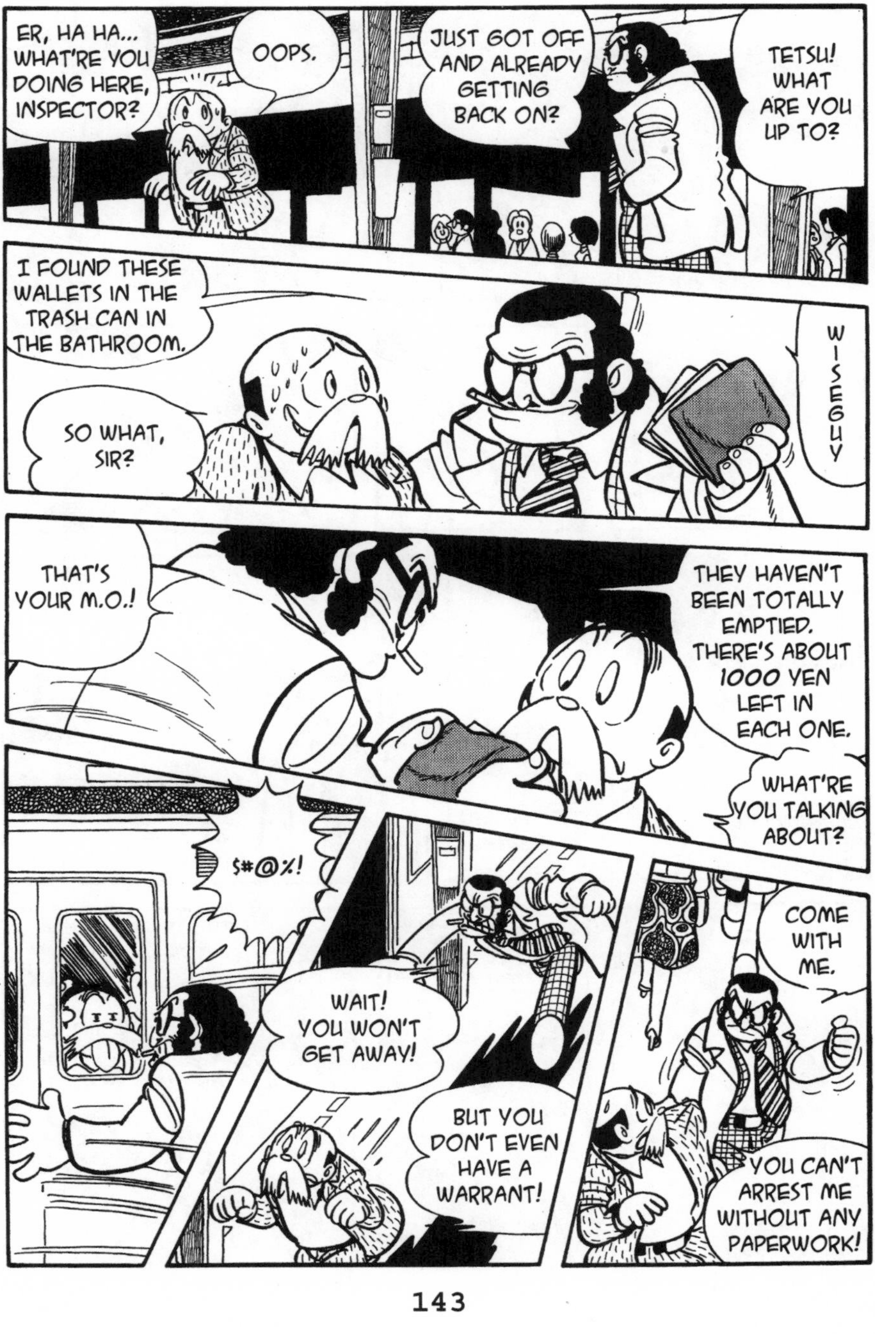
TETSU! WHAT ARE YOU UP TO?
JUST GOT OFF AND ALREADY GETTING BACK ON?
OOPS.
ER, HA HA... WHAT'RE YOU DOING HERE, INSPECTOR?
WISEGUY
I FOUND THESE WALLETS IN THE TRASH CAN IN THE BATHROOM.
SO WHAT, SIR?
THEY HAVEN'T BEEN TOTALLY EMPTIED. THERE'S ABOUT 1000 YEN LEFT IN EACH ONE.
WHAT'RE YOU TALKING ABOUT?
THAT'S YOUR M.O.!
COME WITH ME.
YOU CAN'T ARREST ME WITHOUT ANY PAPERWORK!
WAIT! YOU WON'T GET AWAY!
BUT YOU DON'T EVEN HAVE A WARRANT!
$#@%!

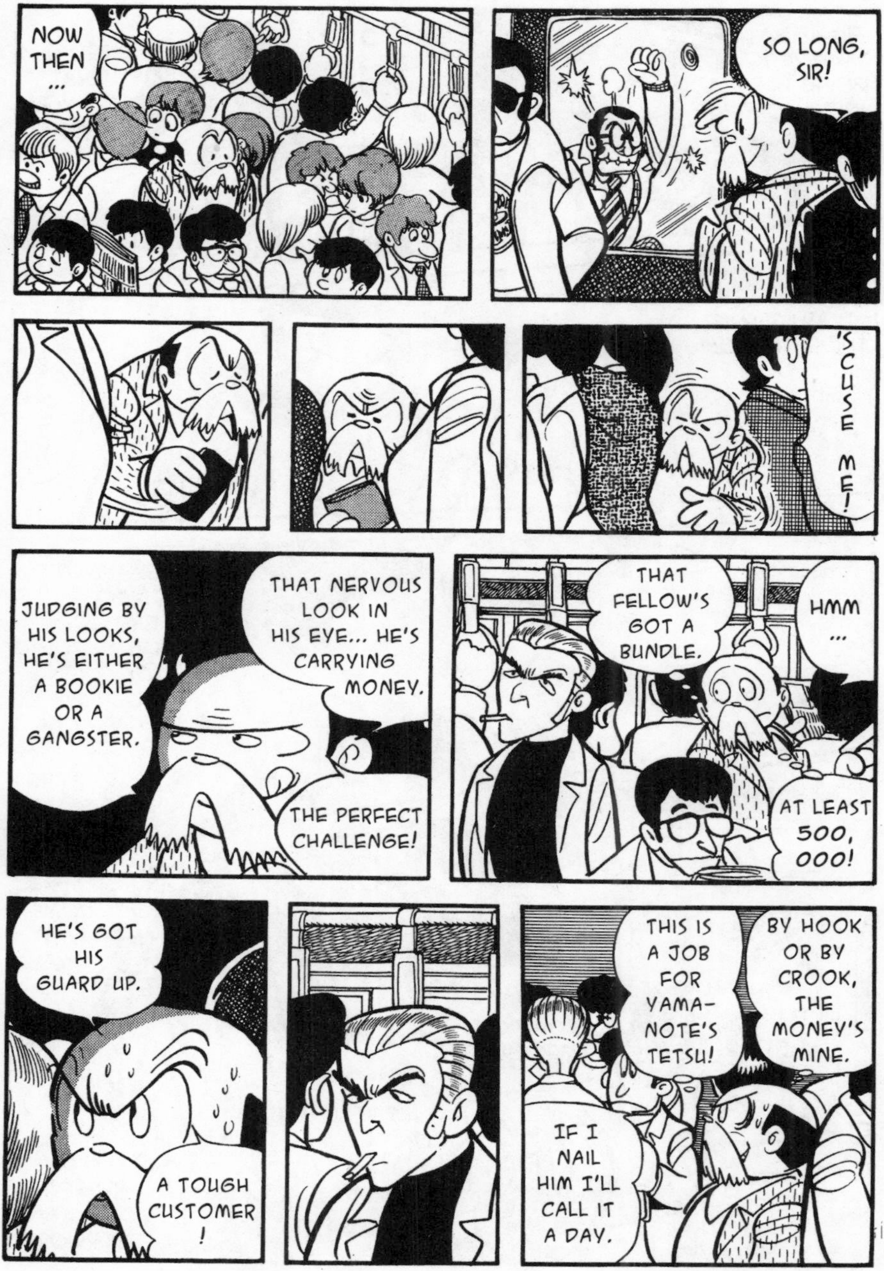
SO LONG, SIR!
NOW THEN ...
'SCUSE ME!
HMM ...
THAT FELLOW'S GOT A BUNDLE.
AT LEAST 500,000!
THAT NERVOUS LOOK IN HIS EYE... HE'S CARRYING MONEY.
JUDGING BY HIS LOOKS, HE'S EITHER A BOOKIE OR A GANGSTER.
THE PERFECT CHALLENGE!
BY HOOK OR BY CROOK, THE MONEY'S MINE.
THIS IS A JOB FOR YAMA-NOTE'S TETSU!
IF I NAIL HIM I'LL CALL IT A DAY.
HE'S GOT HIS GUARD UP.
A TOUGH CUSTOMER!

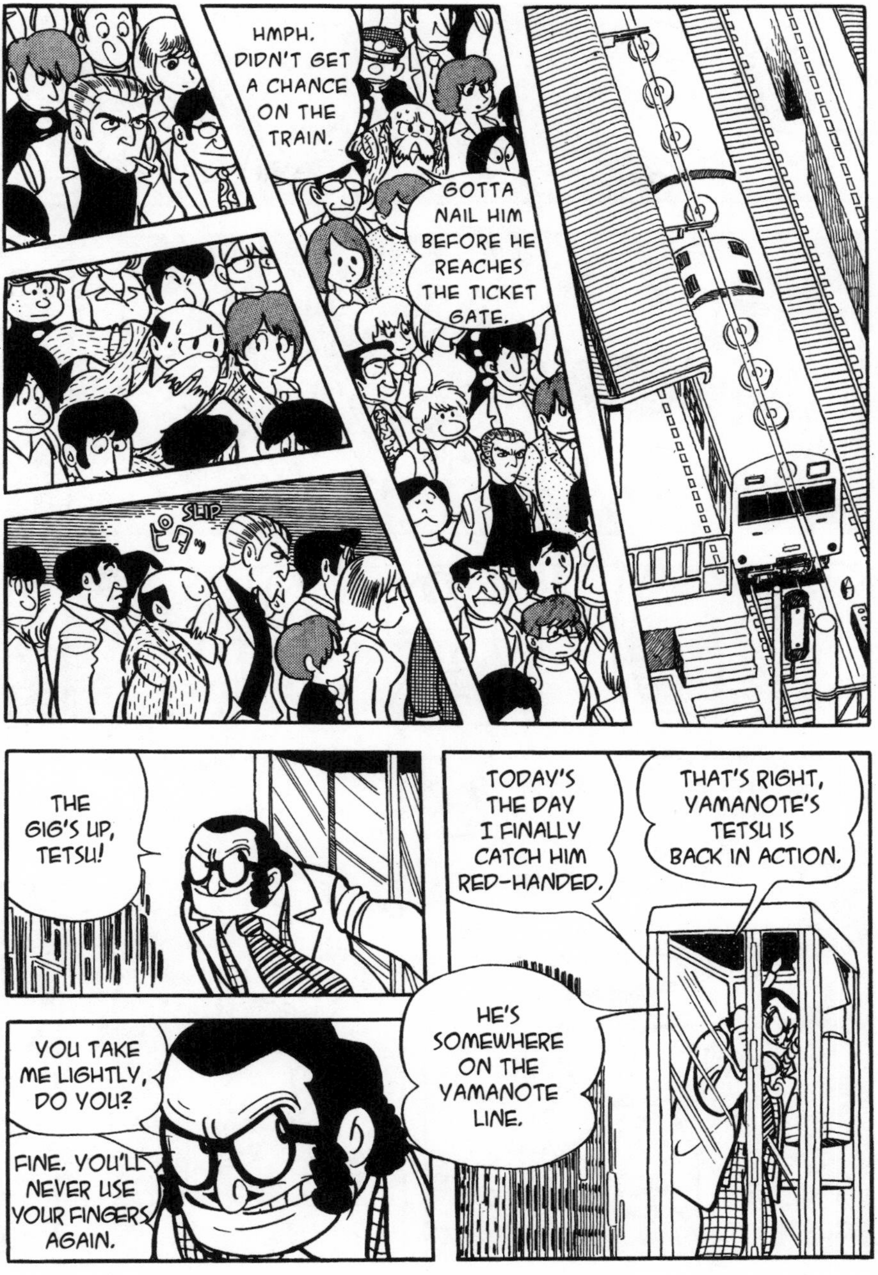
HMPH. DIDN'T GET A CHANCE ON THE TRAIN.
GOTTA NAIL HIM BEFORE HE REACHES THE TICKET GATE.
SLIP
ピタッ
THAT'S RIGHT, YAMANOTE'S TETSU IS BACK IN ACTION.
TODAY'S THE DAY I FINALLY CATCH HIM RED-HANDED.
HE'S SOMEWHERE ON THE YAMANOTE LINE.
THE GIG'S UP, TETSU!
YOU TAKE ME LIGHTLY, DO YOU?
FINE. YOU'LL NEVER USE YOUR FINGERS AGAIN.

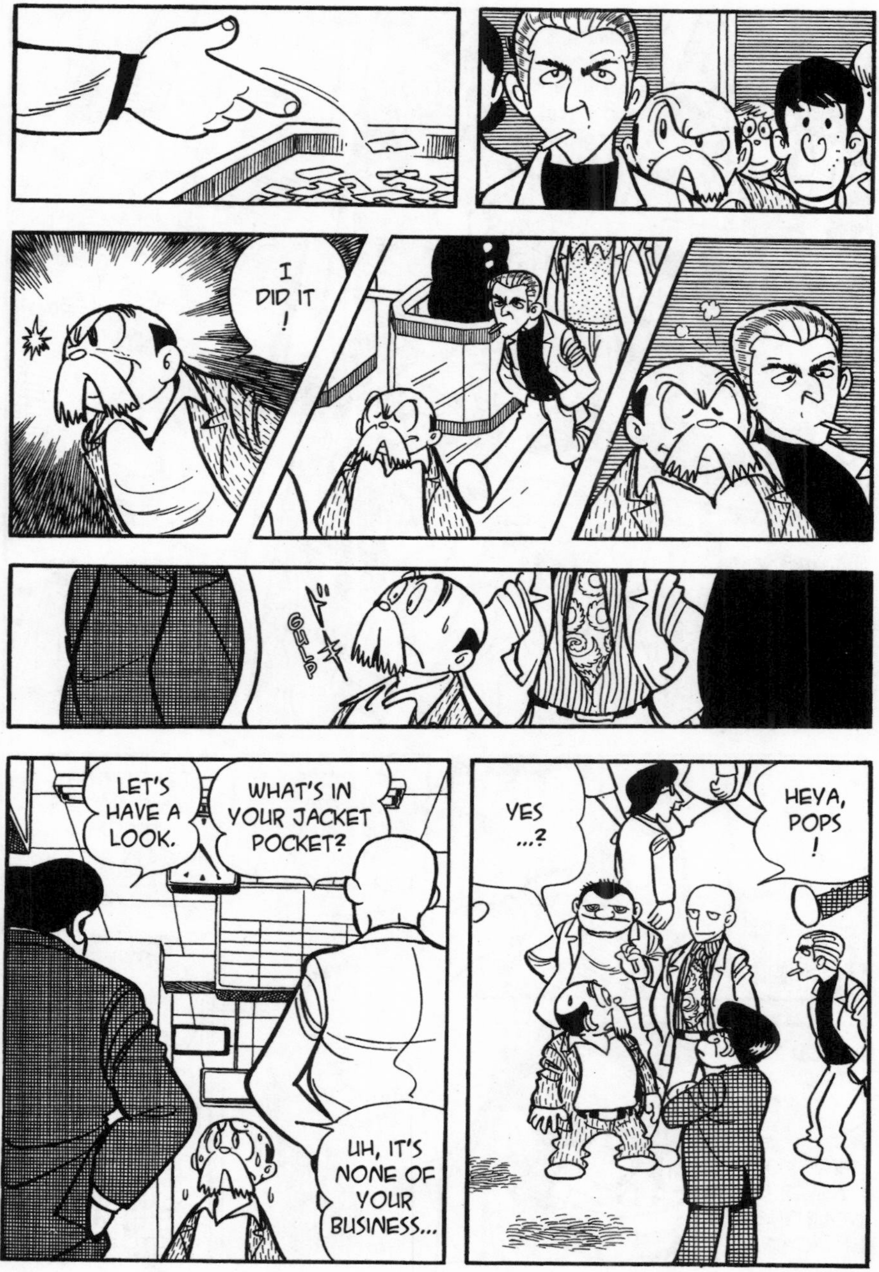
I DID IT !
GULP
HEYA, POPS !
YES ...?
WHAT'S IN YOUR JACKET POCKET?
LET'S HAVE A LOOK.
UH, IT'S NONE OF YOUR BUSINESS...

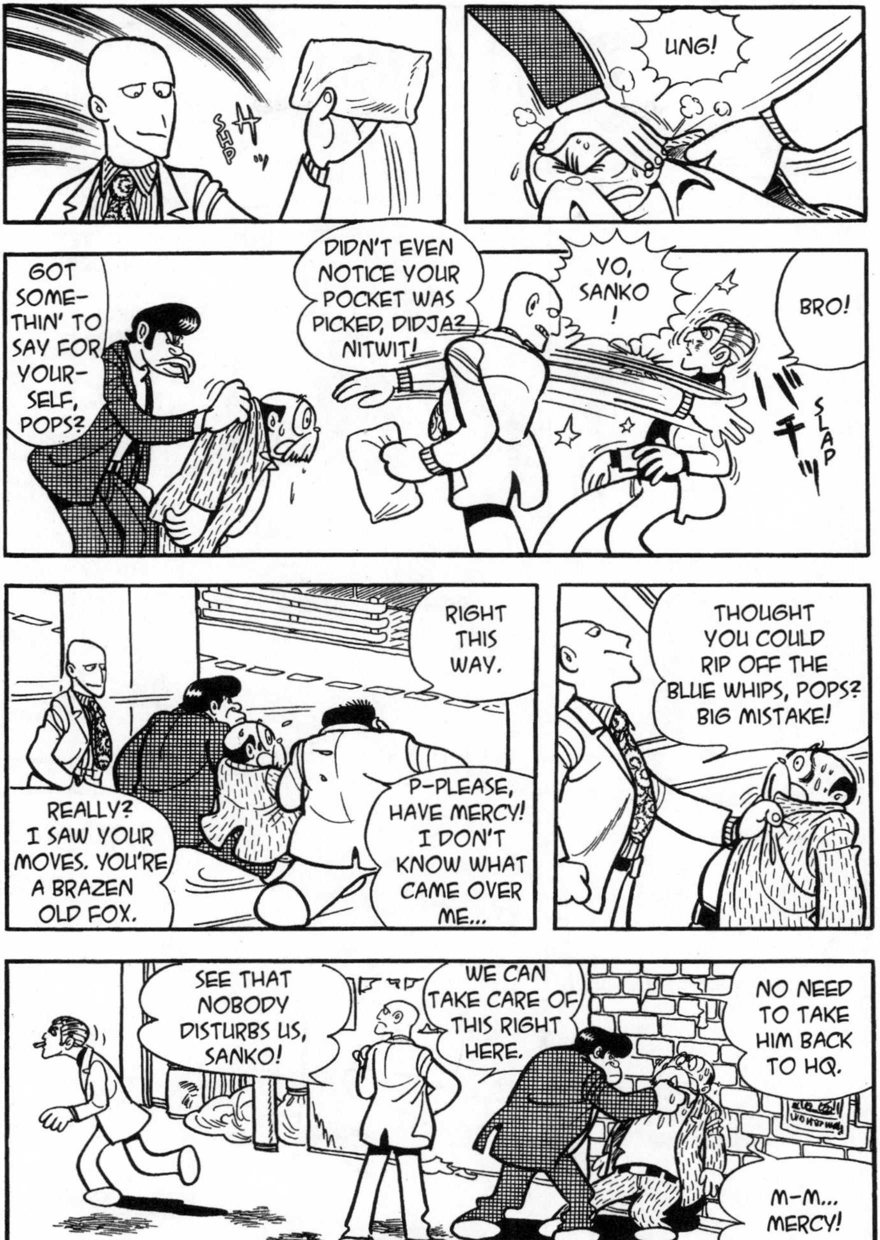
UNG!
SHP
BRO!
SLAP
YO, SANKO!
DIDN'T EVEN NOTICE YOUR POCKET WAS PICKED, DIDJA? NITWIT!
GOT SOME-THIN' TO SAY FOR YOUR-SELF, POPS?
THOUGHT YOU COULD RIP OFF THE BLUE WHIPS, POPS? BIG MISTAKE!
RIGHT THIS WAY.
P-PLEASE, HAVE MERCY! I DON'T KNOW WHAT CAME OVER ME...
REALLY? I SAW YOUR MOVES. YOU'RE A BRAZEN OLD FOX.
NO NEED TO TAKE HIM BACK TO HQ.
M-M... MERCY!
WE CAN TAKE CARE OF THIS RIGHT HERE.
SEE THAT NOBODY DISTURBS US, SANKO!

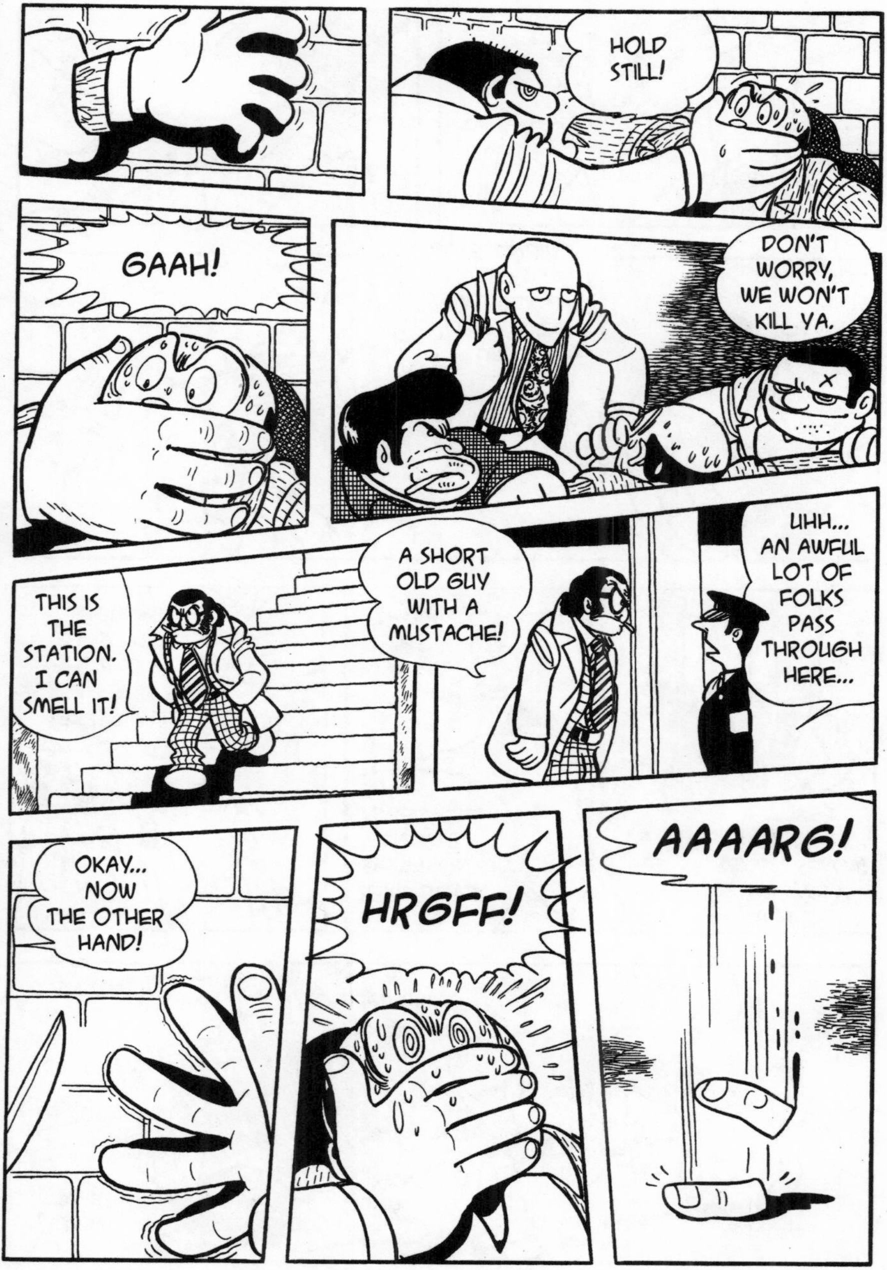

HOLD STILL!
DON'T WORRY, WE WON'T KILL YA.
GAAH!
A SHORT OLD GUY WITH A MUSTACHE!
UHH... AN AWFUL LOT OF FOLKS PASS THROUGH HERE...
THIS IS THE STATION. I CAN SMELL IT!
AAAARG!
HRGFF!
OKAY... NOW THE OTHER HAND!

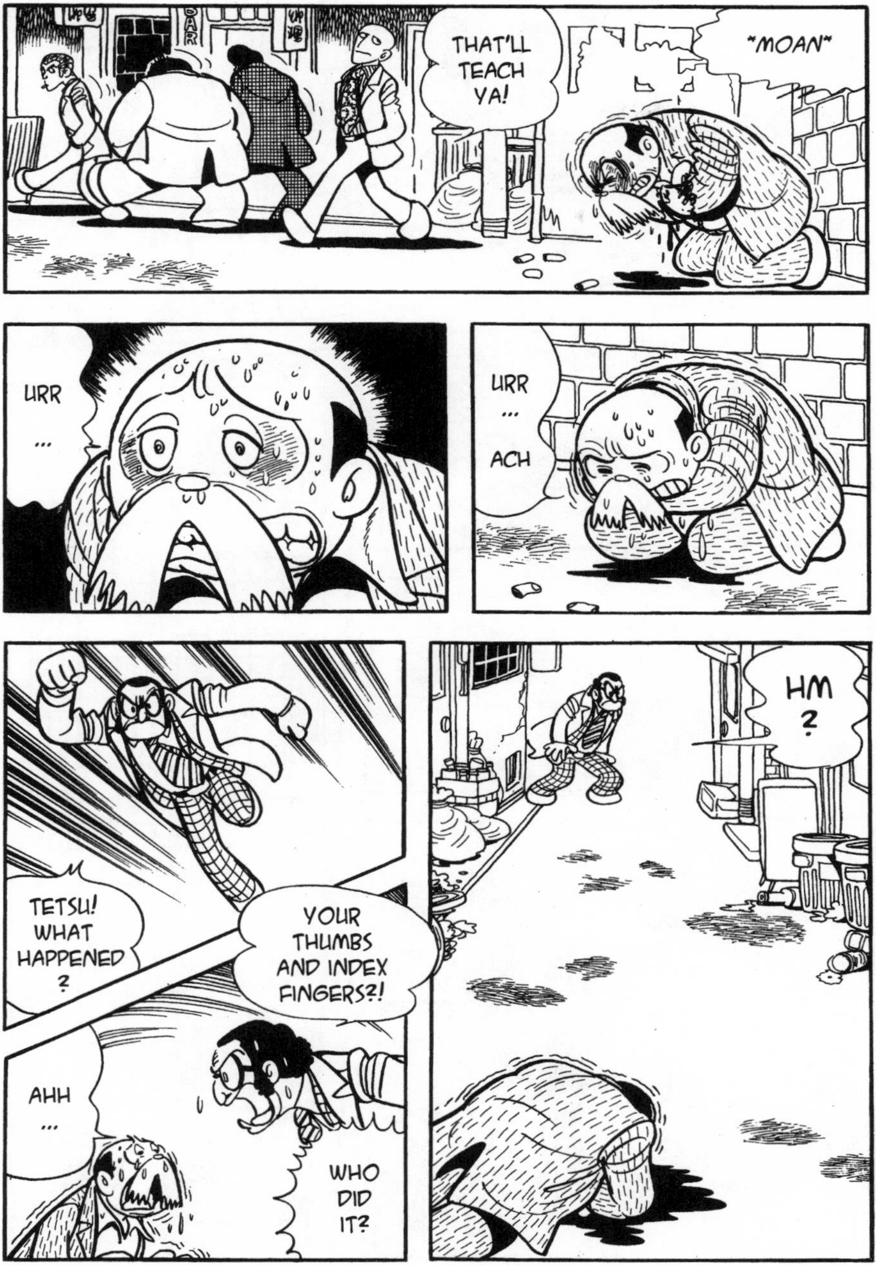
MOAN
THAT'LL TEACH YA!
URR ... ACH
URR ...
HM ?
TETSU! WHAT HAPPENED ?
YOUR THUMBS AND INDEX FINGERS?!
WHO DID IT?
AHH ...

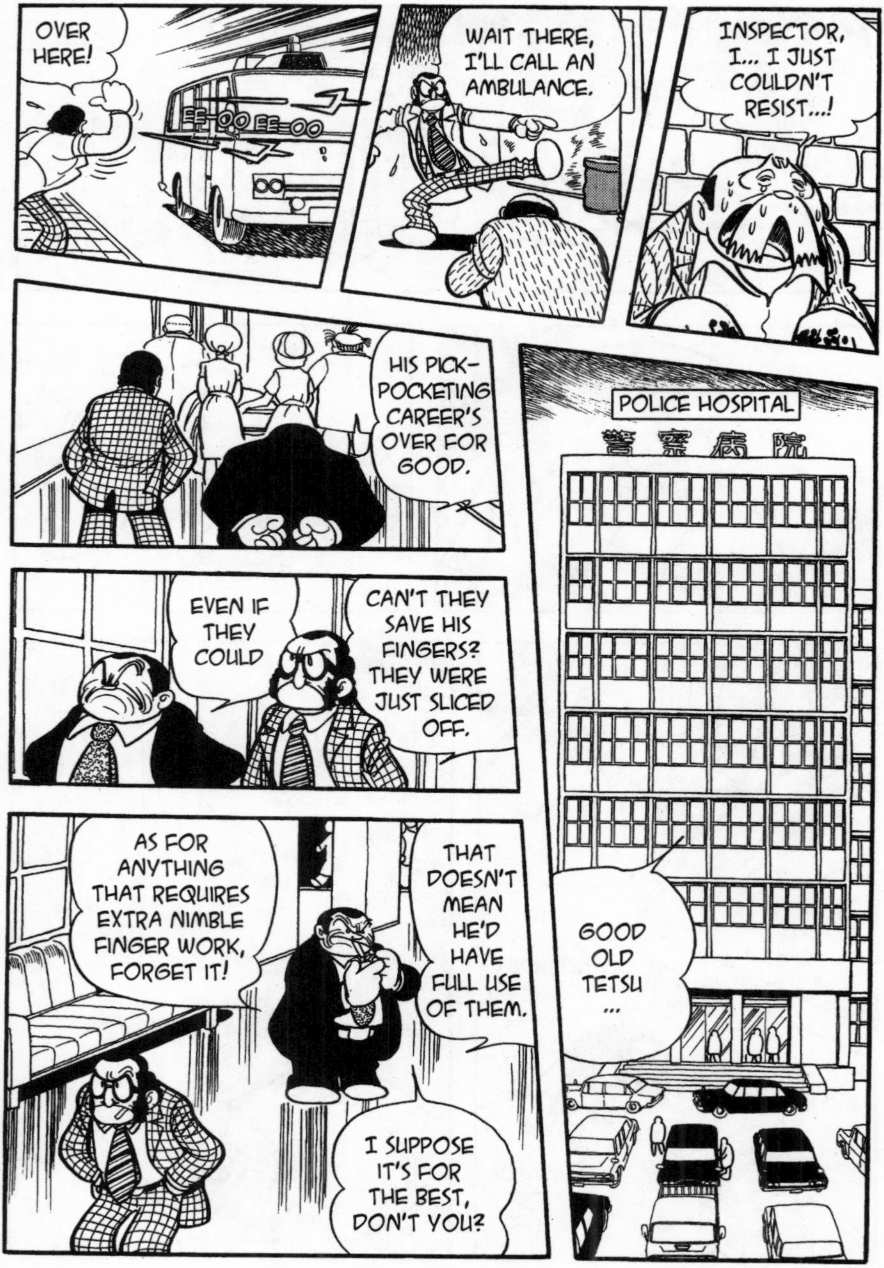
INSPECTOR, I... I JUST COULDN'T RESIST...!
WAIT THERE, I'LL CALL AN AMBULANCE.
OVER HERE!
EE-OO EE-OO
POLICE HOSPITAL
警察病院
GOOD OLD TETSU ...
HIS PICK-POCKETING CAREER'S OVER FOR GOOD.
CAN'T THEY SAVE HIS FINGERS? THEY WERE JUST SLICED OFF.
EVEN IF THEY COULD
THAT DOESN'T MEAN HE'D HAVE FULL USE OF THEM.
AS FOR ANYTHING THAT REQUIRES EXTRA NIMBLE FINGER WORK, FORGET IT!
I SUPPOSE IT'S FOR THE BEST, DON'T YOU?

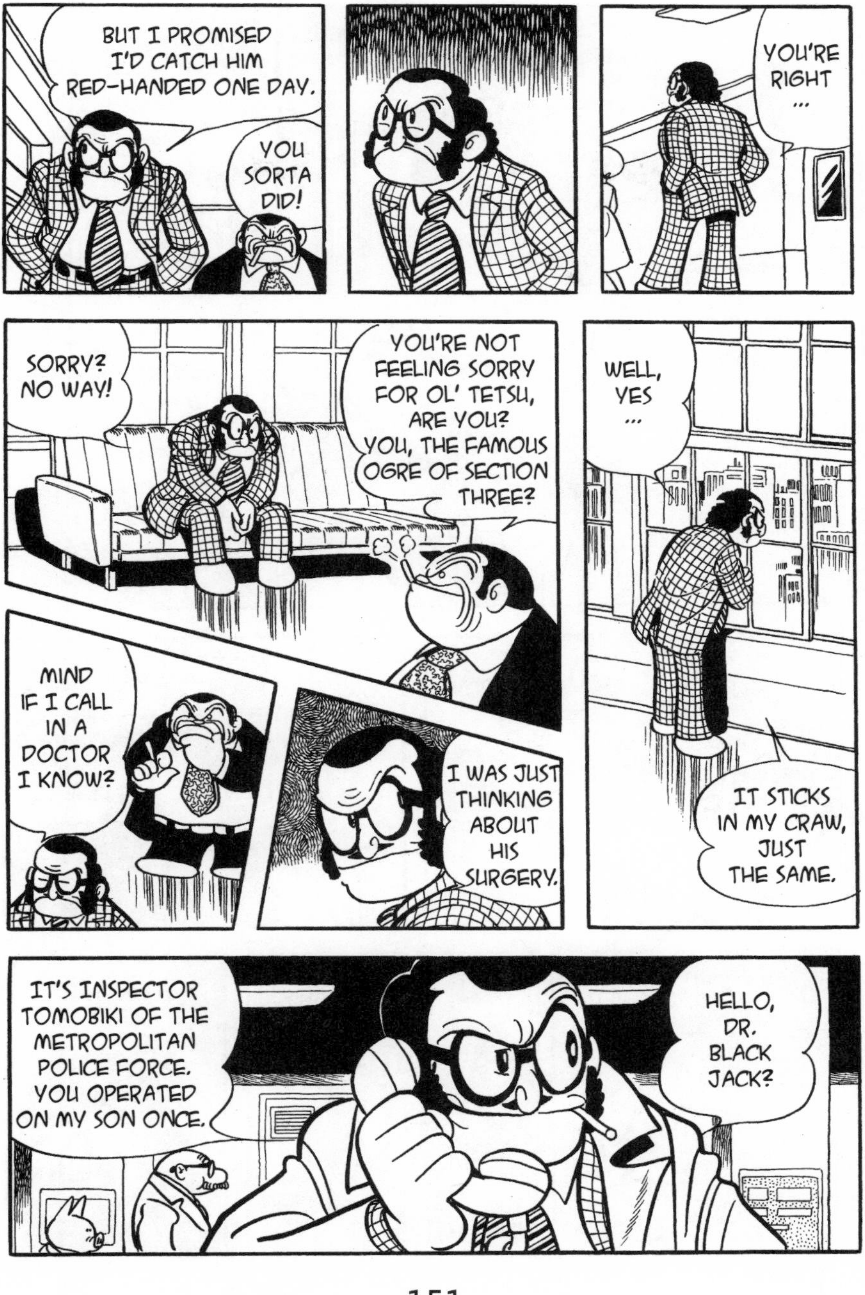
YOU'RE RIGHT ...
BUT I PROMISED I'D CATCH HIM RED-HANDED ONE DAY.
YOU SORTA DID!
WELL, YES ...
IT STICKS IN MY CRAW, JUST THE SAME.
YOU'RE NOT FEELING SORRY FOR OL' TETSU, ARE YOU? YOU, THE FAMOUS OGRE OF SECTION THREE?
SORRY? NO WAY!
I WAS JUST THINKING ABOUT HIS SURGERY.
MIND IF I CALL IN A DOCTOR I KNOW?
HELLO, DR. BLACK JACK?
IT'S INSPECTOR TOMOBIKI OF THE METROPOLITAN POLICE FORCE. YOU OPERATED ON MY SON ONCE.

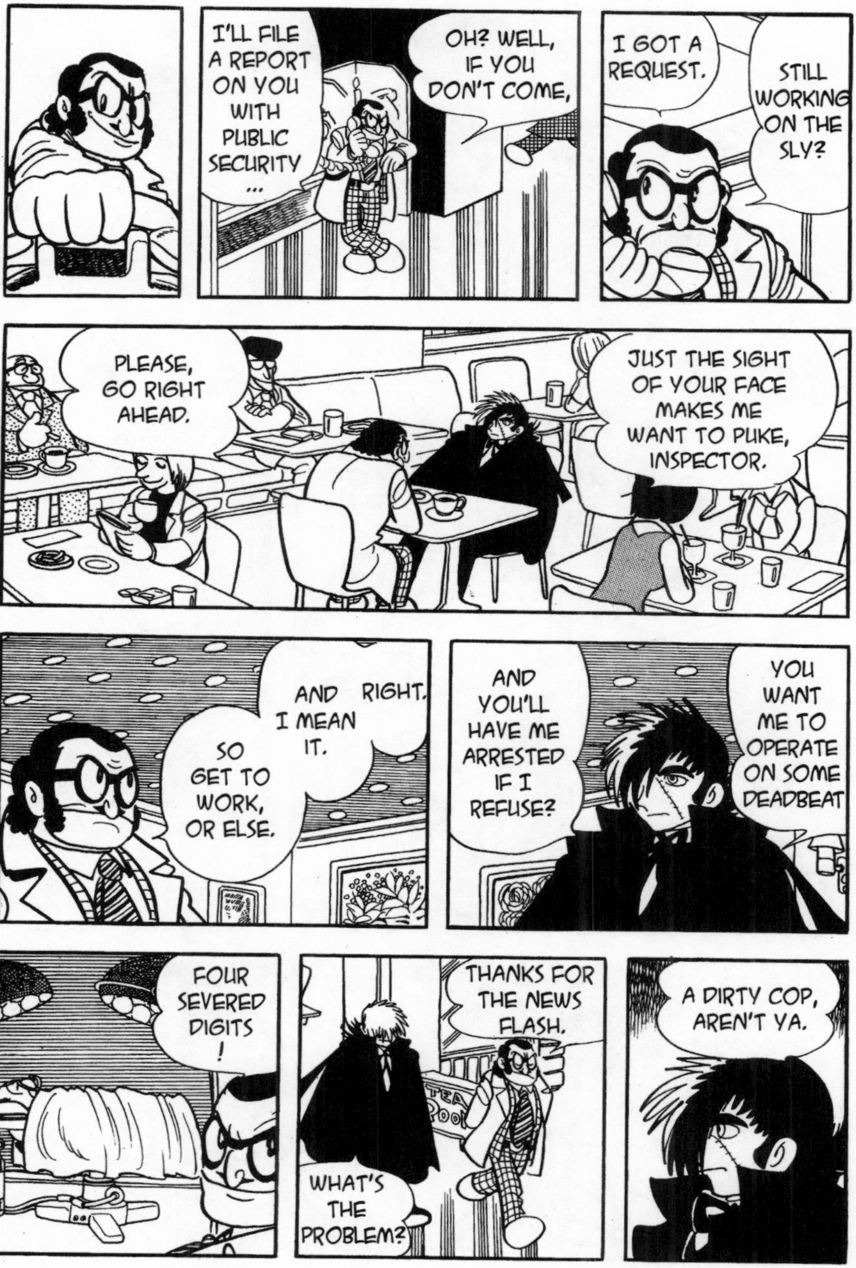
STILL WORKING ON THE SLY?
I GOT A REQUEST.
OH? WELL, IF YOU DON'T COME,
I'LL FILE A REPORT ON YOU WITH PUBLIC SECURITY ...
JUST THE SIGHT OF YOUR FACE MAKES ME WANT TO PUKE, INSPECTOR.
PLEASE, GO RIGHT AHEAD.
YOU WANT ME TO OPERATE ON SOME DEADBEAT
AND YOU'LL HAVE ME ARRESTED IF I REFUSE?
RIGHT.
AND I MEAN IT.
SO GET TO WORK, OR ELSE.
A DIRTY COP, AREN'T YA.
THANKS FOR THE NEWS FLASH.
WHAT'S THE PROBLEM?
FOUR SEVERED DIGITS !

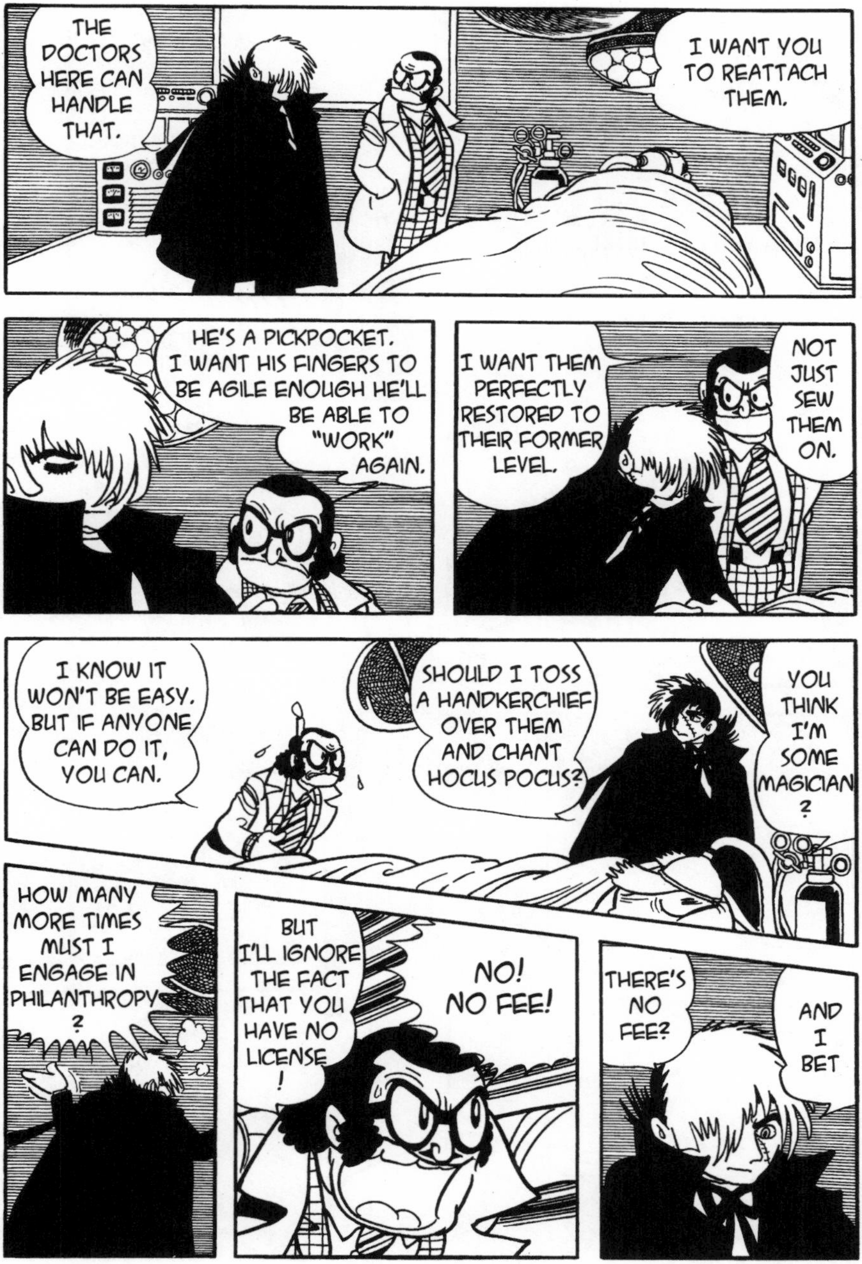
I WANT YOU TO REATTACH THEM.
THE DOCTORS HERE CAN HANDLE THAT.
NOT JUST SEW THEM ON.
I WANT THEM PERFECTLY RESTORED TO THEIR FORMER LEVEL.
HE'S A PICKPOCKET. I WANT HIS FINGERS TO BE AGILE ENOUGH HE'LL BE ABLE TO "WORK" AGAIN.
YOU THINK I'M SOME MAGICIAN?
SHOULD I TOSS A HANDKERCHIEF OVER THEM AND CHANT HOCUS POCUS?
I KNOW IT WON'T BE EASY. BUT IF ANYONE CAN DO IT, YOU CAN.
AND I BET
THERE'S NO FEE?
NO! NO FEE!
BUT I'LL IGNORE THE FACT THAT YOU HAVE NO LICENSE!
HOW MANY MORE TIMES MUST I ENGAGE IN PHILANTHROPY?

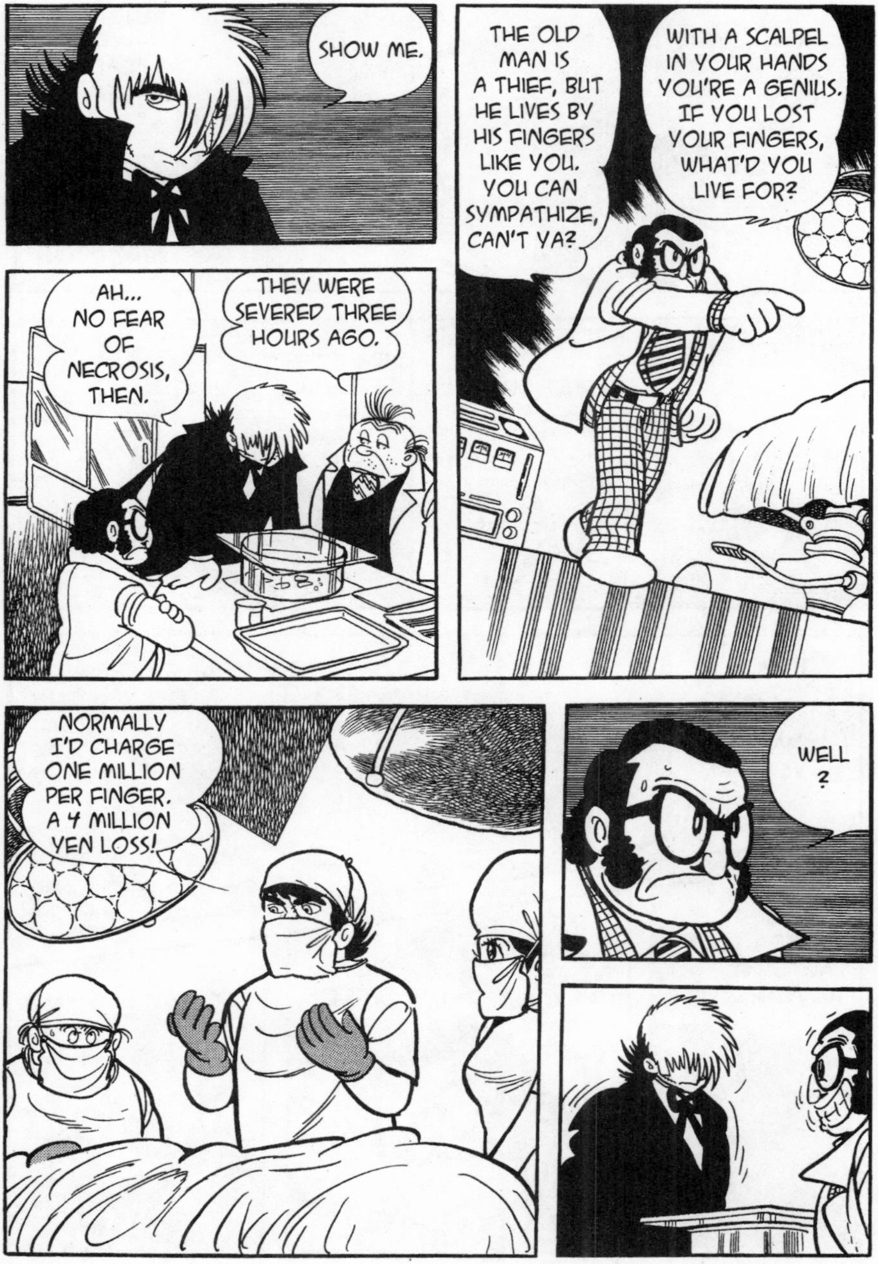
WITH A SCALPEL IN YOUR HANDS YOU'RE A GENIUS. IF YOU LOST YOUR FINGERS, WHAT'D YOU LIVE FOR?
THE OLD MAN IS A THIEF, BUT HE LIVES BY HIS FINGERS LIKE YOU. YOU CAN SYMPATHIZE, CAN'T YA?
SHOW ME.
THEY WERE SEVERED THREE HOURS AGO.
AH... NO FEAR OF NECROSIS, THEN.
WELL ?
NORMALLY I'D CHARGE ONE MILLION PER FINGER. A 4 MILLION YEN LOSS!

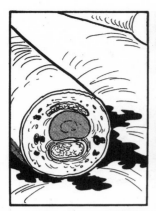
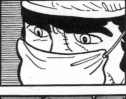
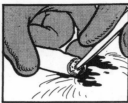
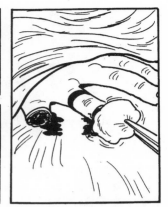
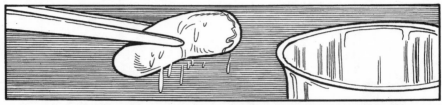
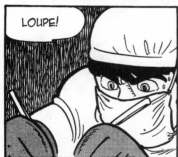

LOUPE!

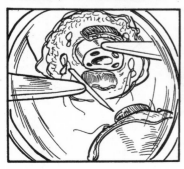
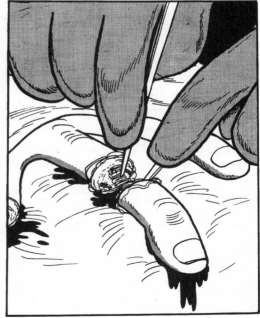

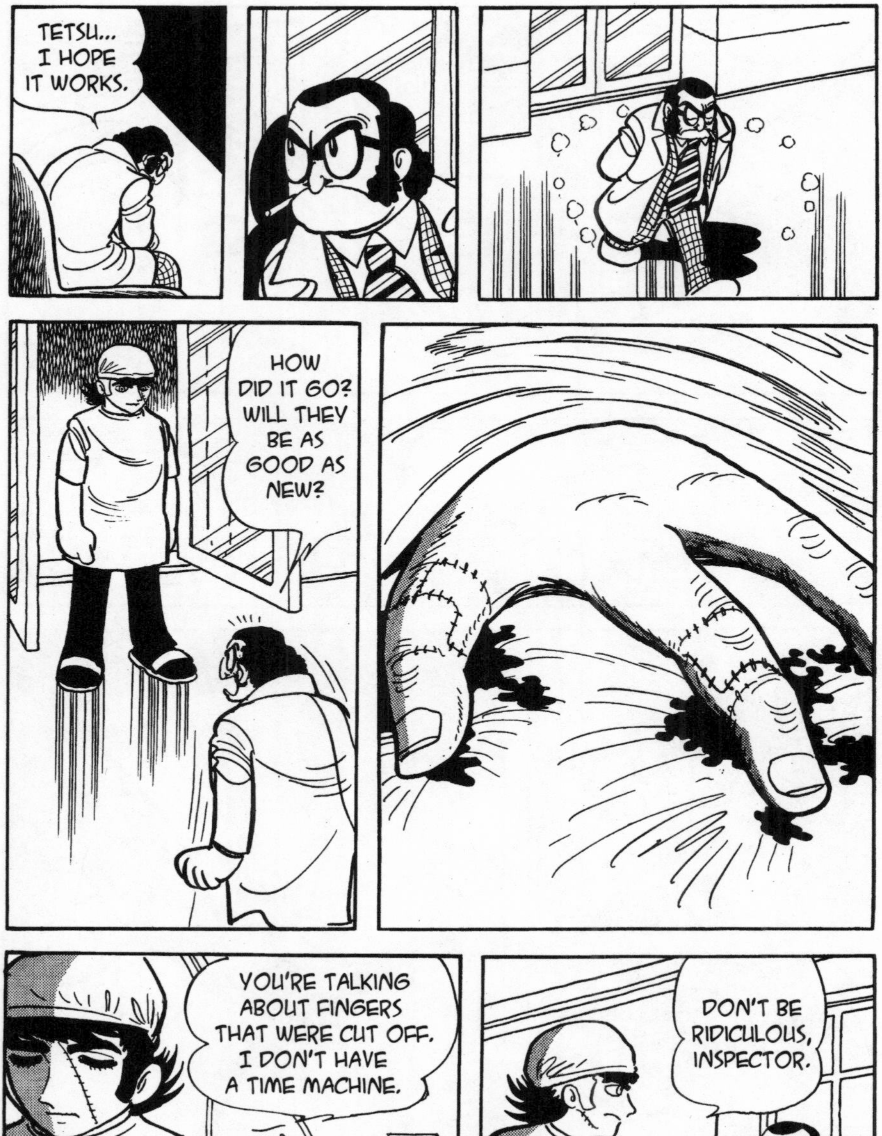
TETSU... I HOPE IT WORKS.
HOW DID IT GO? WILL THEY BE AS GOOD AS NEW?
DON'T BE RIDICULOUS, INSPECTOR.
YOU'RE TALKING ABOUT FINGERS THAT WERE CUT OFF. I DON'T HAVE A TIME MACHINE.

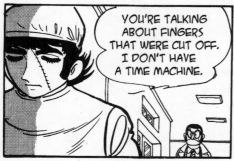

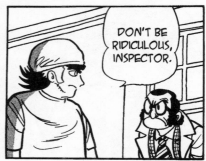

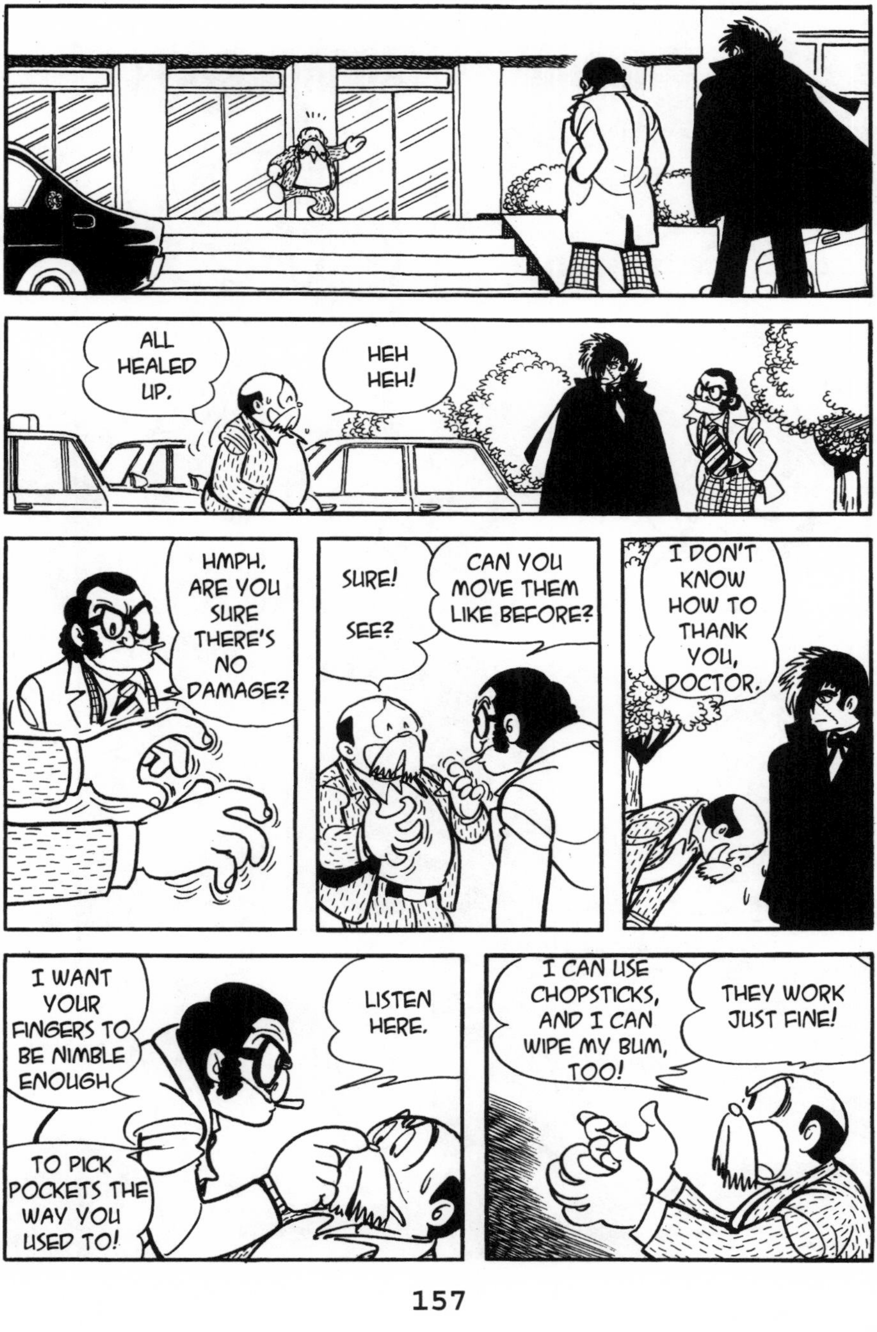
HEH HEH!
ALL HEALED UP.
I DON'T KNOW HOW TO THANK YOU, DOCTOR.
CAN YOU MOVE THEM LIKE BEFORE?
SURE!
SEE?
HMPH. ARE YOU SURE THERE'S NO DAMAGE?
THEY WORK JUST FINE!
I CAN USE CHOPSTICKS, AND I CAN WIPE MY BUM, TOO!
LISTEN HERE.
I WANT YOUR FINGERS TO BE NIMBLE ENOUGH
TO PICK POCKETS THE WAY YOU USED TO!

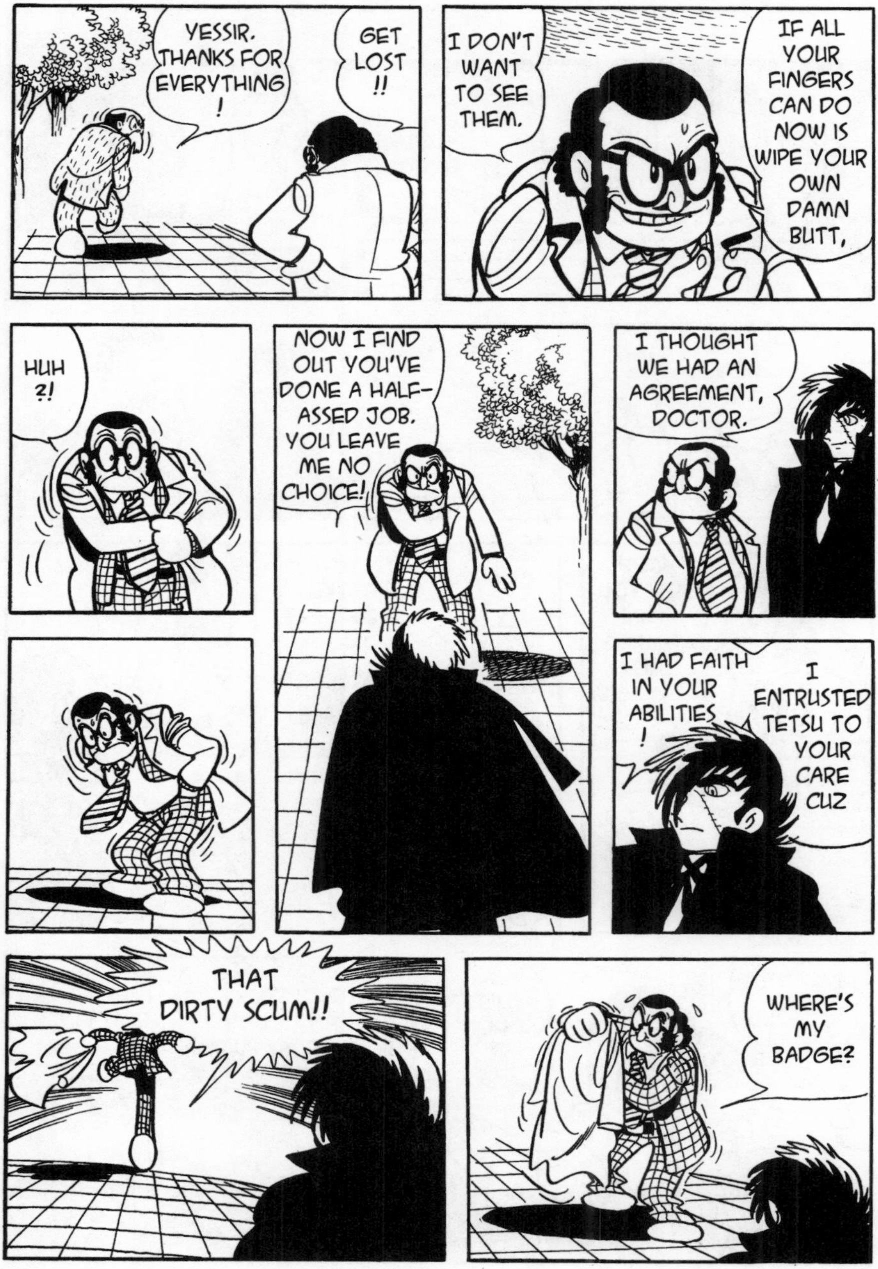
IF ALL YOUR FINGERS CAN DO NOW IS WIPE YOUR OWN DAMN BUTT,
I DON'T WANT TO SEE THEM.
GET LOST !!
YESSIR. THANKS FOR EVERYTHING !
I THOUGHT WE HAD AN AGREEMENT, DOCTOR.
I ENTRUSTED TETSU TO YOUR CARE CUZ
I HAD FAITH IN YOUR ABILITIES !
NOW I FIND OUT YOU'VE DONE A HALF-ASSED JOB. YOU LEAVE ME NO CHOICE!
HUH ?!
WHERE'S MY BADGE?
THAT DIRTY SCUM!!

TETSU !!
YOU FILTHY ...!
VOILA! YOUR BADGE!
YOUR PEN!
AND YOUR WALLET!
Y-YOU'RE UNDER ARREST!
AW, I WAS JUST SHOWIN' YA!
SEE? MY FINGERS ARE GOOD AS NEW!
OH ...
WHADDYA SAY WE TIP A FEW BACK AND TOAST THE GREAT DOCTOR BLACK JACK, INSPECTOR?
WELL, THAT'S JUST... GREAT!
ONE OF THESE DAYS, I'LL NAB YOU.
EH, NONE OF THAT TONIGHT, SIR.

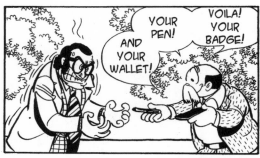

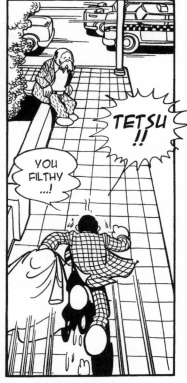

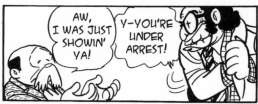

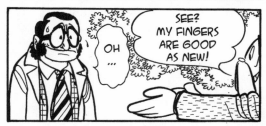

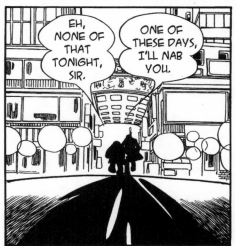

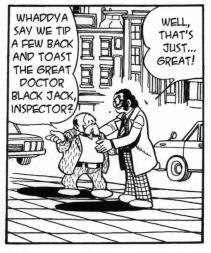

TITLES

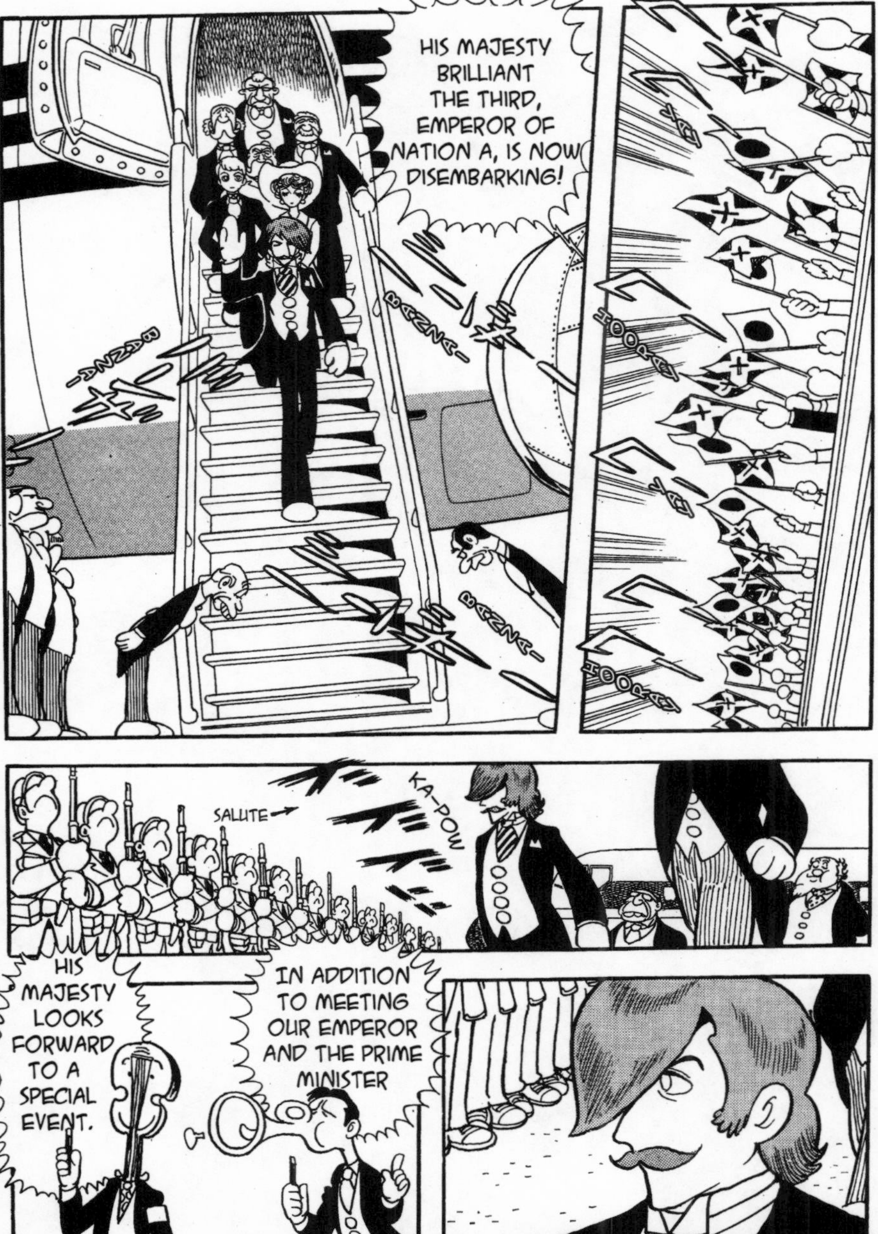
HOORAY
HOORAY
HIS MAJESTY BRILLIANT THE THIRD, EMPEROR OF NATION A, IS NOW DISEMBARKING!
BANZAI-
BANZAI-
BANZAI-
KA-POW
SALUTE
IN ADDITION TO MEETING OUR EMPEROR AND THE PRIME MINISTER
HIS MAJESTY LOOKS FORWARD TO A SPECIAL EVENT.

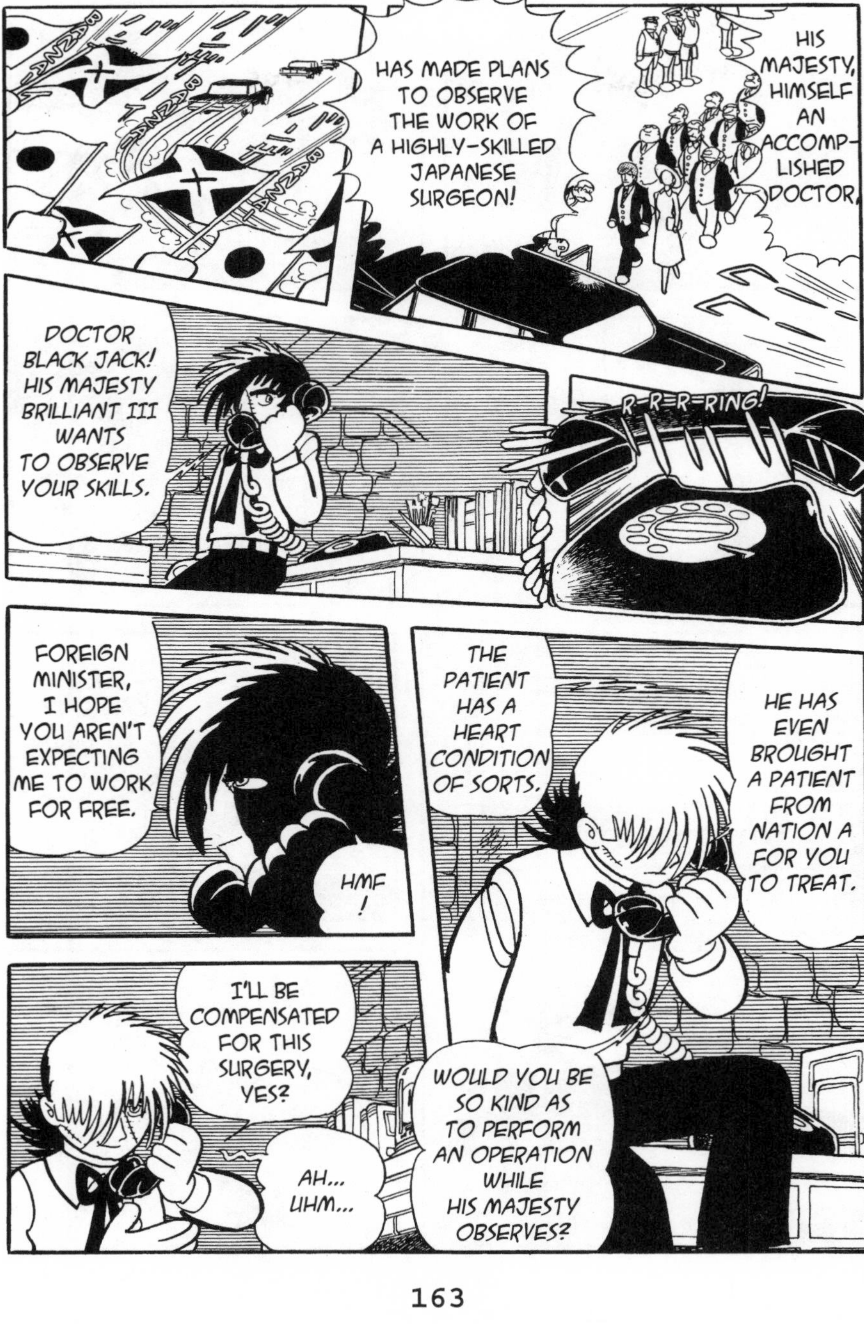
HIS MAJESTY, HIMSELF AN ACCOMPLISHED DOCTOR,
HAS MADE PLANS TO OBSERVE THE WORK OF A HIGHLY-SKILLED JAPANESE SURGEON!
R-R-R-RING!
DOCTOR BLACK JACK! HIS MAJESTY BRILLIANT III WANTS TO OBSERVE YOUR SKILLS.
HE HAS EVEN BROUGHT A PATIENT FROM NATION A FOR YOU TO TREAT.
THE PATIENT HAS A HEART CONDITION OF SORTS.
FOREIGN MINISTER, I HOPE YOU AREN'T EXPECTING ME TO WORK FOR FREE.
HMF!
WOULD YOU BE SO KIND AS TO PERFORM AN OPERATION WHILE HIS MAJESTY OBSERVES?
I'LL BE COMPENSATED FOR THIS SURGERY, YES?
AH... UHM...

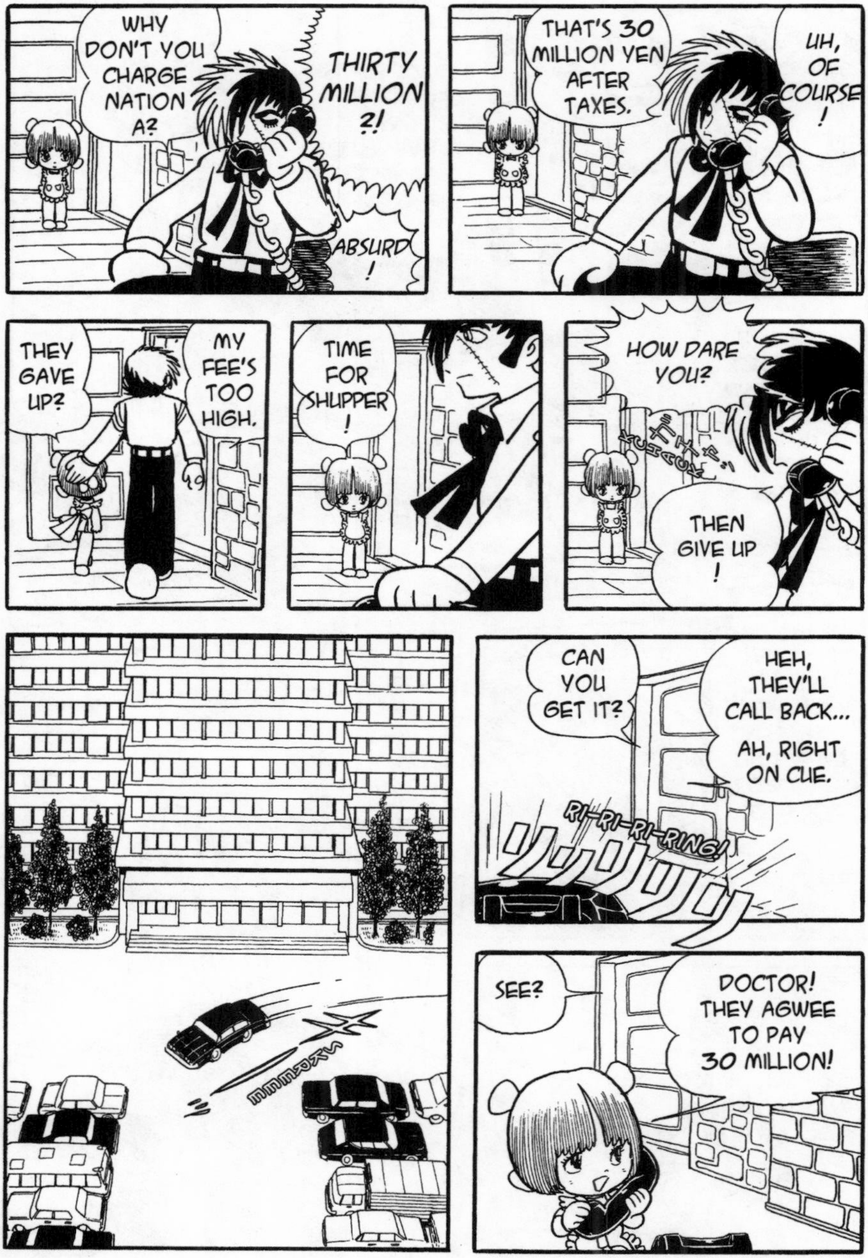
UH, OF COURSE!
THAT'S 30 MILLION YEN AFTER TAXES.
THIRTY MILLION ?!
ABSURD!
WHY DON'T YOU CHARGE NATION A?
HOW DARE YOU?
THEN GIVE UP!
TIME FOR SHUPPER!
MY FEE'S TOO HIGH.
THEY GAVE UP?
HEH, THEY'LL CALL BACK...
AH, RIGHT ON CUE.
CAN YOU GET IT?
RI-RI-RI-RING!
DOCTOR! THEY AGWEE TO PAY 30 MILLION!
SEE?

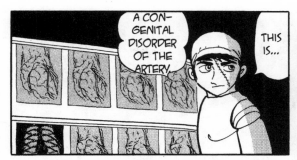

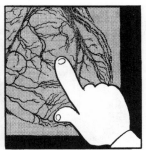

THIS IS...
A CON-GENITAL DISORDER OF THE ARTERY.
YES, ANOMALOUS ORIGIN, CORO-NARY AND PULMONARY.
THE ONLY JAPANESE DOCTOR TO EVER CURE IT IS PROF. SUZUKI OF J UNIVERSITY.
THIS SHOULDN'T BE HARD.
I HOPE YOU REALIZE WHAT A RARE HONOR IT IS TO OPERATE HERE AT T UNIVERSITY.
DON'T FORGET THAT YOU AREN'T EVEN LICENSED.
JAPAN MARITIME CLUB
PRESENTING HIS MAJESTY BRILLIANT THE THIRD!

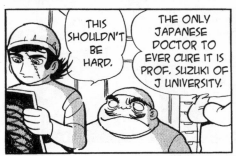

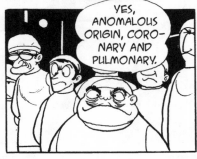

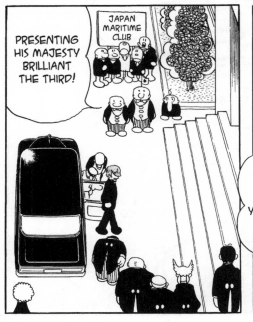

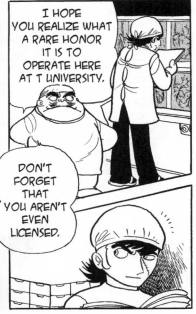

AHEM! WE ARE PLEASED TO HUMBLY WELCOME YOUR IMPERIAL MAJESTY TO THE T UNIVERSITY HOSPITAL!
WHAT IS THE STATUS OF THE PATIENT?
ANESTHETIZED AND IN THE OPERATING ROOM, YOUR MAJESTY!
LET US PROCEED THEN.
WHERE IS DOCTOR BLACK JACK?
EH, I'M AFRAID THAT DR. BLACK JACK IS AN UNLICENSED SURGEON...
YES, I AM AWARE OF THAT. BUT I WISH TO OBSERVE HIS TECHNIQUE.
HA HA HA... YES, WELL, HE'S THE SECOND DOCTOR FROM THE RIGHT.

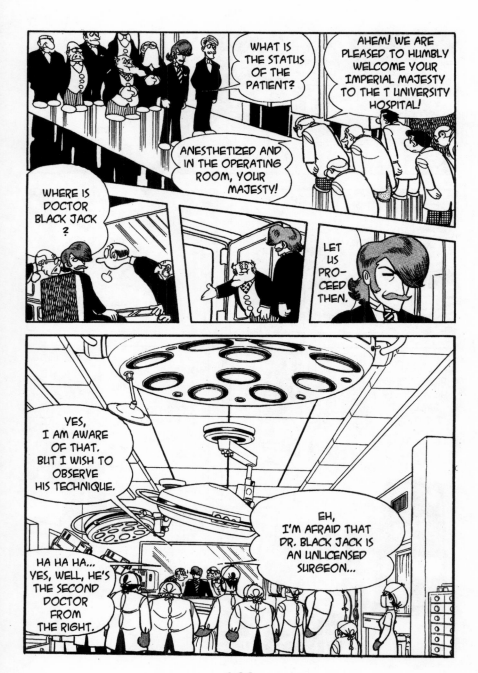

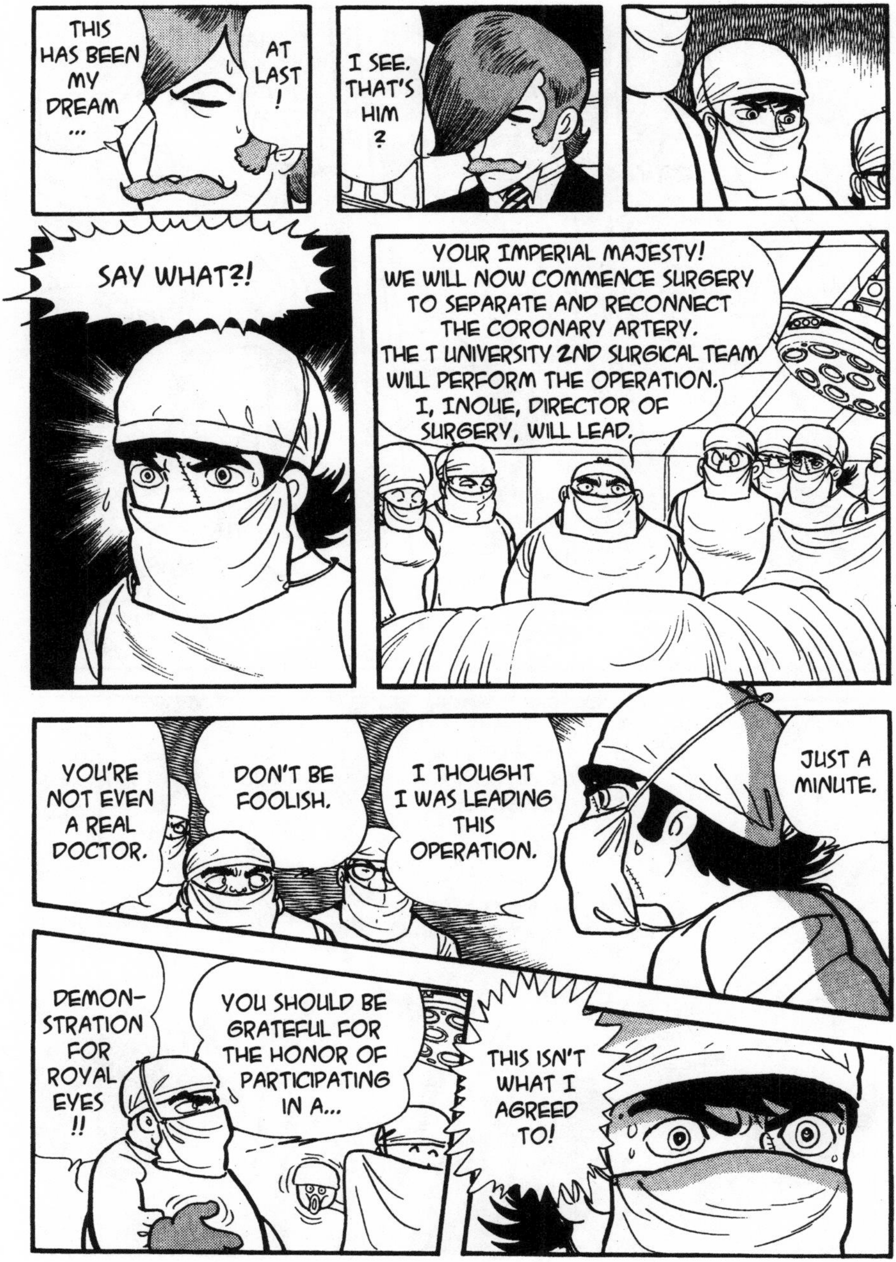
I SEE. THAT'S HIM ?
AT LAST !
THIS HAS BEEN MY DREAM ...
YOUR IMPERIAL MAJESTY! WE WILL NOW COMMENCE SURGERY TO SEPARATE AND RECONNECT THE CORONARY ARTERY. THE T UNIVERSITY 2ND SURGICAL TEAM WILL PERFORM THE OPERATION. I, INOUE, DIRECTOR OF SURGERY, WILL LEAD.
SAY WHAT?!
JUST A MINUTE.
I THOUGHT I WAS LEADING THIS OPERATION.
DON'T BE FOOLISH.
YOU'RE NOT EVEN A REAL DOCTOR.
THIS ISN'T WHAT I AGREED TO!
YOU SHOULD BE GRATEFUL FOR THE HONOR OF PARTICIPATING IN A...
DEMON-STRATION FOR ROYAL EYES !!

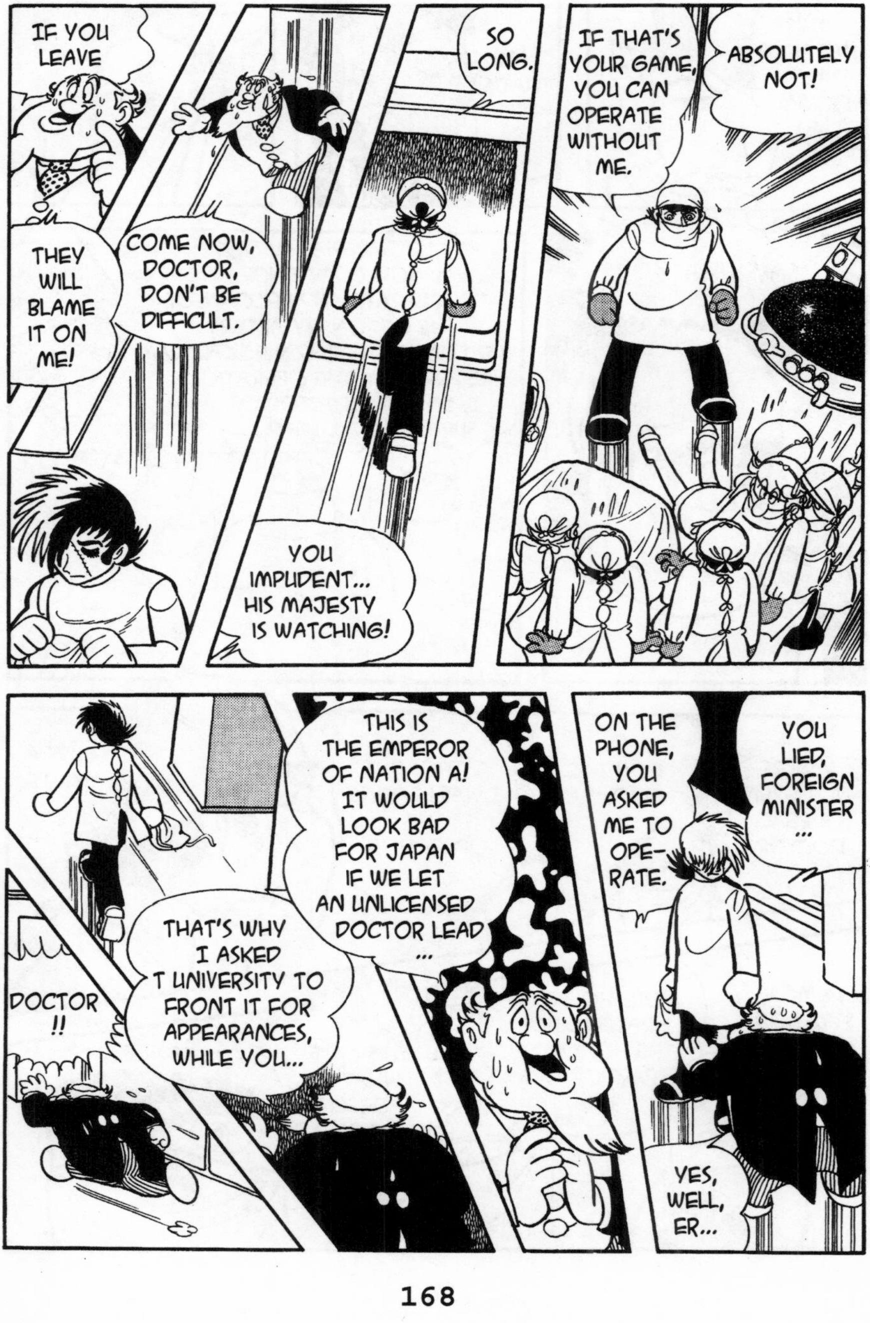
ABSOLUTELY NOT!
IF THAT'S YOUR GAME, YOU CAN OPERATE WITHOUT ME.
SO LONG.
YOU IMPUDENT... HIS MAJESTY IS WATCHING!
COME NOW, DOCTOR, DON'T BE DIFFICULT.
IF YOU LEAVE
THEY WILL BLAME IT ON ME!
YOU LIED, FOREIGN MINISTER ...
ON THE PHONE, YOU ASKED ME TO OPE-RATE.
YES, WELL, ER...
THIS IS THE EMPEROR OF NATION A! IT WOULD LOOK BAD FOR JAPAN IF WE LET AN UNLICENSED DOCTOR LEAD ...
THAT'S WHY I ASKED T UNIVERSITY TO FRONT IT FOR APPEARANCES, WHILE YOU...
DOCTOR !!

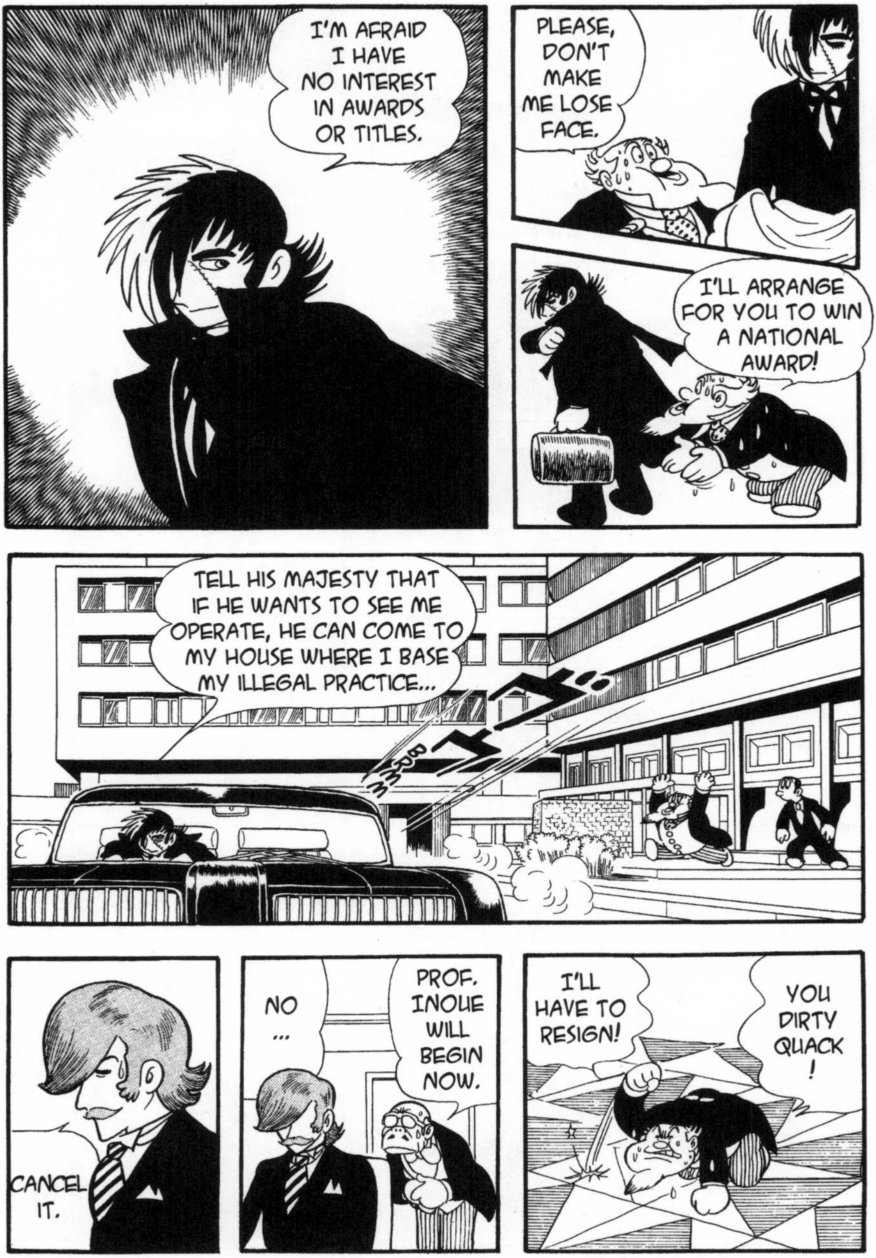
PLEASE, DON'T MAKE ME LOSE FACE.
I'LL ARRANGE FOR YOU TO WIN A NATIONAL AWARD!
I'M AFRAID I HAVE NO INTEREST IN AWARDS OR TITLES.
TELL HIS MAJESTY THAT IF HE WANTS TO SEE ME OPERATE, HE CAN COME TO MY HOUSE WHERE I BASE MY ILLEGAL PRACTICE...
BRMM
YOU DIRTY QUACK!
I'LL HAVE TO RESIGN!
PROF. INOUE WILL BEGIN NOW.
NO ...
CANCEL IT.

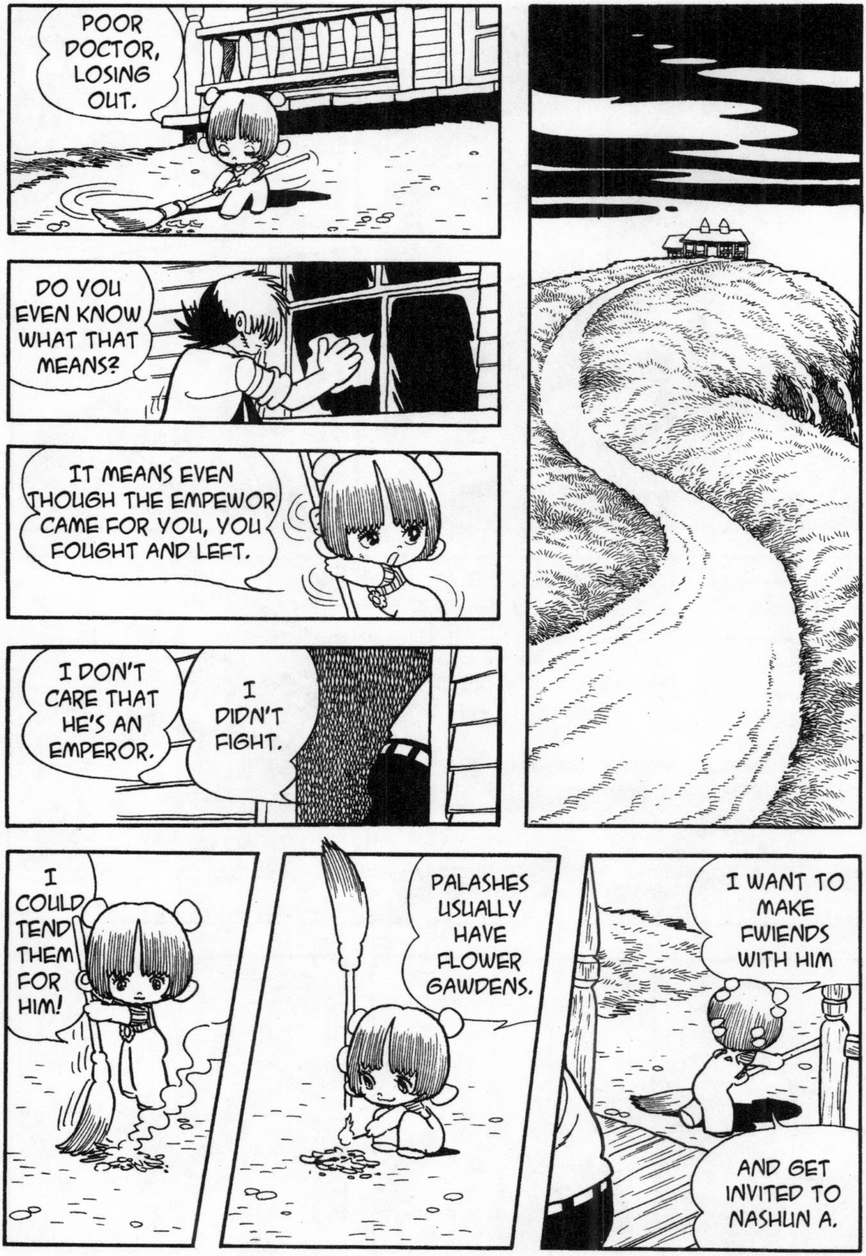
POOR DOCTOR, LOSING OUT.
DO YOU EVEN KNOW WHAT THAT MEANS?
IT MEANS EVEN THOUGH THE EMPEWOR CAME FOR YOU, YOU FOUGHT AND LEFT.
I DIDN'T FIGHT.
I DON'T CARE THAT HE'S AN EMPEROR.
I WANT TO MAKE FWIENDS WITH HIM
AND GET INVITED TO NASHUN A.
PALASHES USUALLY HAVE FLOWER GAWDENS.
I COULD TEND THEM FOR HIM!

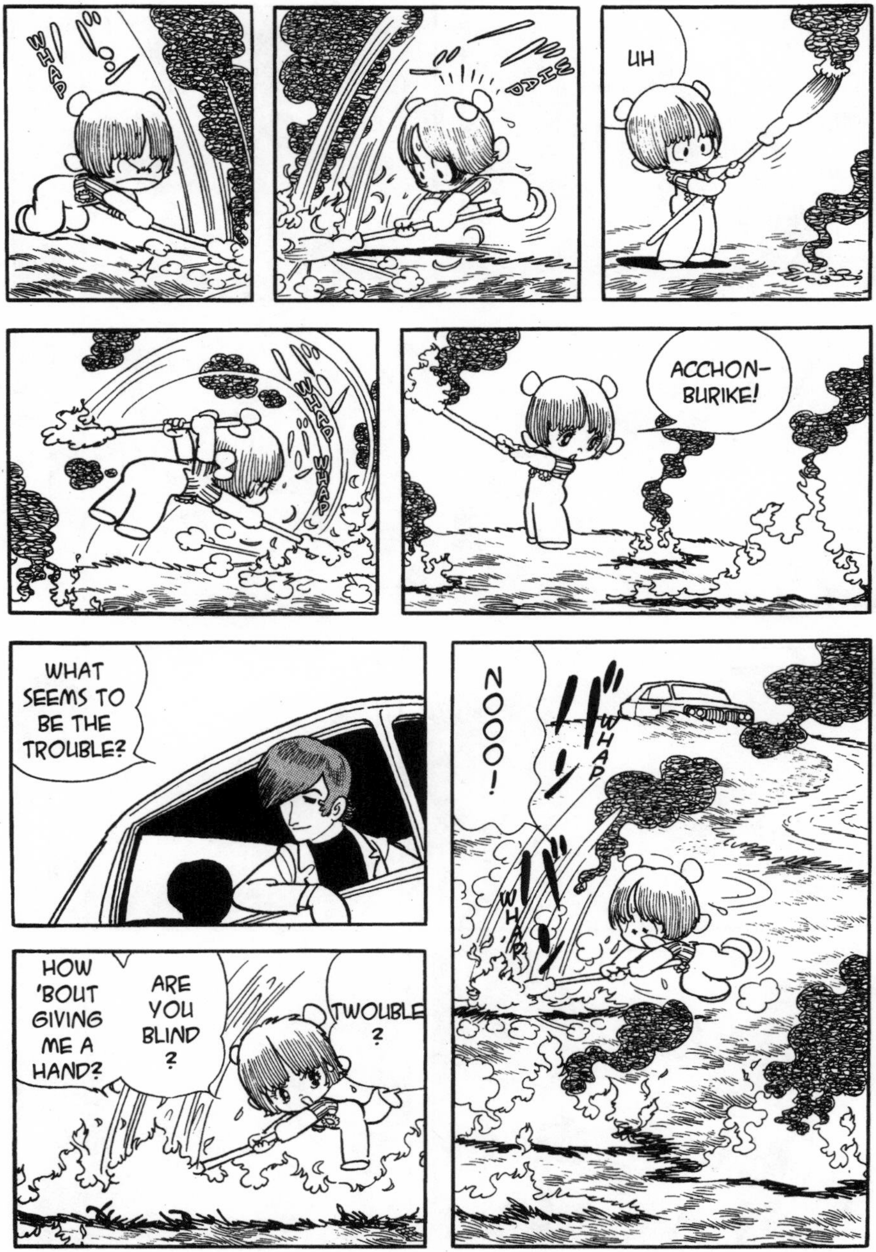
UH
WHAP
WHAP
ACCHON-BURIKE!
WHAP
WHAP
NOOOO!
WHAP
WHAP
WHAT SEEMS TO BE THE TROUBLE?
TWOUBLE?
ARE YOU BLIND?
HOW 'BOUT GIVING ME A HAND?

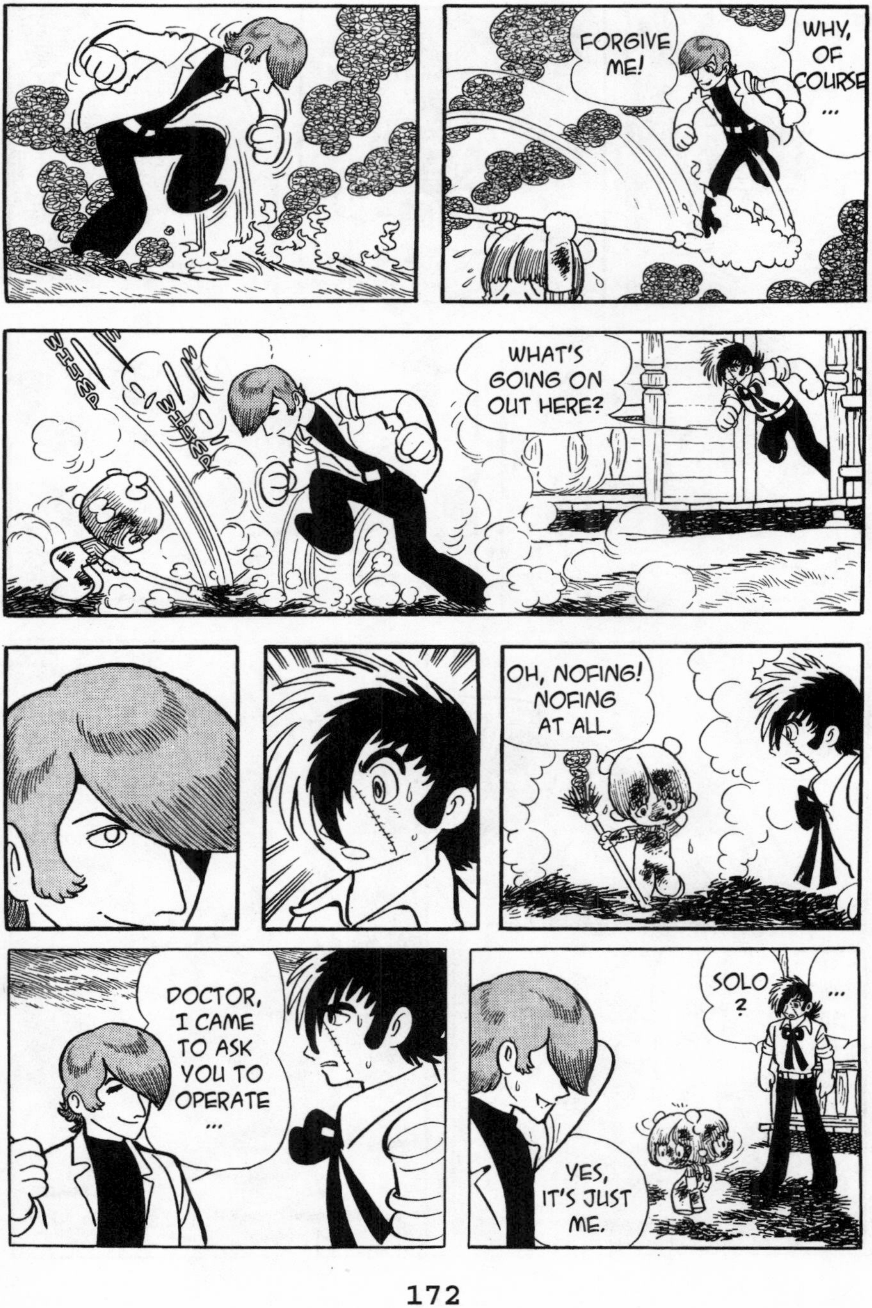
WHY, OF COURSE ...
FORGIVE ME!
WHAT'S GOING ON OUT HERE?
WHUMP
WHUMP
OH, NOFING! NOFING AT ALL.
SOLO ?
...
YES, IT'S JUST ME.
DOCTOR, I CAME TO ASK YOU TO OPERATE ...

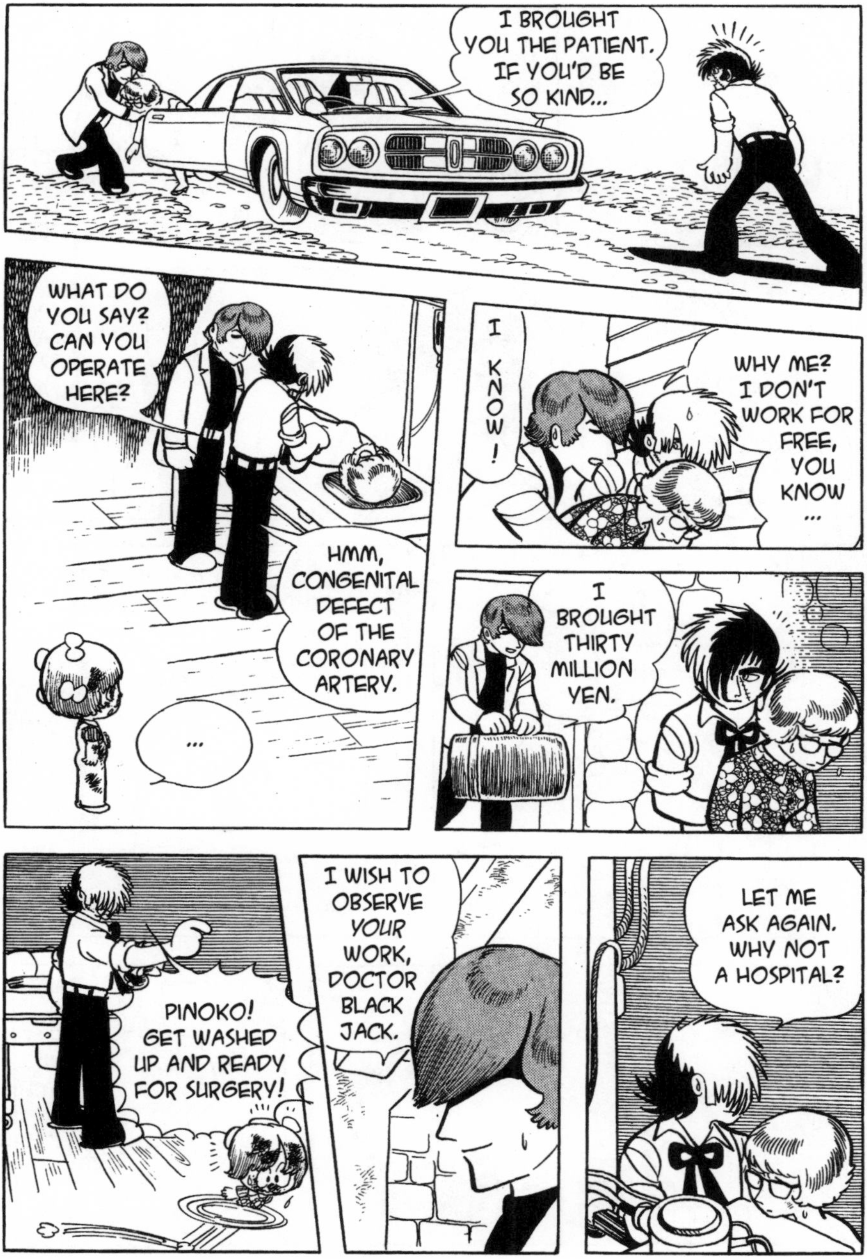
I BROUGHT YOU THE PATIENT. IF YOU'D BE SO KIND...
WHY ME? I DON'T WORK FOR FREE, YOU KNOW ...
I KNOW!
I BROUGHT THIRTY MILLION YEN.
WHAT DO YOU SAY? CAN YOU OPERATE HERE?
HMM, CONGENITAL DEFECT OF THE CORONARY ARTERY.
...
LET ME ASK AGAIN. WHY NOT A HOSPITAL?
I WISH TO OBSERVE *YOUR* WORK, DOCTOR BLACK JACK.
PINOKO! GET WASHED UP AND READY FOR SURGERY!

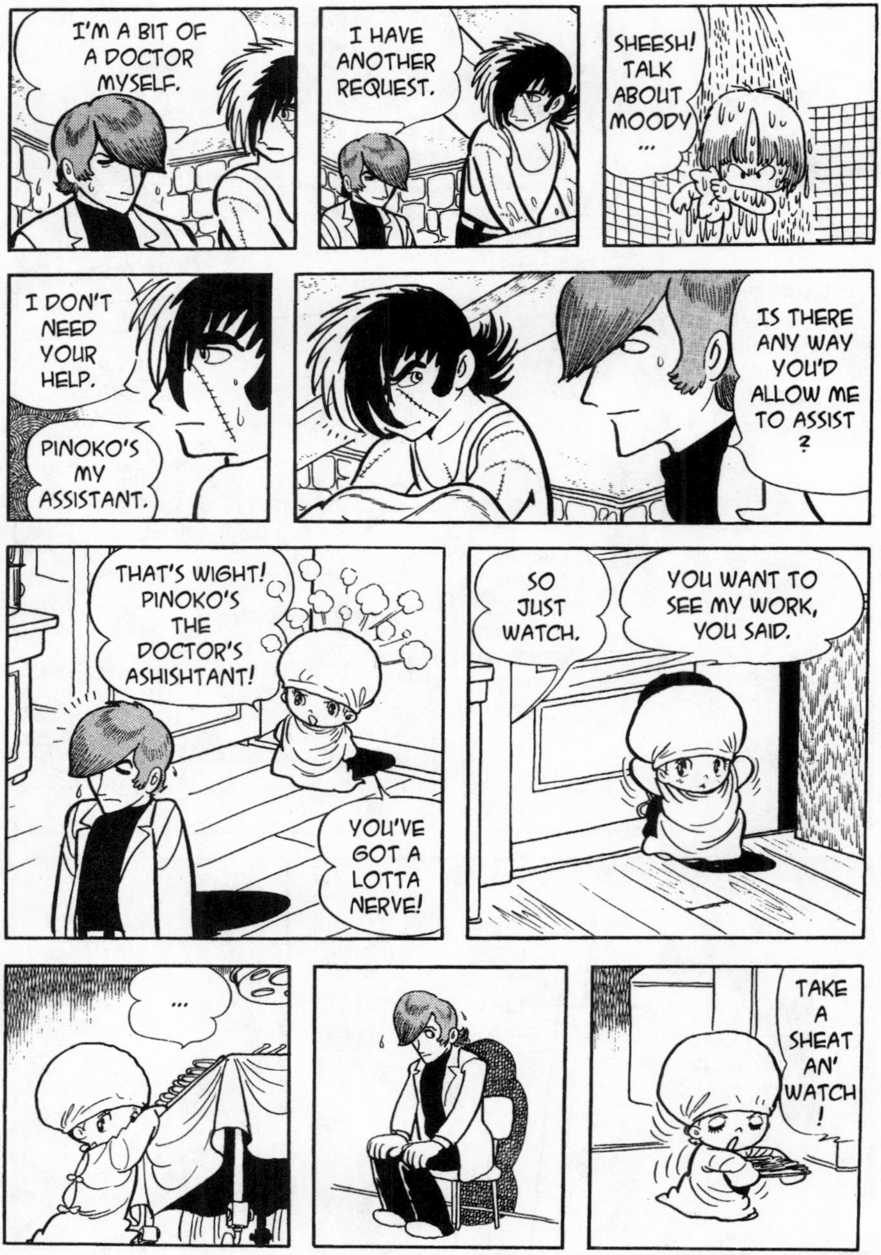
SHEESH! TALK ABOUT MOODY...
I HAVE ANOTHER REQUEST.
I'M A BIT OF A DOCTOR MYSELF.
IS THERE ANY WAY YOU'D ALLOW ME TO ASSIST?
I DON'T NEED YOUR HELP.
PINOKO'S MY ASSISTANT.
YOU WANT TO SEE MY WORK, YOU SAID.
SO JUST WATCH.
THAT'S WIGHT! PINOKO'S THE DOCTOR'S ASHISHTANT!
YOU'VE GOT A LOTTA NERVE!
TAKE A SHEAT AN' WATCH!
...

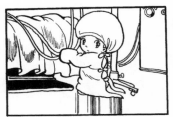

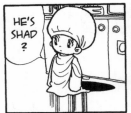

HE'S SHAD?
HEY, DOCTOR?
UHM ...
NO!
I DIDN'T ASHK ANYFING ...
HE LOOKS PWETTY SHAD.
MAYBE YOU COULD LET HIM HELP.
NO WAY!
HE WON'T MEDDLE WITH MY WORK!
BUT DOCTOR, HE'S HAND-SHOME!
HE'D PWOBABLY DO FINE!
MAYBE NOT AS GOOD AS PINOKO...
BUT I FINK HE'S OKAY.
IF YOU WANT HIM TO ASSIST SO MUCH
YOU USE HIM!
I DON'T CARE IF HE HELPS YOU.

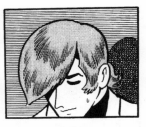

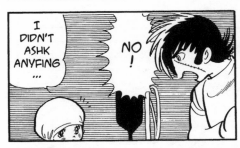

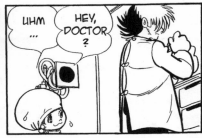

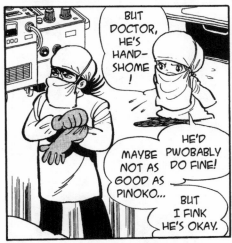

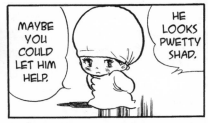

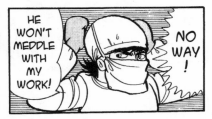

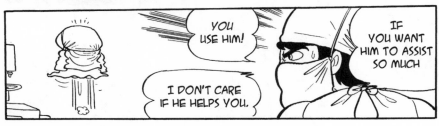

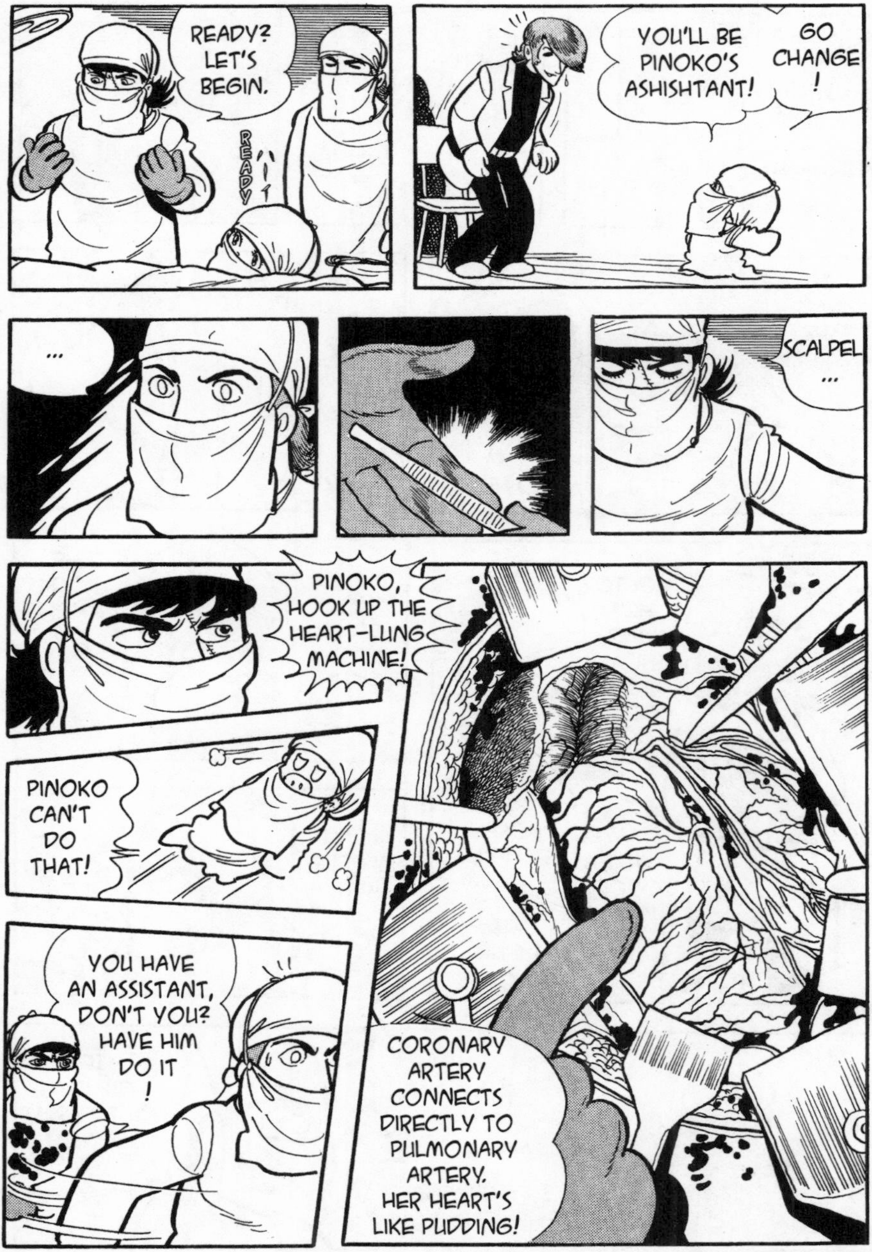
GO CHANGE !
YOU'LL BE PINOKO'S ASHISHTANT!
READY? LET'S BEGIN.
READY
SCALPEL ...
...
CORONARY ARTERY CONNECTS DIRECTLY TO PULMONARY ARTERY. HER HEART'S LIKE PUDDING!
PINOKO, HOOK UP THE HEART-LUNG MACHINE!
PINOKO CAN'T DO THAT!
YOU HAVE AN ASSISTANT, DON'T YOU? HAVE HIM DO IT !

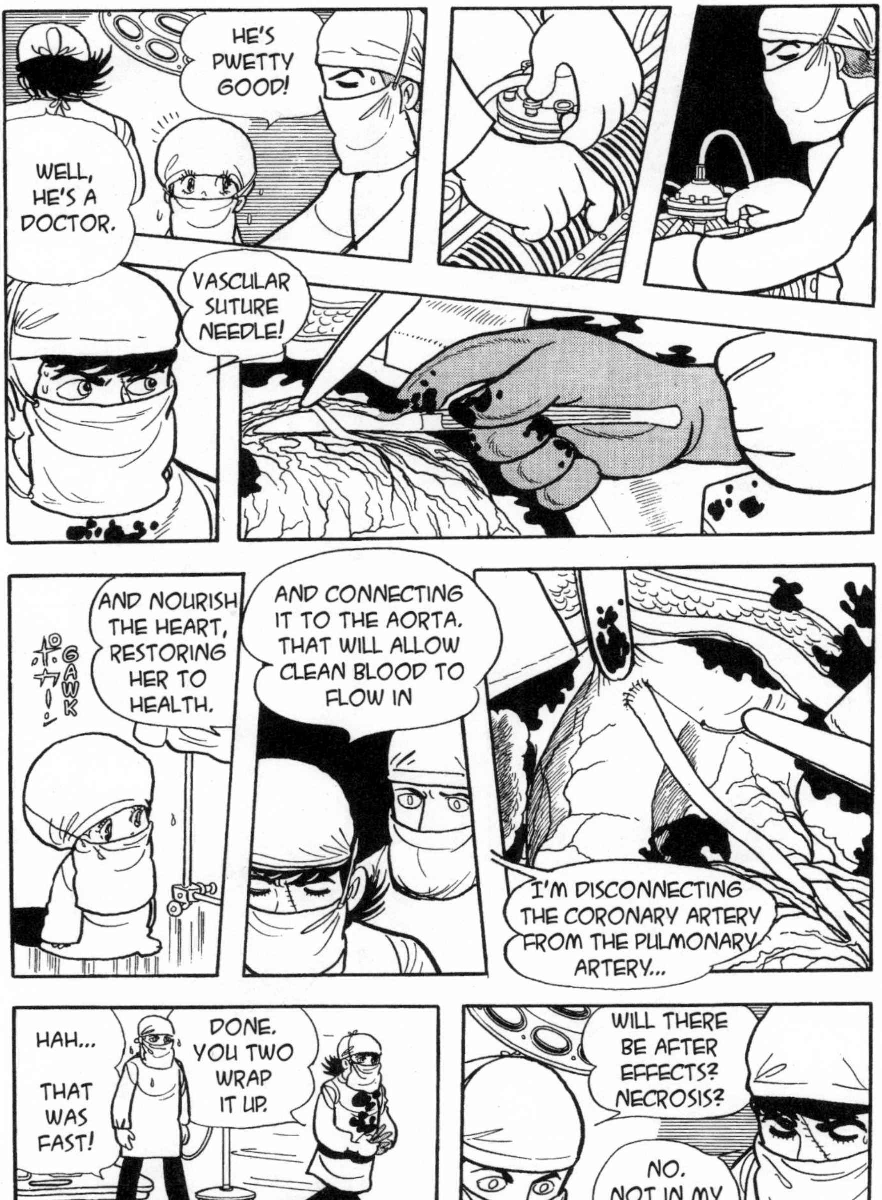
HE'S PWETTY GOOD!
WELL, HE'S A DOCTOR.
VASCULAR SUTURE NEEDLE!
I'M DISCONNECTING THE CORONARY ARTERY FROM THE PULMONARY ARTERY...
AND CONNECTING IT TO THE AORTA. THAT WILL ALLOW CLEAN BLOOD TO FLOW IN
AND NOURISH THE HEART, RESTORING HER TO HEALTH.
GAWK
WILL THERE BE AFTER EFFECTS? NECROSIS?
NO. NOT IN MY EXPERIENCE.
DONE. YOU TWO WRAP IT UP.
HAH... THAT WAS FAST!

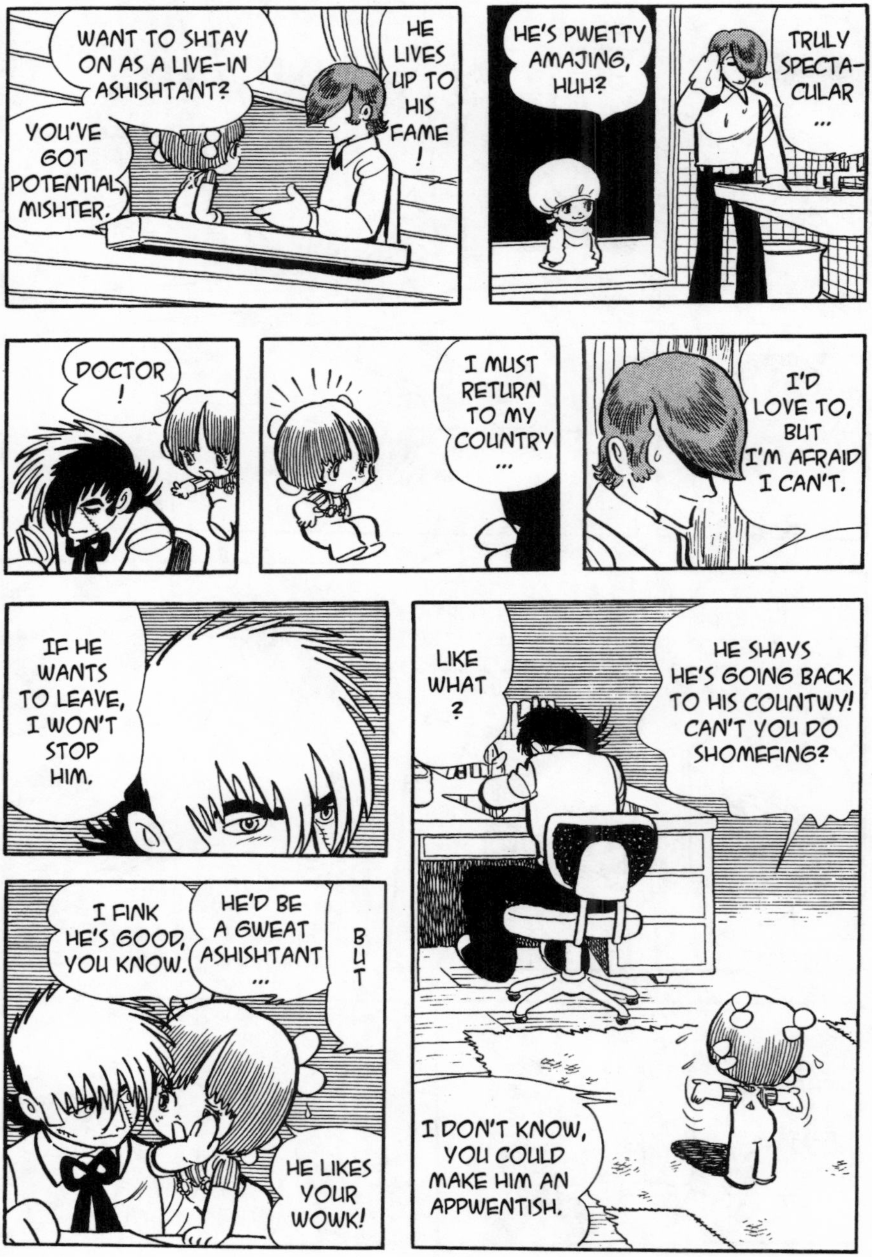
TRULY SPECTACULAR ...
HE'S PWETTY AMAJING, HUH?
HE LIVES UP TO HIS FAME!
WANT TO SHTAY ON AS A LIVE-IN ASHISHTANT?
YOU'VE GOT POTENTIAL, MISHTER.
I'D LOVE TO, BUT I'M AFRAID I CAN'T.
I MUST RETURN TO MY COUNTRY ...
DOCTOR!
HE SHAYS HE'S GOING BACK TO HIS COUNTWY! CAN'T YOU DO SHOMEFING?
LIKE WHAT?
I DON'T KNOW, YOU COULD MAKE HIM AN APPWENTISH.
IF HE WANTS TO LEAVE, I WON'T STOP HIM.
BUT
HE'D BE A GWEAT ASHISHTANT ...
I FINK HE'S GOOD, YOU KNOW.
HE LIKES YOUR WOWK!

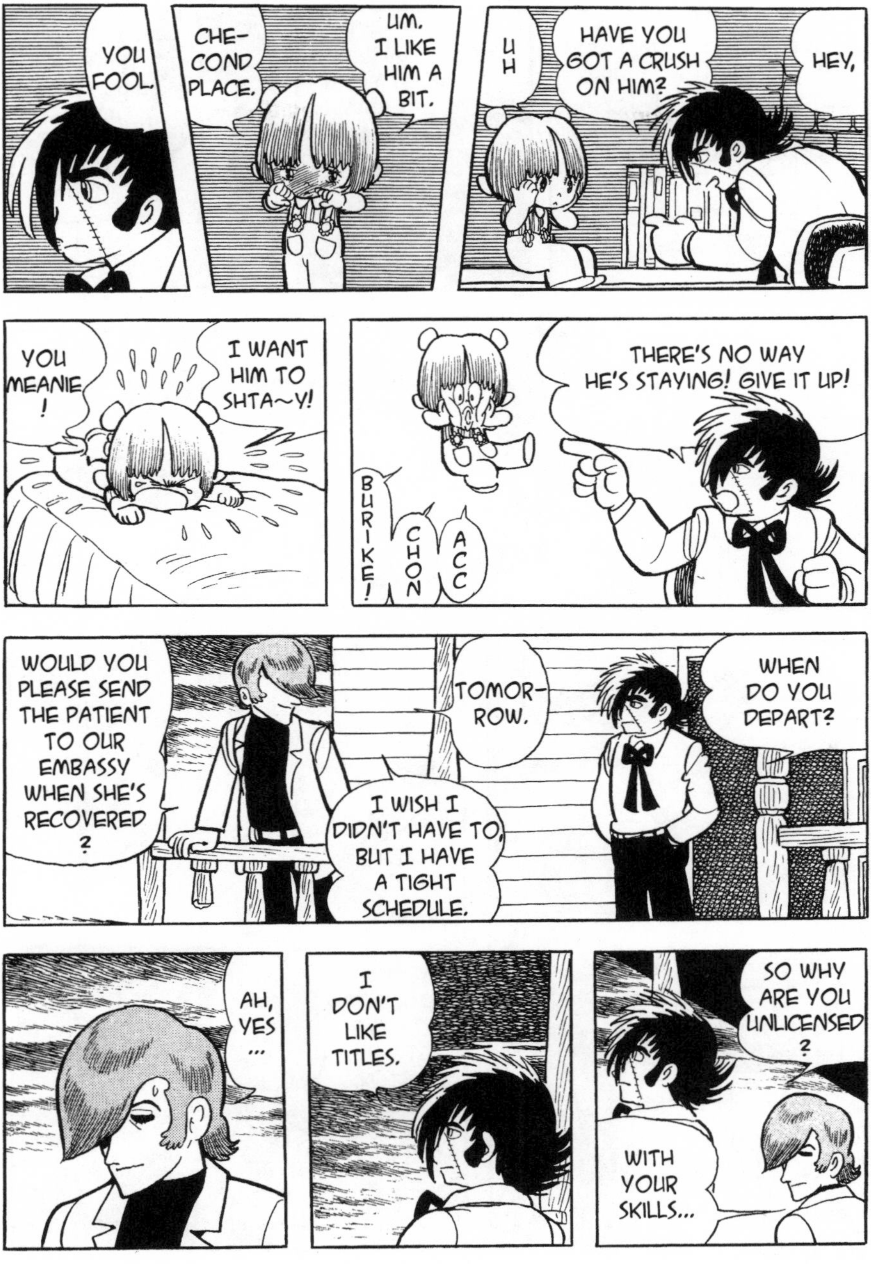
HEY,
HAVE YOU GOT A CRUSH ON HIM?
UH
UM. I LIKE HIM A BIT.
CHE-COND PLACE.
YOU FOOL.
THERE'S NO WAY HE'S STAYING! GIVE IT UP!
ACC
CHON
BURIKE!
I WANT HIM TO SHTA~Y!
YOU MEANIE!
WHEN DO YOU DEPART?
TOMOR-ROW.
I WISH I DIDN'T HAVE TO, BUT I HAVE A TIGHT SCHEDULE.
WOULD YOU PLEASE SEND THE PATIENT TO OUR EMBASSY WHEN SHE'S RECOVERED?
SO WHY ARE YOU UNLICENSED?
WITH YOUR SKILLS...
I DON'T LIKE TITLES.
AH, YES...

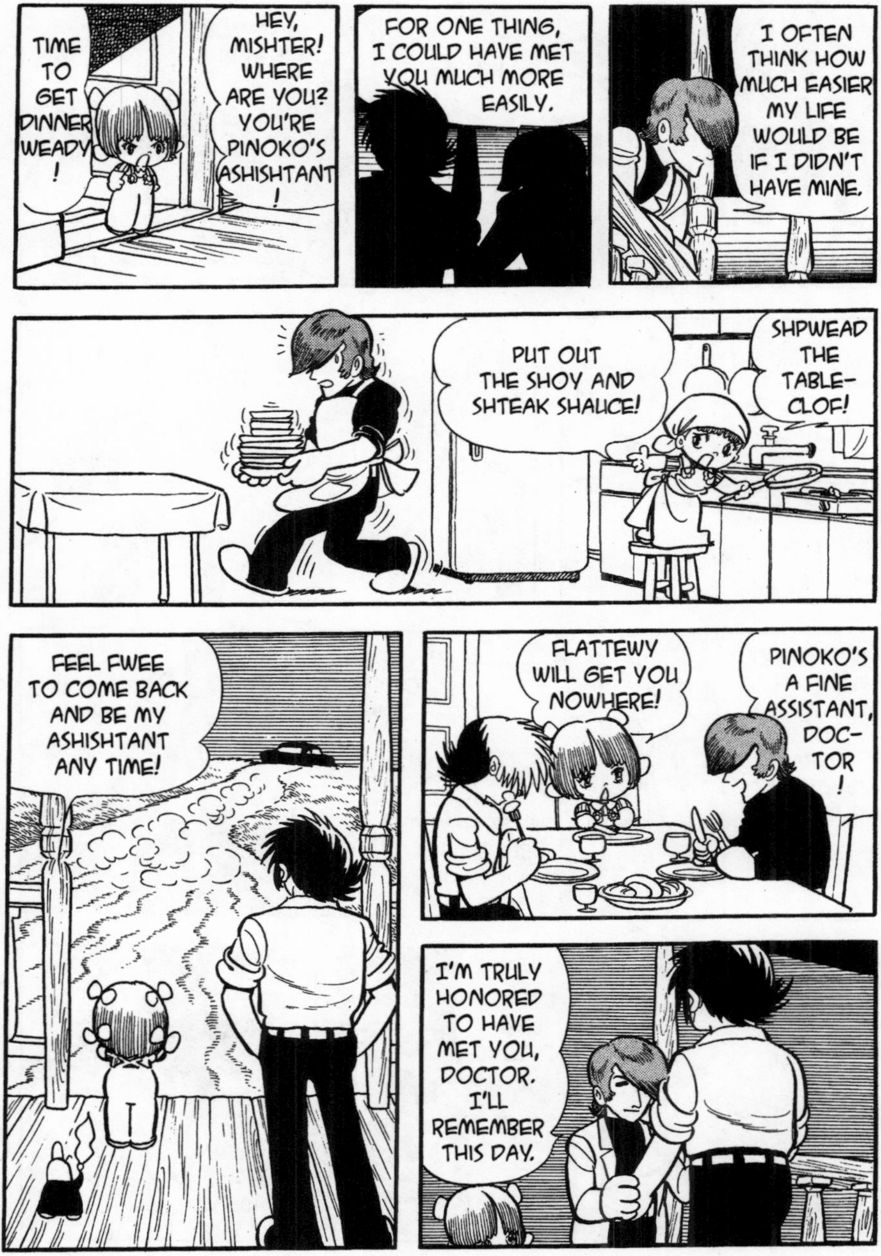
I OFTEN THINK HOW MUCH EASIER MY LIFE WOULD BE IF I DIDN'T HAVE MINE.
FOR ONE THING, I COULD HAVE MET YOU MUCH MORE EASILY.
HEY, MISHTER! WHERE ARE YOU? YOU'RE PINOKO'S ASHISHTANT!
TIME TO GET DINNER WEADY!
SHPWEAD THE TABLE-CLOF!
PUT OUT THE SHOY AND SHTEAK SHAUCE!
PINOKO'S A FINE ASSISTANT, DOCTOR!
FLATTEWY WILL GET YOU NOWHERE!
I'M TRULY HONORED TO HAVE MET YOU, DOCTOR. I'LL REMEMBER THIS DAY.
FEEL FWEE TO COME BACK AND BE MY ASHISHTANT ANY TIME!

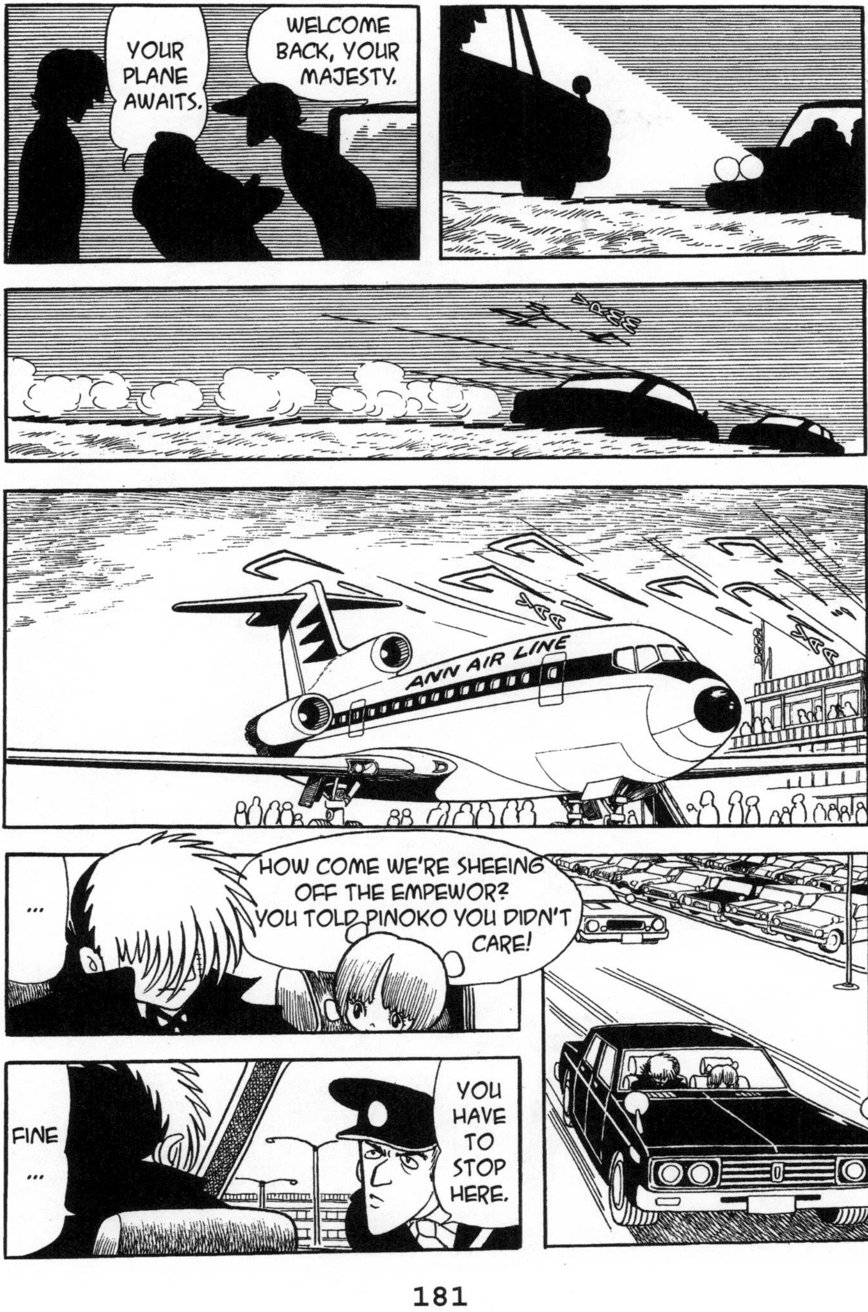
WELCOME BACK, YOUR MAJESTY.
YOUR PLANE AWAITS.
ANN AIR LINE
HOW COME WE'RE SHEEING OFF THE EMPEWOR? YOU TOLD PINOKO YOU DIDN'T CARE!
...
YOU HAVE TO STOP HERE.
FINE ...

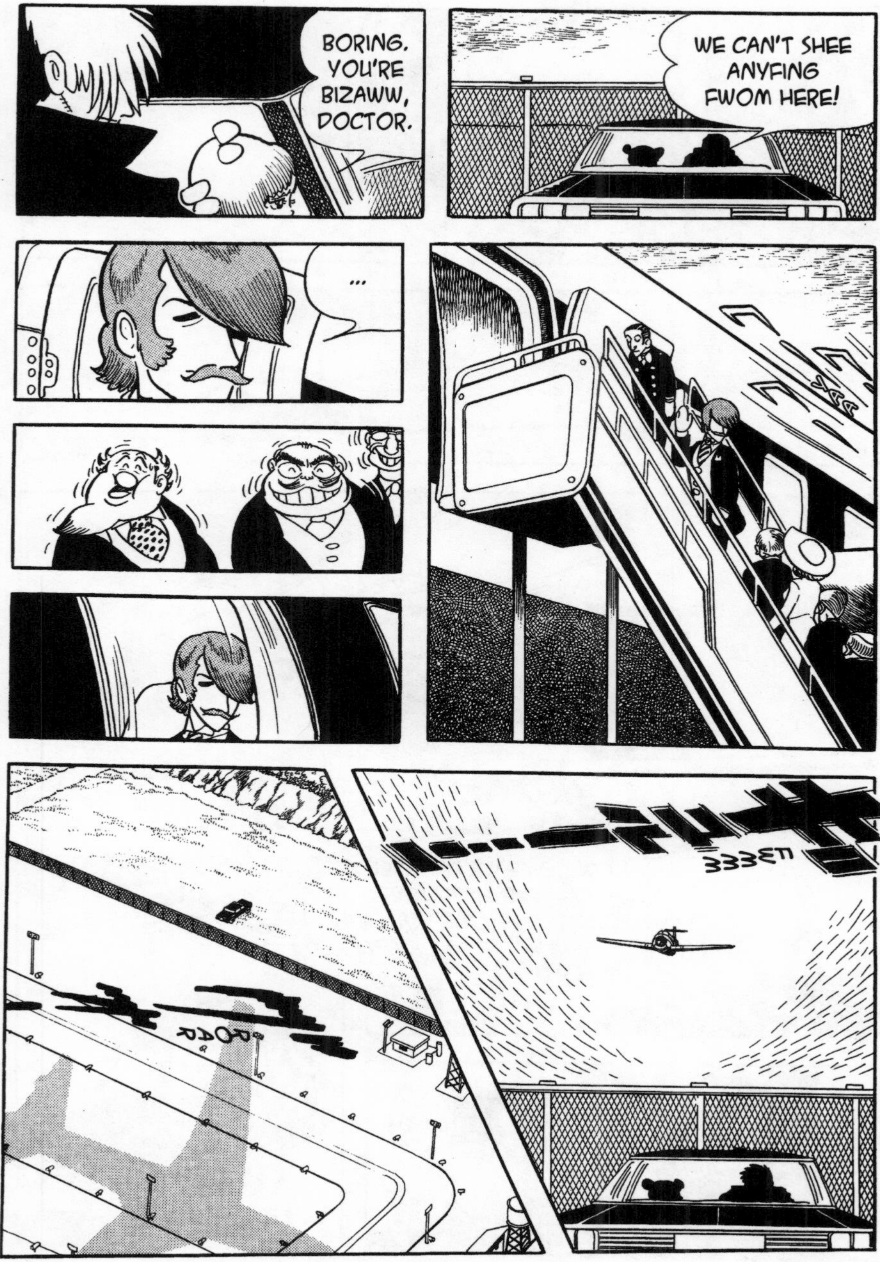
WE CAN'T SHEE ANYFING FWOM HERE!
BORING. YOU'RE BIZAWW, DOCTOR.
...
ROAR

LOST AND FOUND

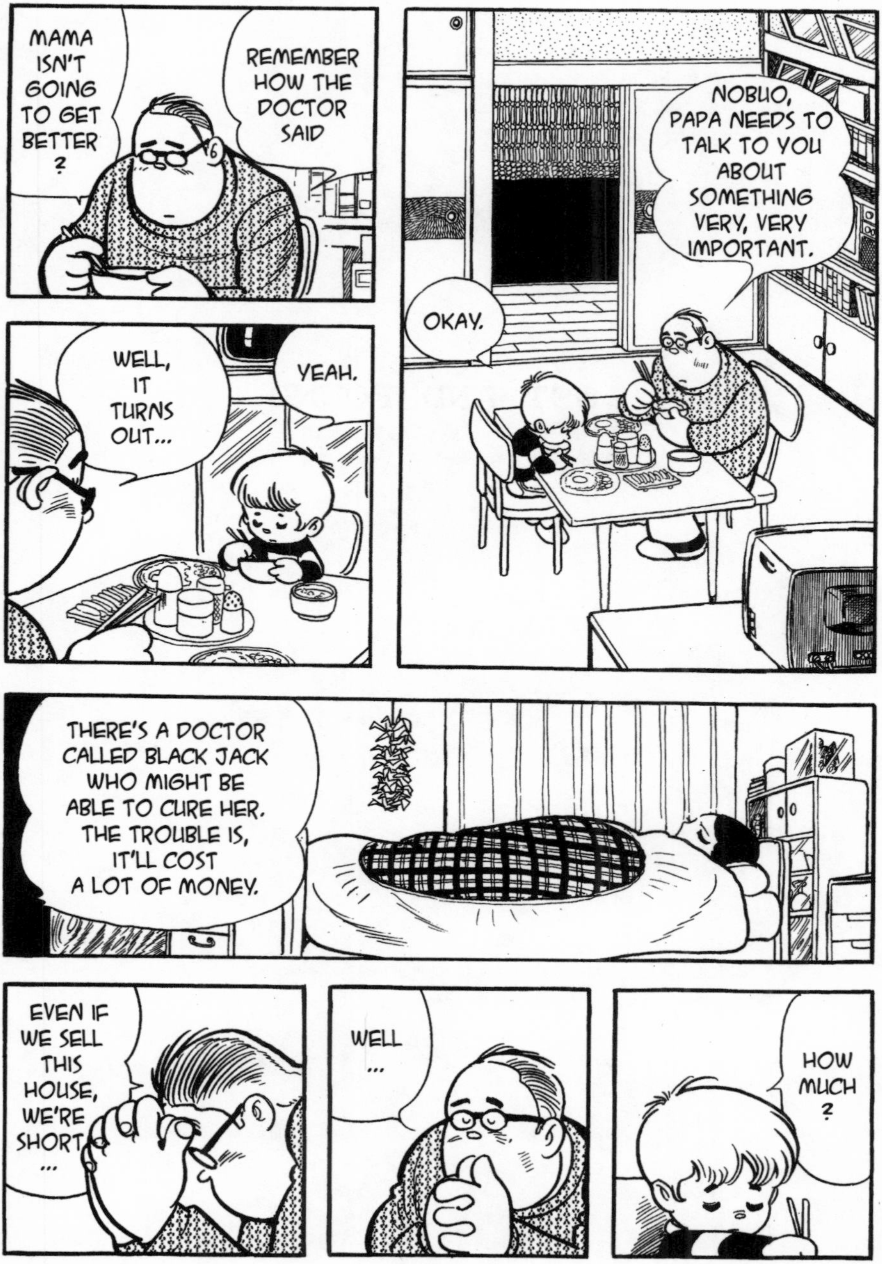
NOBUO, PAPA NEEDS TO TALK TO YOU ABOUT SOMETHING VERY, VERY IMPORTANT.
OKAY.
REMEMBER HOW THE DOCTOR SAID
MAMA ISN'T GOING TO GET BETTER?
YEAH.
WELL, IT TURNS OUT...
THERE'S A DOCTOR CALLED BLACK JACK WHO MIGHT BE ABLE TO CURE HER. THE TROUBLE IS, IT'LL COST A LOT OF MONEY.
HOW MUCH?
WELL...
EVEN IF WE SELL THIS HOUSE, WE'RE SHORT...

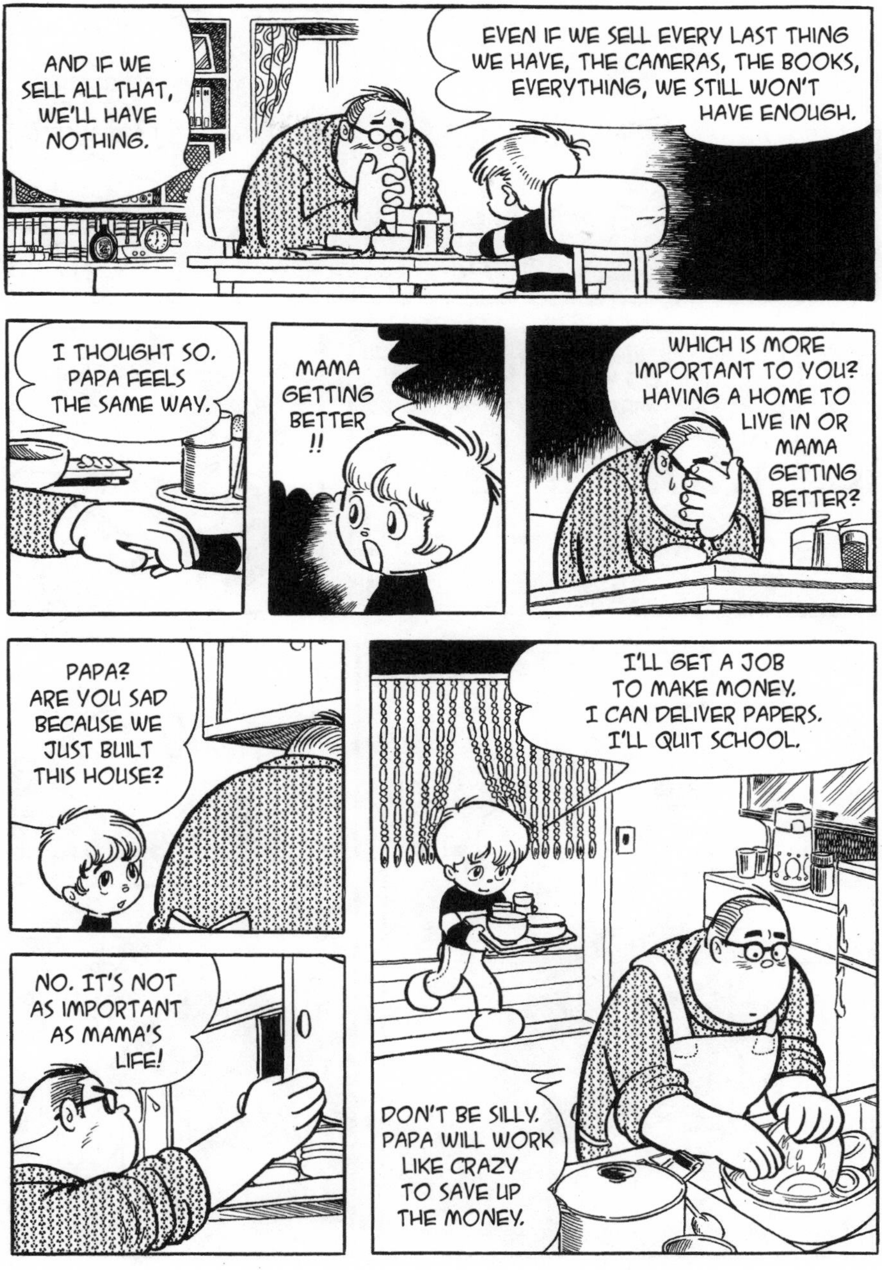
EVEN IF WE SELL EVERY LAST THING WE HAVE, THE CAMERAS, THE BOOKS, EVERYTHING, WE STILL WON'T HAVE ENOUGH.
AND IF WE SELL ALL THAT, WE'LL HAVE NOTHING.
WHICH IS MORE IMPORTANT TO YOU? HAVING A HOME TO LIVE IN OR MAMA GETTING BETTER?
MAMA GETTING BETTER !!
I THOUGHT SO. PAPA FEELS THE SAME WAY.
I'LL GET A JOB TO MAKE MONEY. I CAN DELIVER PAPERS. I'LL QUIT SCHOOL.
DON'T BE SILLY. PAPA WILL WORK LIKE CRAZY TO SAVE UP THE MONEY.
PAPA? ARE YOU SAD BECAUSE WE JUST BUILT THIS HOUSE?
NO. IT'S NOT AS IMPORTANT AS MAMA'S LIFE!

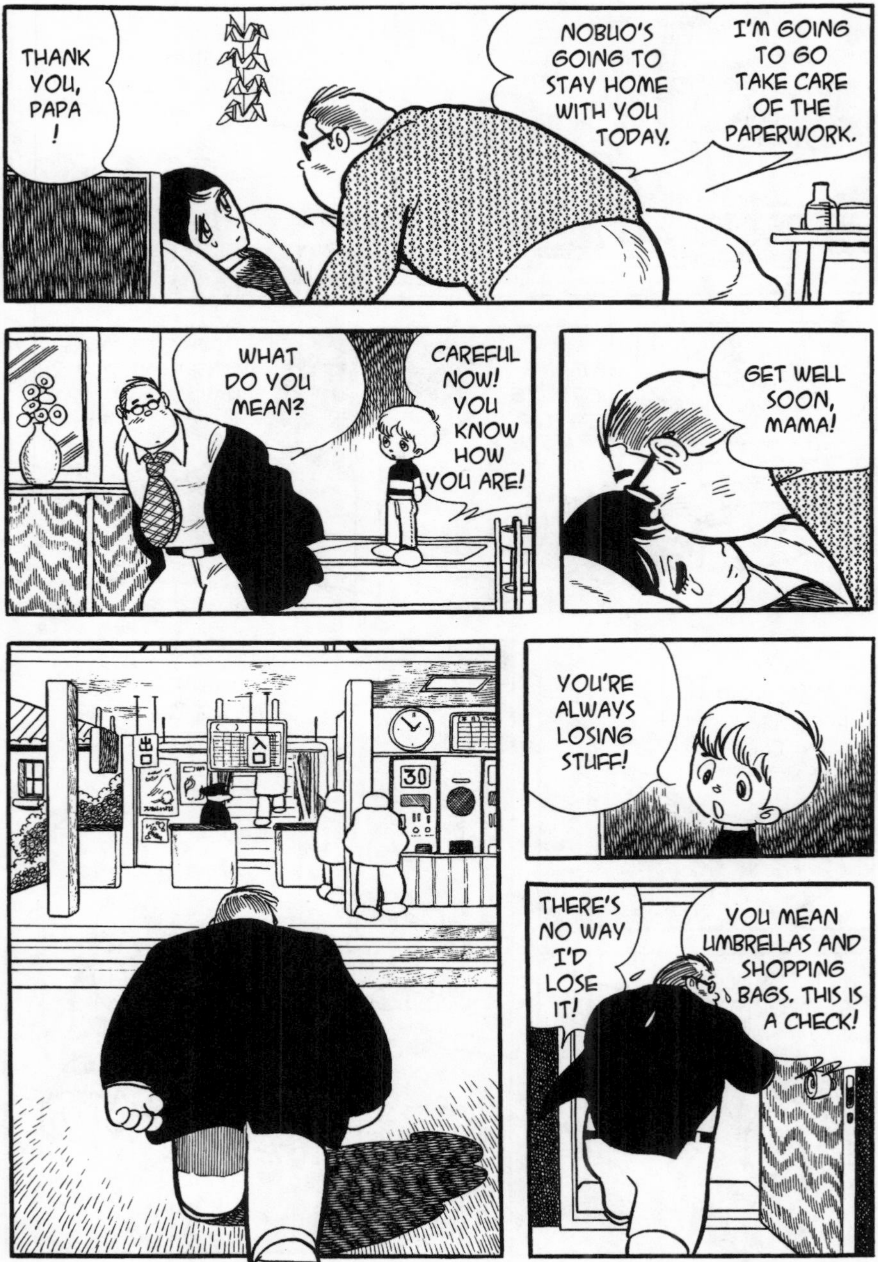
I'M GOING TO GO TAKE CARE OF THE PAPERWORK.
NOBUO'S GOING TO STAY HOME WITH YOU TODAY.
THANK YOU, PAPA!
GET WELL SOON, MAMA!
CAREFUL NOW! YOU KNOW HOW YOU ARE!
WHAT DO YOU MEAN?
YOU'RE ALWAYS LOSING STUFF!
YOU MEAN UMBRELLAS AND SHOPPING BAGS. THIS IS A CHECK!
THERE'S NO WAY I'D LOSE IT!

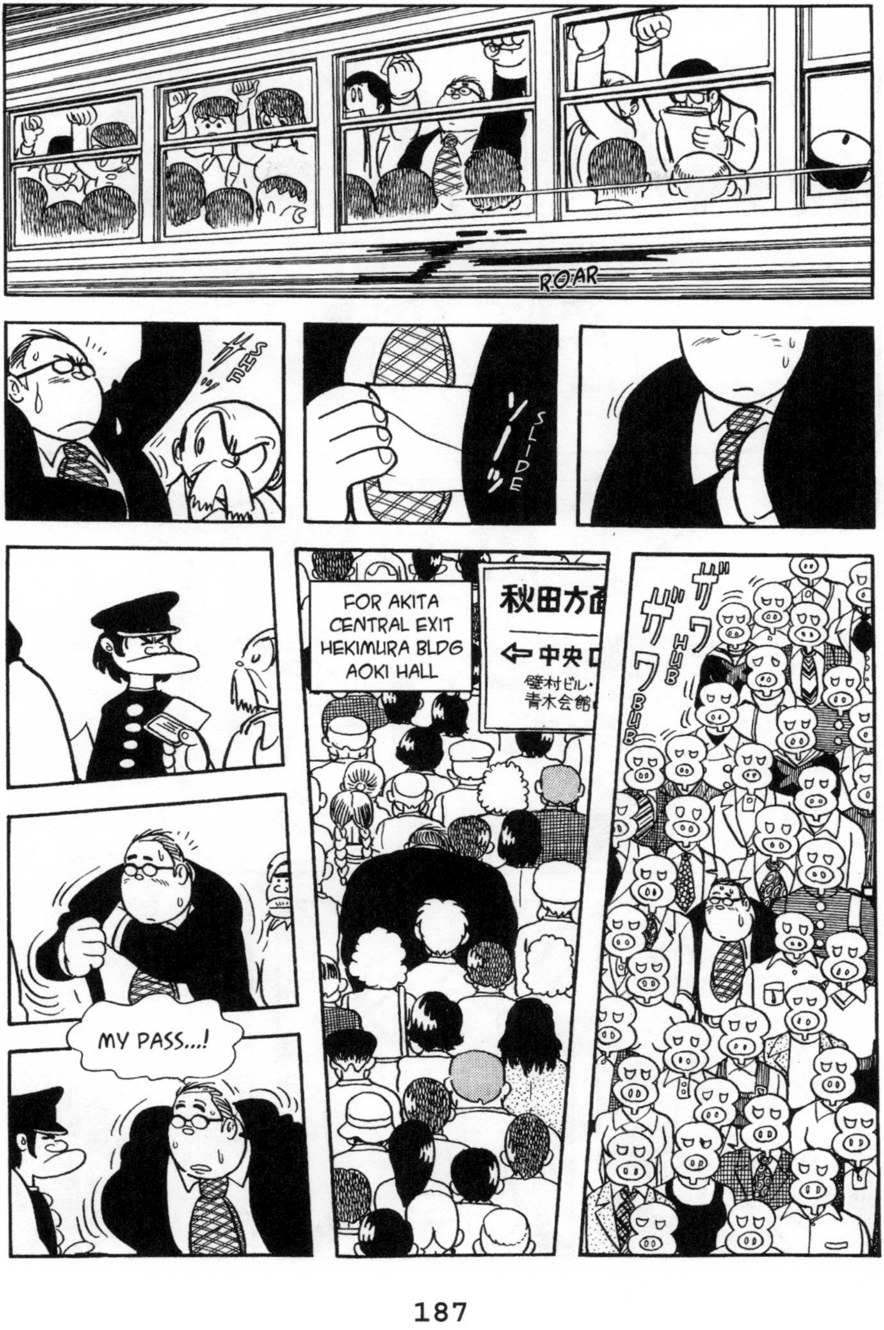
ROAR
ソーッ
SLIDE
SHE
ザワ
ザワ
ワ
HUB
BUB
FOR AKITA
CENTRAL EXIT
HEKIMURA BLDG
AOKI HALL
秋田方面
⇦中央口
MY PASS...!

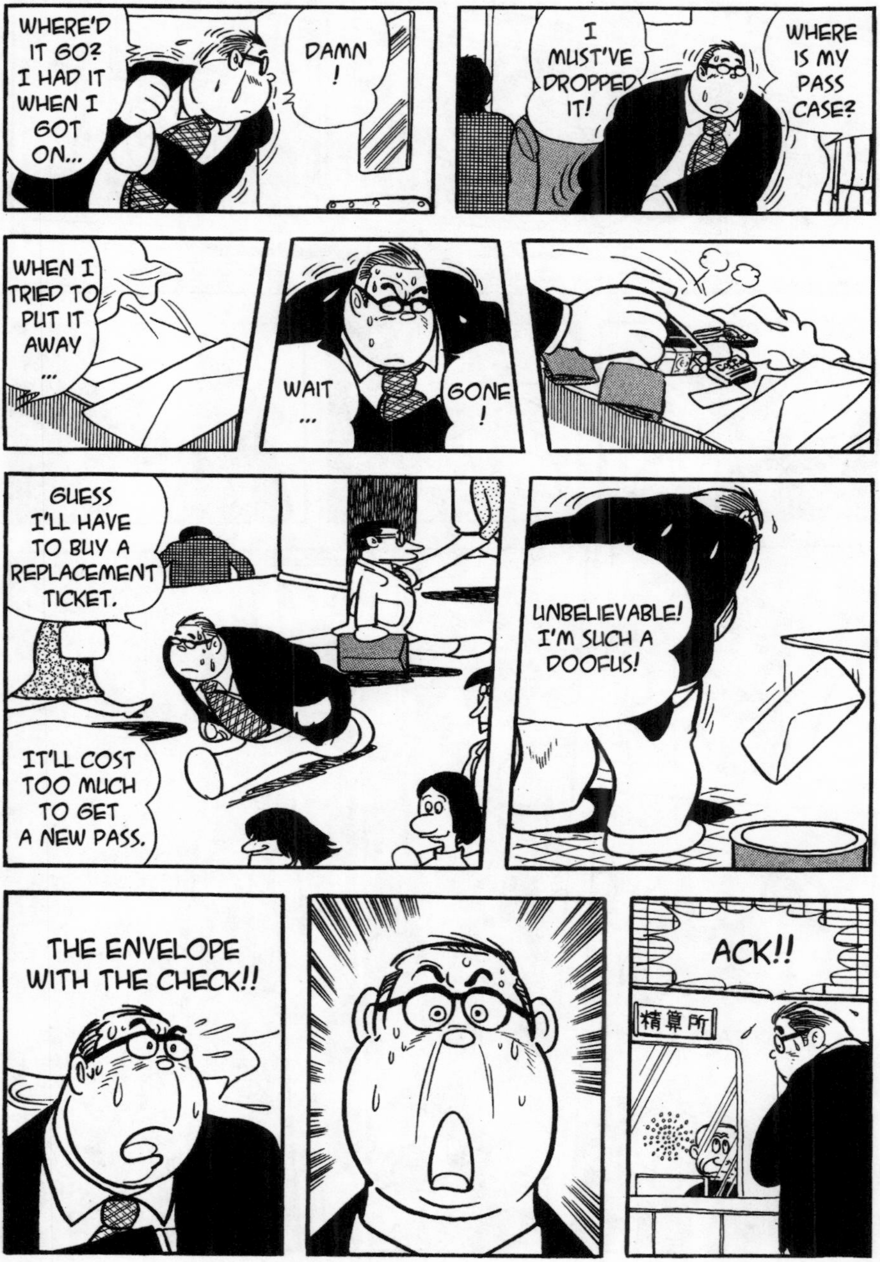
WHERE IS MY PASS CASE?
I MUST'VE DROPPED IT!
DAMN!
WHERE'D IT GO? I HAD IT WHEN I GOT ON...
GONE!
WAIT...
WHEN I TRIED TO PUT IT AWAY...
UNBELIEVABLE! I'M SUCH A DOOFUS!
GUESS I'LL HAVE TO BUY A REPLACEMENT TICKET.
IT'LL COST TOO MUCH TO GET A NEW PASS.
ACK!!
精算所
THE ENVELOPE WITH THE CHECK!!

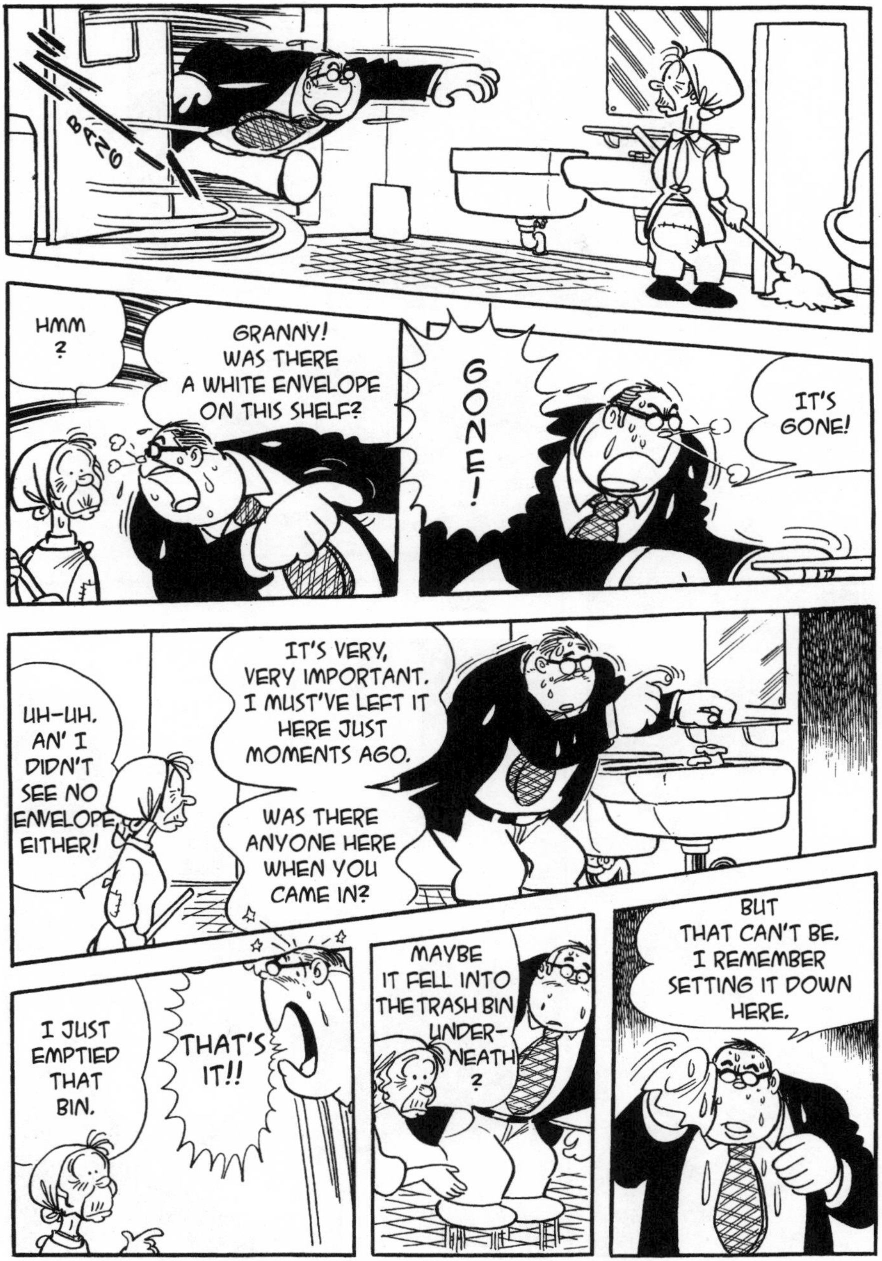
BRZO
IT'S GONE!
GONE!
GRANNY! WAS THERE A WHITE ENVELOPE ON THIS SHELF?
HMM ?
IT'S VERY, VERY IMPORTANT. I MUST'VE LEFT IT HERE JUST MOMENTS AGO.
WAS THERE ANYONE HERE WHEN YOU CAME IN?
UH-UH. AN' I DIDN'T SEE NO ENVELOPE EITHER!
BUT THAT CAN'T BE. I REMEMBER SETTING IT DOWN HERE.
MAYBE IT FELL INTO THE TRASH BIN UNDER-NEATH ?
THAT'S IT!!
I JUST EMPTIED THAT BIN.

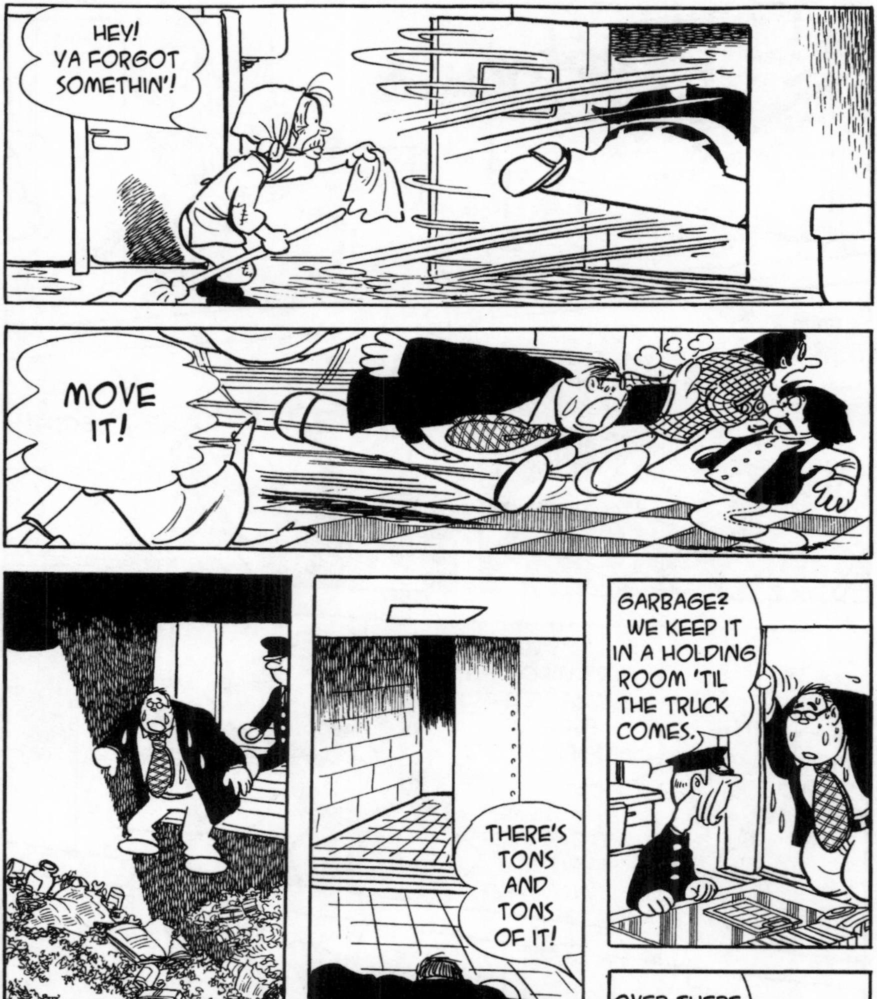
HEY! YA FORGOT SOMETHIN'!
MOVE IT!
GARBAGE? WE KEEP IT IN A HOLDING ROOM 'TIL THE TRUCK COMES.
OVER THERE. BUT I'M AFRAID IT'S HOPELESS.
THERE'S TONS AND TONS OF IT!

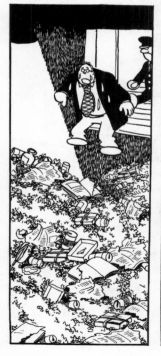

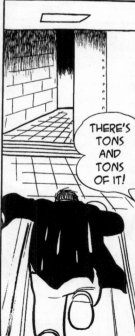

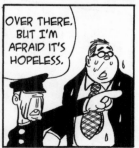

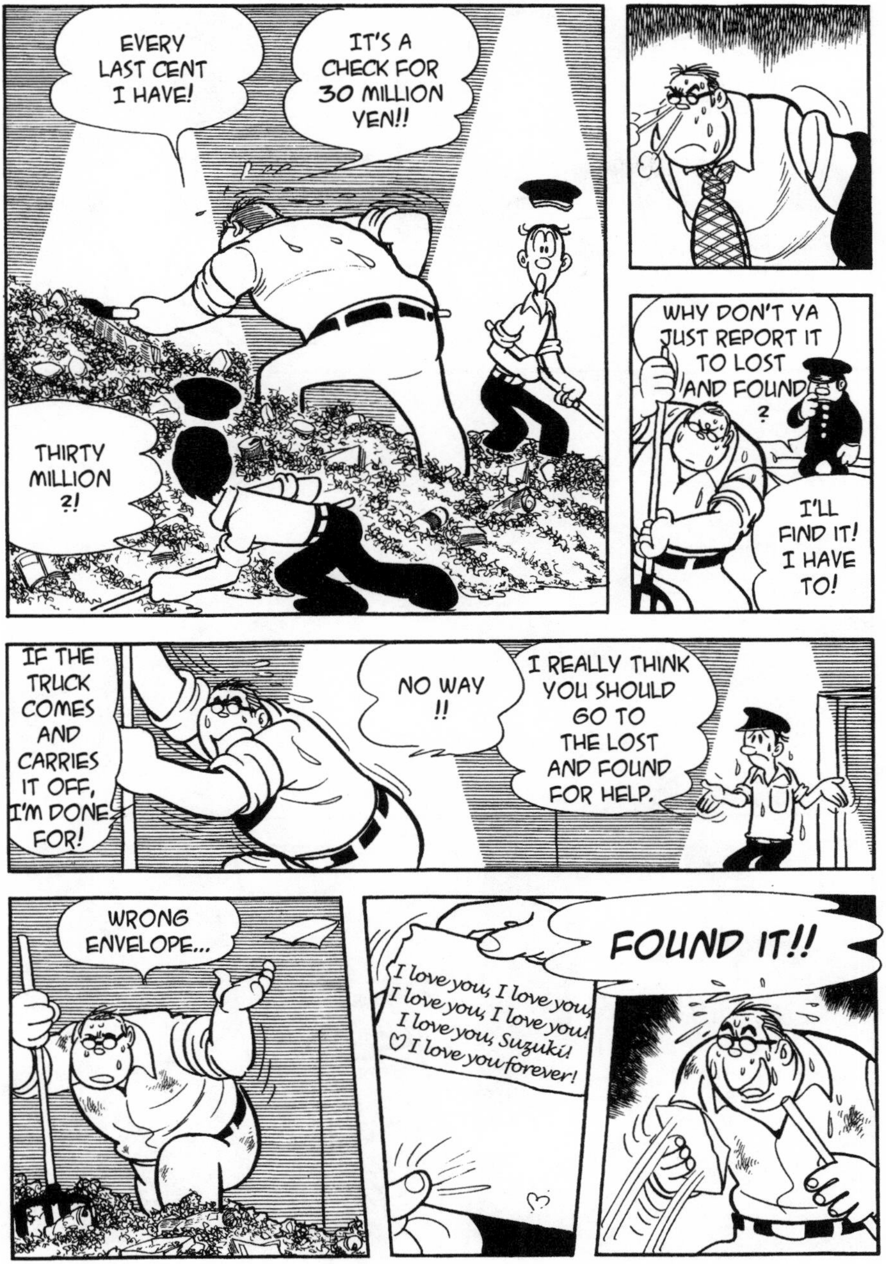
WHY DON'T YA JUST REPORT IT TO LOST AND FOUND?
I'LL FIND IT! I HAVE TO!
IT'S A CHECK FOR 30 MILLION YEN!!
EVERY LAST CENT I HAVE!
THIRTY MILLION ?!
I REALLY THINK YOU SHOULD GO TO THE LOST AND FOUND FOR HELP.
NO WAY !!
IF THE TRUCK COMES AND CARRIES IT OFF, I'M DONE FOR!
FOUND IT!!
I love you, I love you, I love you, I love you, I love you! I love you, Suzuki! ♡ I love you forever!
WRONG ENVELOPE...

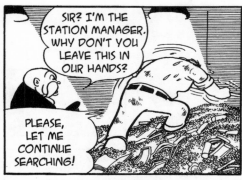

SIR? I'M THE STATION MANAGER. WHY DON'T YOU LEAVE THIS IN OUR HANDS?

PLEASE, LET ME CONTINUE SEARCHING!

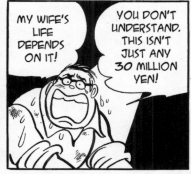

MY WIFE'S LIFE DEPENDS ON IT!

YOU DON'T UNDERSTAND. THIS ISN'T JUST ANY 30 MILLION YEN!

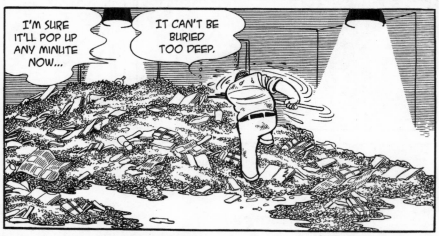

I'M SURE IT'LL POP UP ANY MINUTE NOW...

IT CAN'T BE BURIED TOO DEEP.

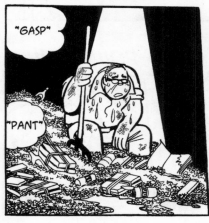

"GASP"

"PANT"

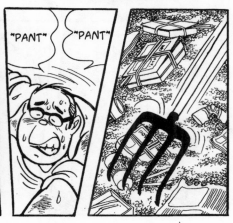

"PANT"

"PANT"

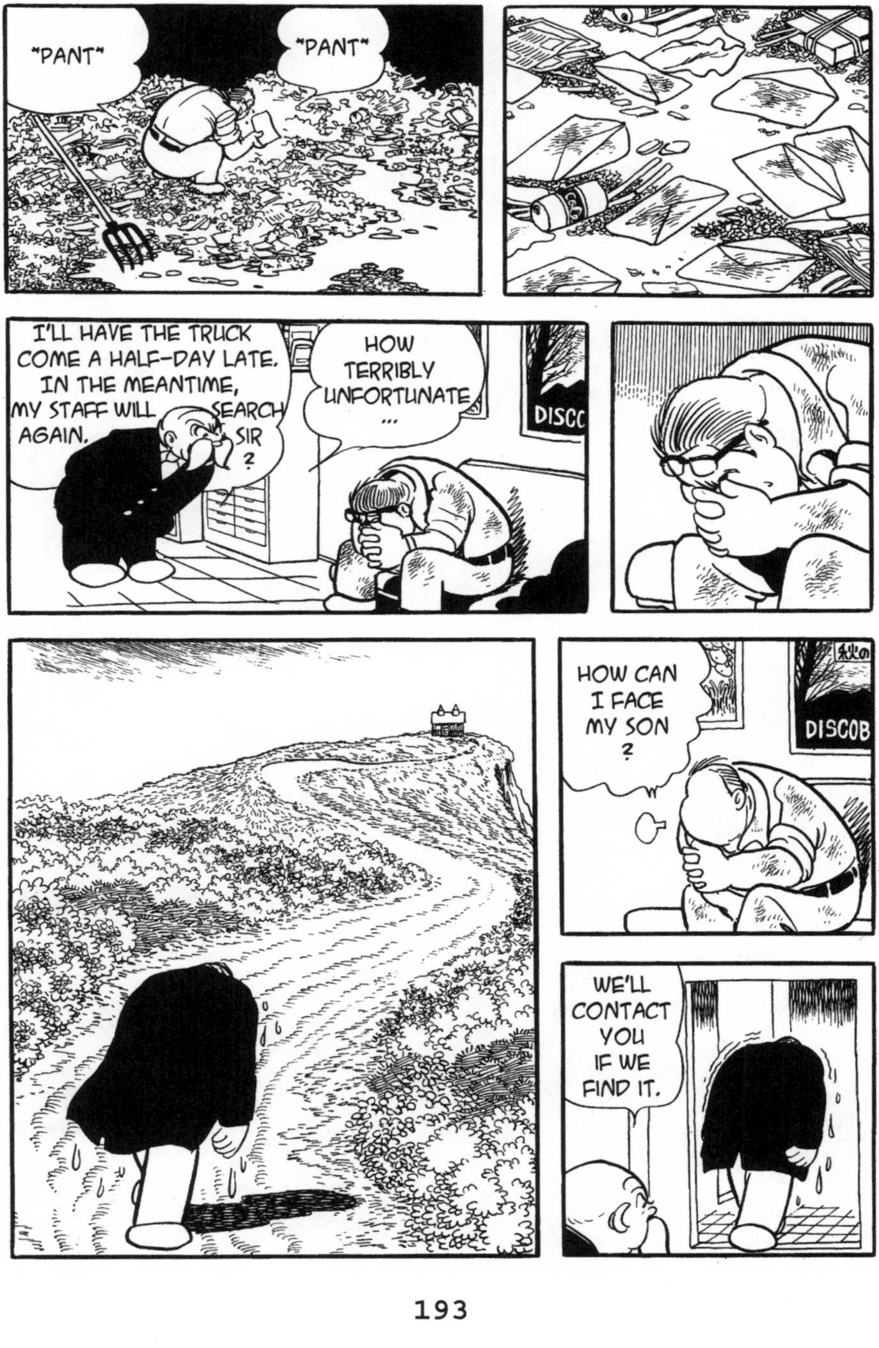
PANT
PANT
DISCO
HOW TERRIBLY UNFORTUNATE ...
SIR ?
I'LL HAVE THE TRUCK COME A HALF-DAY LATE. IN THE MEANTIME, MY STAFF WILL SEARCH AGAIN.
DISCOB
HOW CAN I FACE MY SON ?
WE'LL CONTACT YOU IF WE FIND IT.

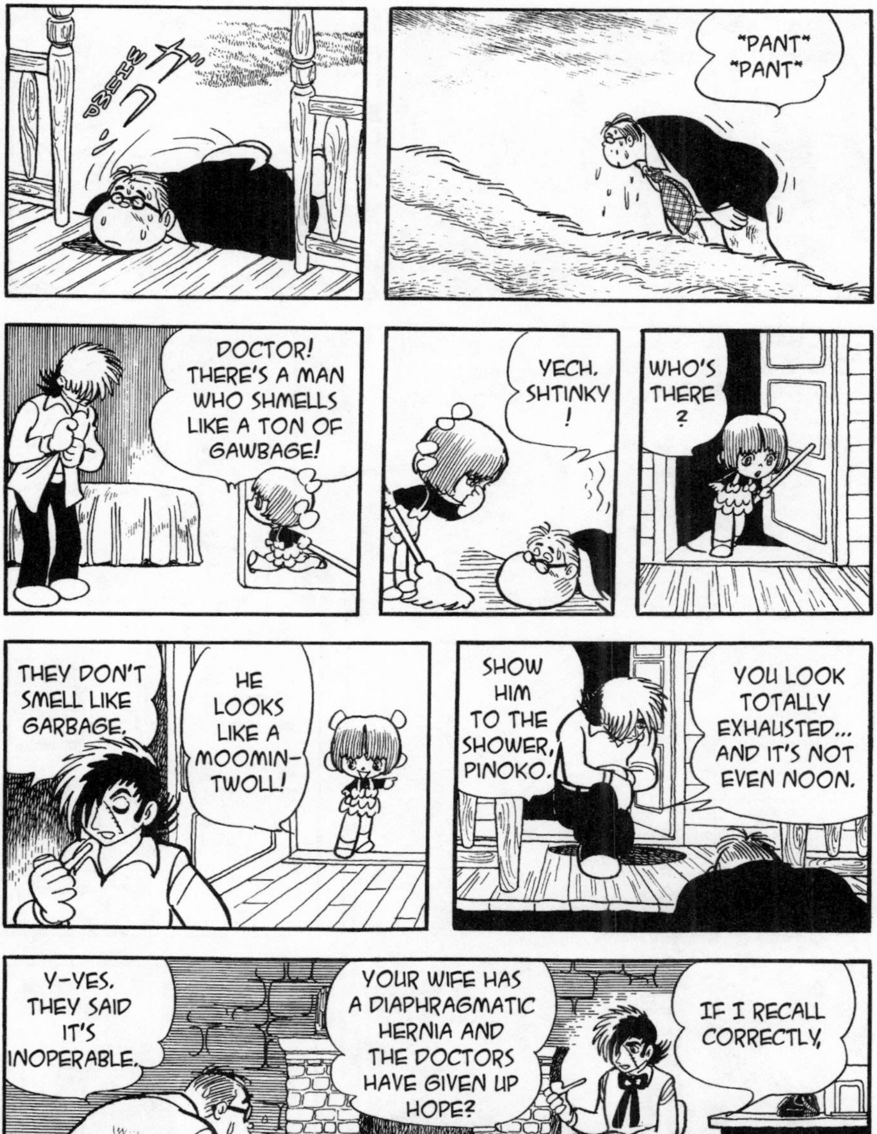
PANT *PANT*
WHUMP
ガクッ
WHO'S THERE?
YECH. SHTINKY!
DOCTOR! THERE'S A MAN WHO SHMELLS LIKE A TON OF GAWBAGE!
YOU LOOK TOTALLY EXHAUSTED... AND IT'S NOT EVEN NOON.
SHOW HIM TO THE SHOWER, PINOKO.
HE LOOKS LIKE A MOOMIN-TWOLL!
THEY DON'T SMELL LIKE GARBAGE.
IF I RECALL CORRECTLY,
YOUR WIFE HAS A DIAPHRAGMATIC HERNIA AND THE DOCTORS HAVE GIVEN UP HOPE?
Y-YES. THEY SAID IT'S INOPERABLE.

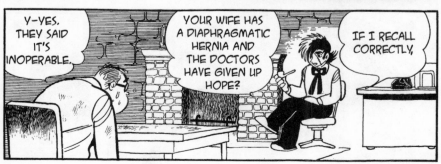

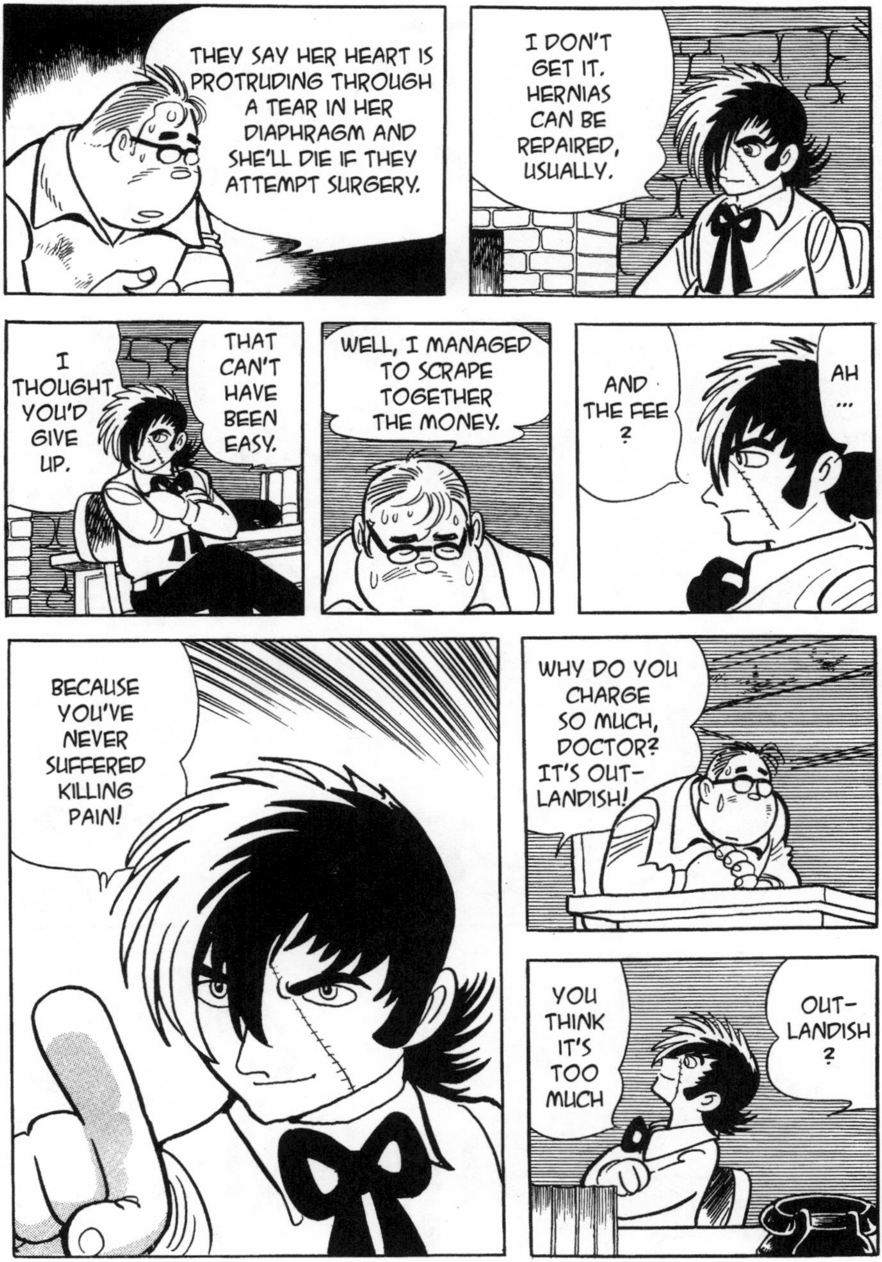
I DON'T GET IT. HERNIAS CAN BE REPAIRED, USUALLY.
THEY SAY HER HEART IS PROTRUDING THROUGH A TEAR IN HER DIAPHRAGM AND SHE'LL DIE IF THEY ATTEMPT SURGERY.
AH ...
AND THE FEE?
WELL, I MANAGED TO SCRAPE TOGETHER THE MONEY.
THAT CAN'T HAVE BEEN EASY.
I THOUGHT YOU'D GIVE UP.
WHY DO YOU CHARGE SO MUCH, DOCTOR? IT'S OUT-LANDISH!
OUT-LANDISH?
YOU THINK IT'S TOO MUCH
BECAUSE YOU'VE NEVER SUFFERED KILLING PAIN!

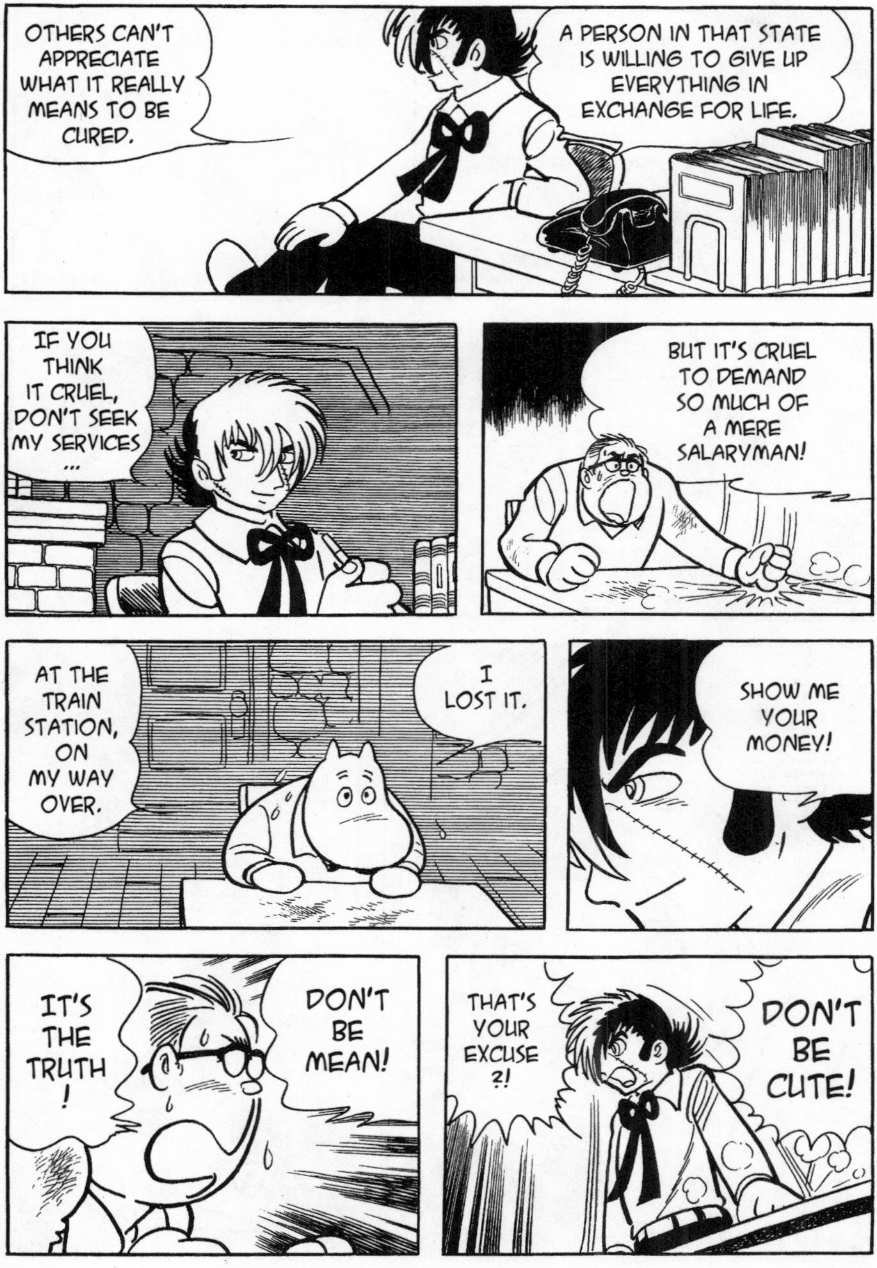
A PERSON IN THAT STATE IS WILLING TO GIVE UP EVERYTHING IN EXCHANGE FOR LIFE.
OTHERS CAN'T APPRECIATE WHAT IT REALLY MEANS TO BE CURED.
BUT IT'S CRUEL TO DEMAND SO MUCH OF A MERE SALARYMAN!
IF YOU THINK IT CRUEL, DON'T SEEK MY SERVICES ...
SHOW ME YOUR MONEY!
I LOST IT.
AT THE TRAIN STATION, ON MY WAY OVER.
DON'T BE CUTE!
THAT'S YOUR EXCUSE ?!
DON'T BE MEAN!
IT'S THE TRUTH !

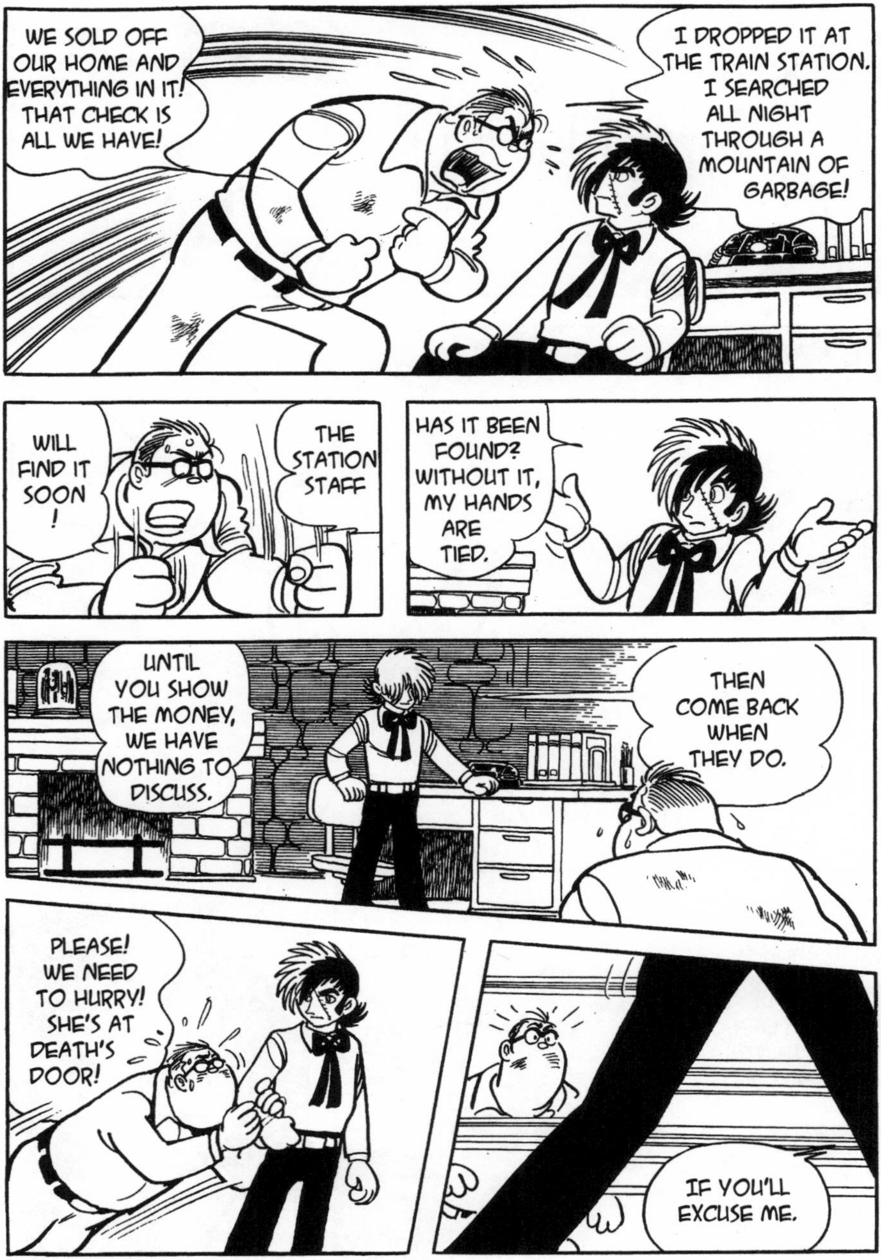
I DROPPED IT AT THE TRAIN STATION. I SEARCHED ALL NIGHT THROUGH A MOUNTAIN OF GARBAGE!
WE SOLD OFF OUR HOME AND EVERYTHING IN IT! THAT CHECK IS ALL WE HAVE!
HAS IT BEEN FOUND? WITHOUT IT, MY HANDS ARE TIED.
THE STATION STAFF
WILL FIND IT SOON!
UNTIL YOU SHOW THE MONEY, WE HAVE NOTHING TO DISCUSS.
THEN COME BACK WHEN THEY DO.
IF YOU'LL EXCUSE ME.
PLEASE! WE NEED TO HURRY! SHE'S AT DEATH'S DOOR!

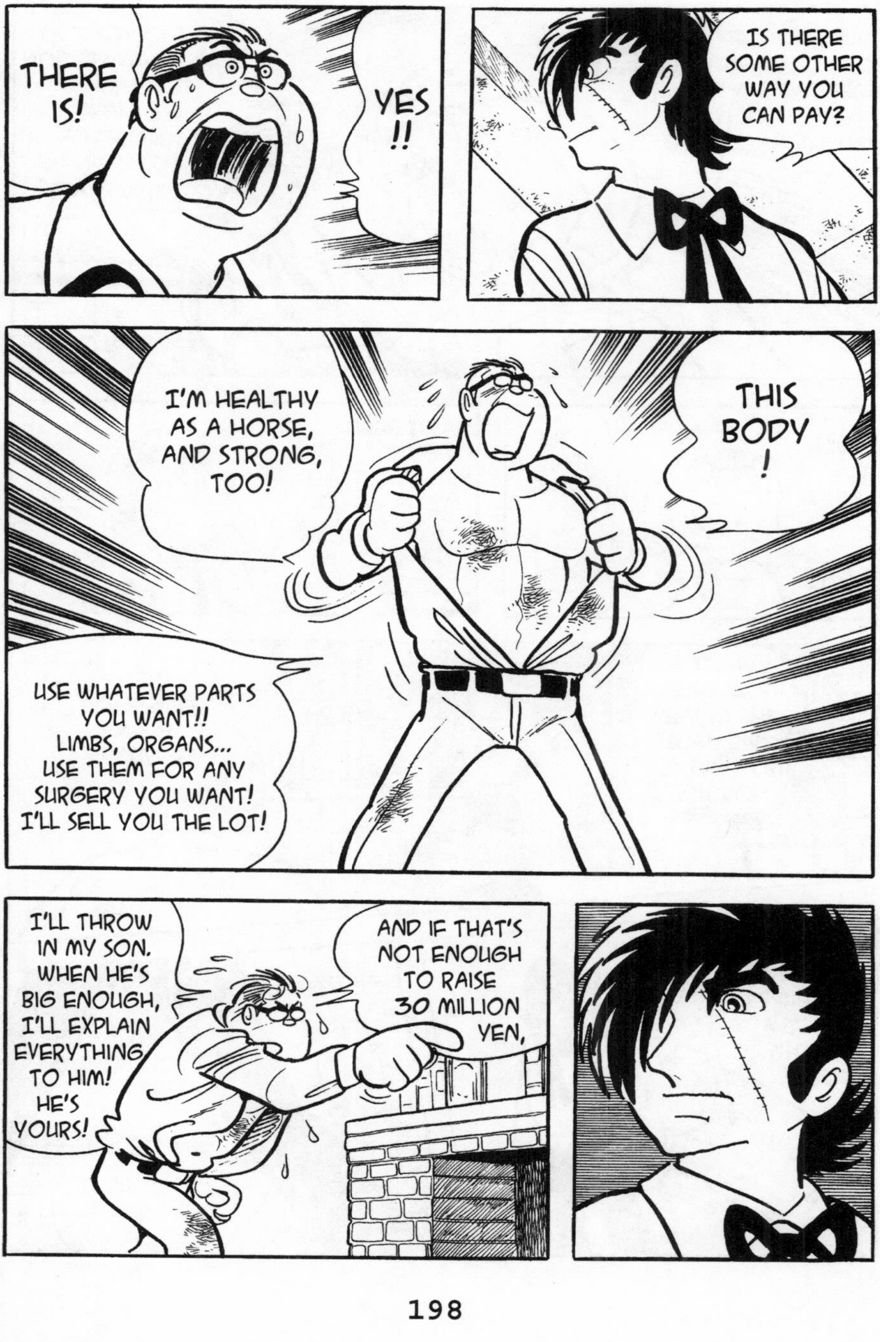
IS THERE SOME OTHER WAY YOU CAN PAY?
YES!!
THERE IS!
THIS BODY!
I'M HEALTHY AS A HORSE, AND STRONG, TOO!
USE WHATEVER PARTS YOU WANT!! LIMBS, ORGANS... USE THEM FOR ANY SURGERY YOU WANT! I'LL SELL YOU THE LOT!
AND IF THAT'S NOT ENOUGH TO RAISE 30 MILLION YEN,
I'LL THROW IN MY SON. WHEN HE'S BIG ENOUGH, I'LL EXPLAIN EVERYTHING TO HIM! HE'S YOURS!

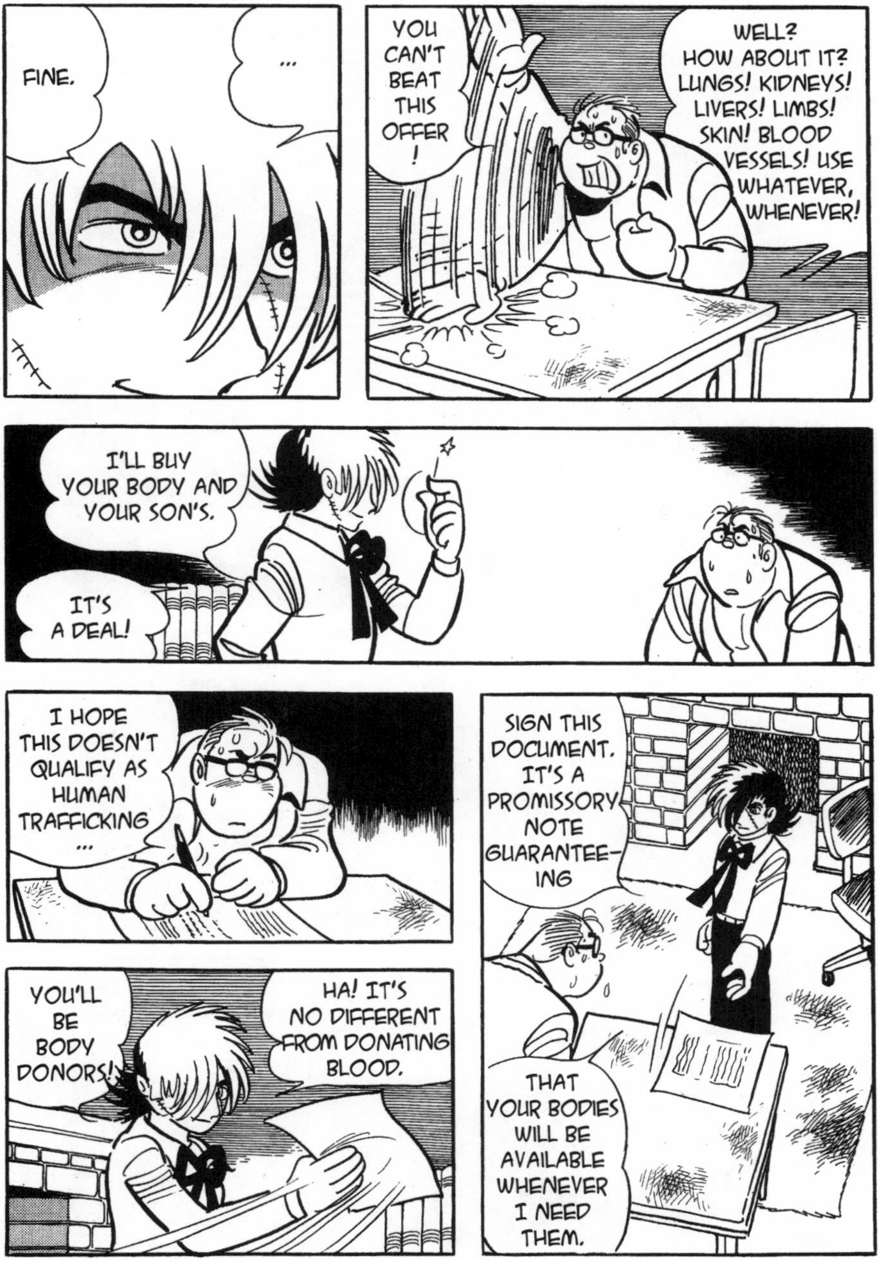
WELL? HOW ABOUT IT? LUNGS! KIDNEYS! LIVERS! LIMBS! SKIN! BLOOD VESSELS! USE WHATEVER, WHENEVER!
YOU CAN'T BEAT THIS OFFER!
...
FINE.
I'LL BUY YOUR BODY AND YOUR SON'S.
IT'S A DEAL!
SIGN THIS DOCUMENT. IT'S A PROMISSORY NOTE GUARANTEEING
THAT YOUR BODIES WILL BE AVAILABLE WHENEVER I NEED THEM.
I HOPE THIS DOESN'T QUALIFY AS HUMAN TRAFFICKING ...
HA! IT'S NO DIFFERENT FROM DONATING BLOOD.
YOU'LL BE BODY DONORS!

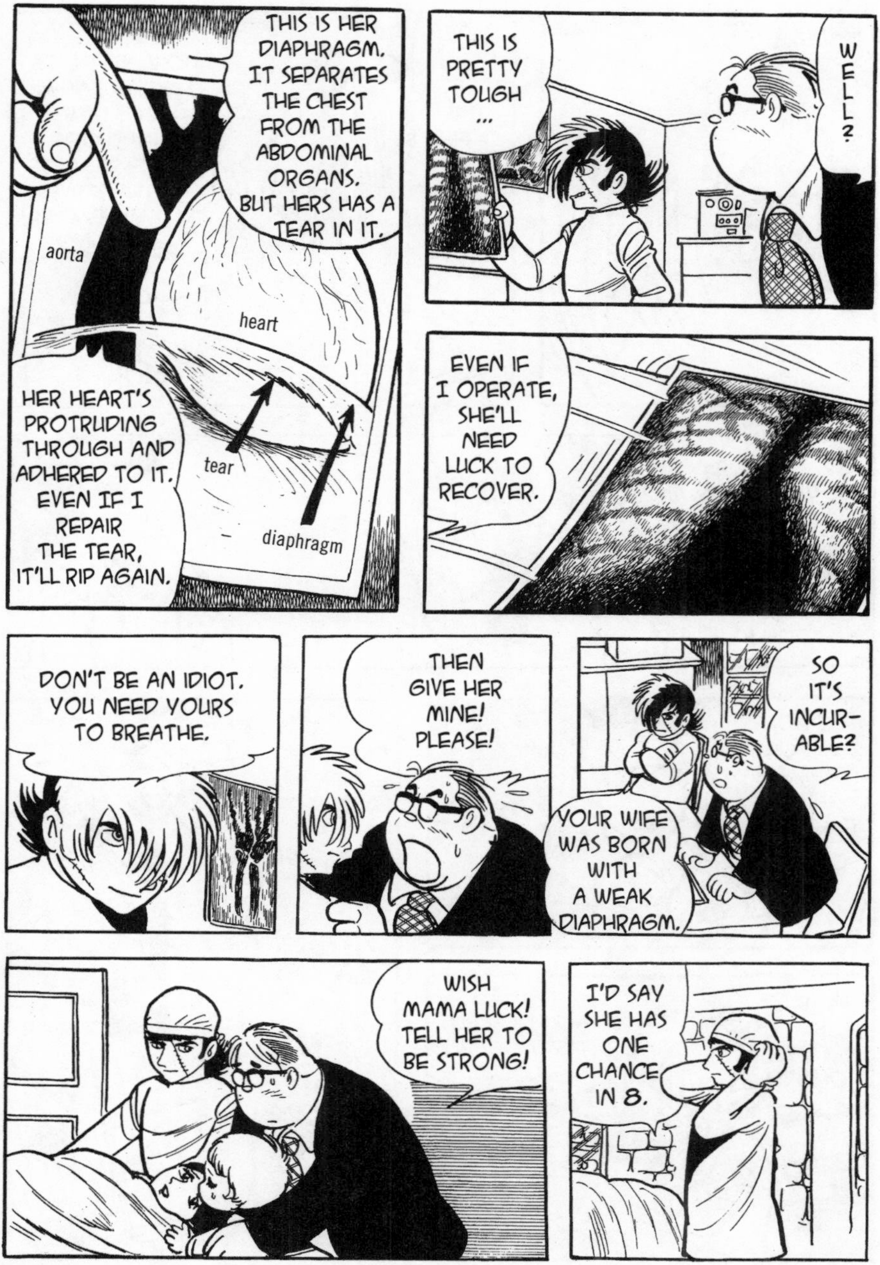
WELL?
THIS IS PRETTY TOUGH ...
EVEN IF I OPERATE, SHE'LL NEED LUCK TO RECOVER.
THIS IS HER DIAPHRAGM. IT SEPARATES THE CHEST FROM THE ABDOMINAL ORGANS. BUT HERS HAS A TEAR IN IT.
aorta
heart
tear
diaphragm
HER HEART'S PROTRUDING THROUGH AND ADHERED TO IT. EVEN IF I REPAIR THE TEAR, IT'LL RIP AGAIN.
SO IT'S INCUR-ABLE?
YOUR WIFE WAS BORN WITH A WEAK DIAPHRAGM.
THEN GIVE HER MINE! PLEASE!
DON'T BE AN IDIOT. YOU NEED YOURS TO BREATHE.
I'D SAY SHE HAS ONE CHANCE IN 8.
WISH MAMA LUCK! TELL HER TO BE STRONG!

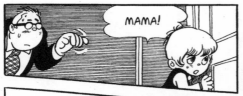

MAMA!

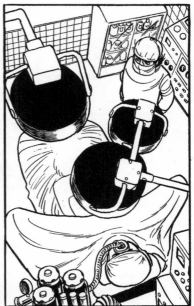

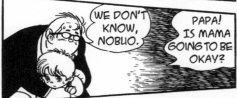

WE DON'T KNOW, NOBUO.

PAPA! IS MAMA GOING TO BE OKAY?

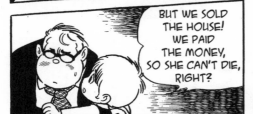

BUT WE SOLD THE HOUSE! WE PAID THE MONEY, SO SHE CAN'T DIE, RIGHT?

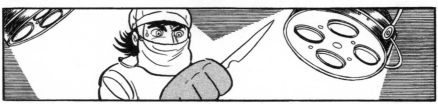

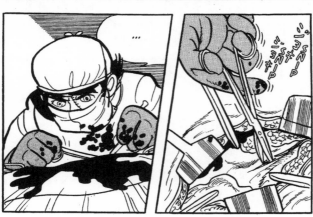

...

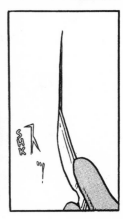

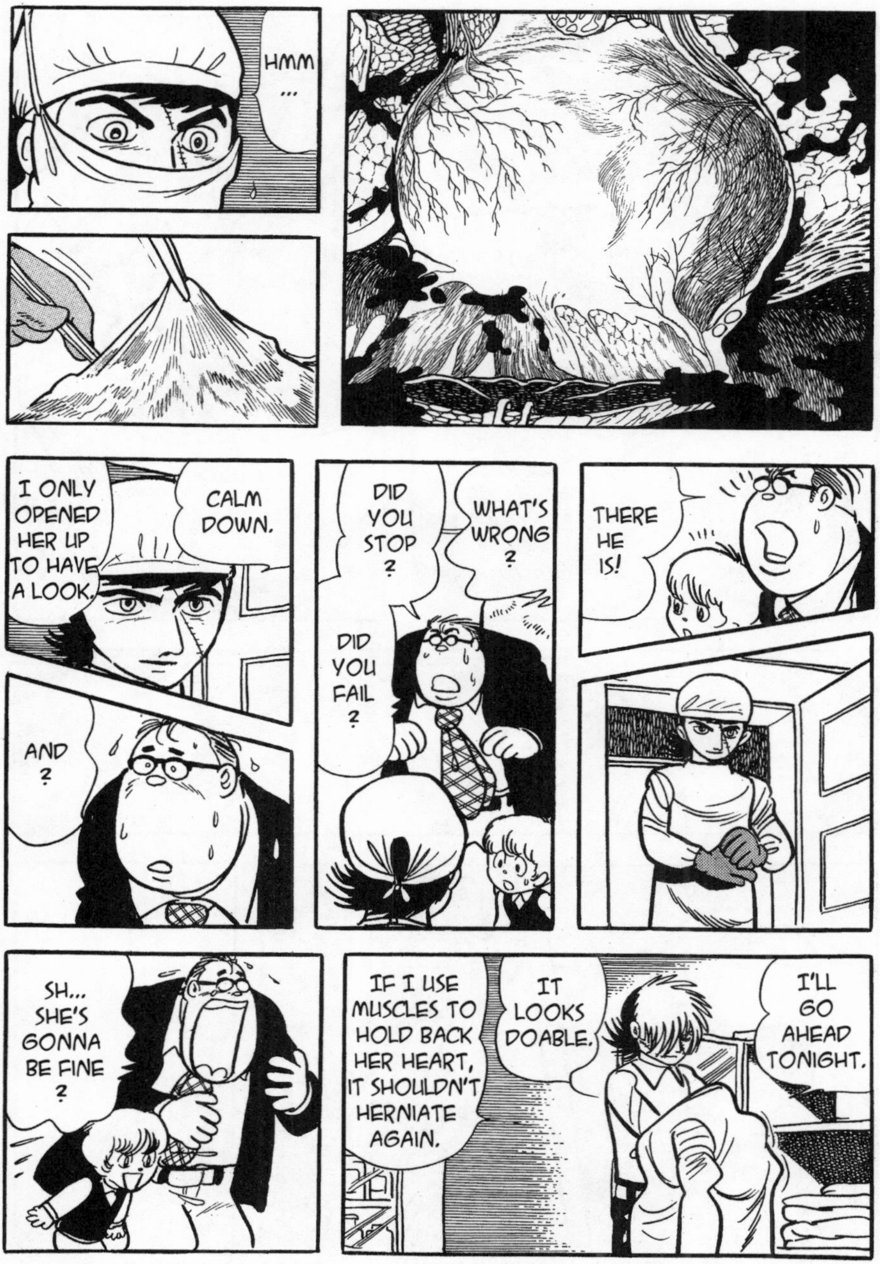
HMM ...
THERE HE IS!
WHAT'S WRONG?
DID YOU STOP?
DID YOU FAIL?
CALM DOWN.
I ONLY OPENED HER UP TO HAVE A LOOK.
AND?
I'LL GO AHEAD TONIGHT.
IT LOOKS DOABLE.
IF I USE MUSCLES TO HOLD BACK HER HEART, IT SHOULDN'T HERNIATE AGAIN.
SH... SHE'S GONNA BE FINE?

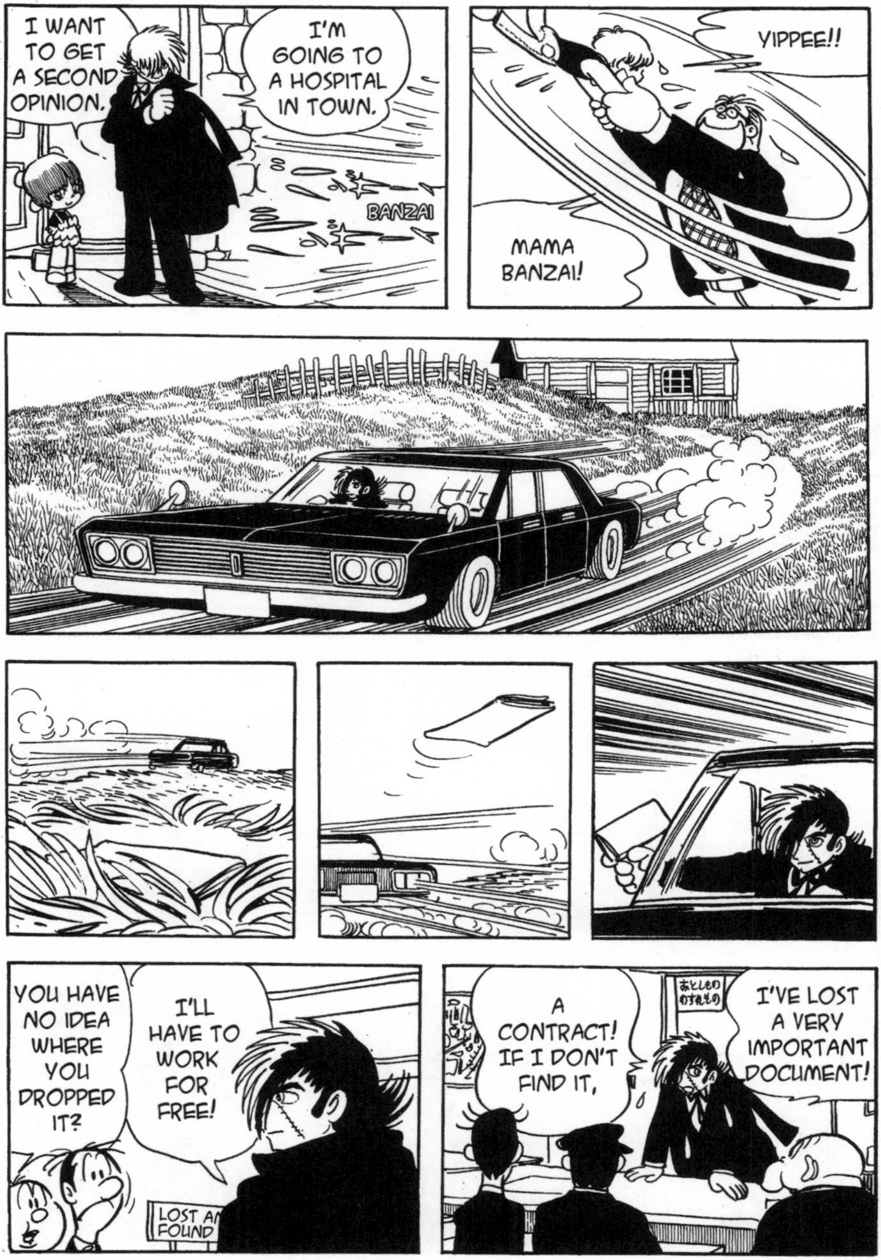
YIPPEE!!
MAMA BANZAI!
I'M GOING TO A HOSPITAL IN TOWN.
I WANT TO GET A SECOND OPINION.
BANZAI
I'VE LOST A VERY IMPORTANT DOCUMENT!
A CONTRACT! IF I DON'T FIND IT,
おとしもの わすれもの
I'LL HAVE TO WORK FOR FREE!
YOU HAVE NO IDEA WHERE YOU DROPPED IT?

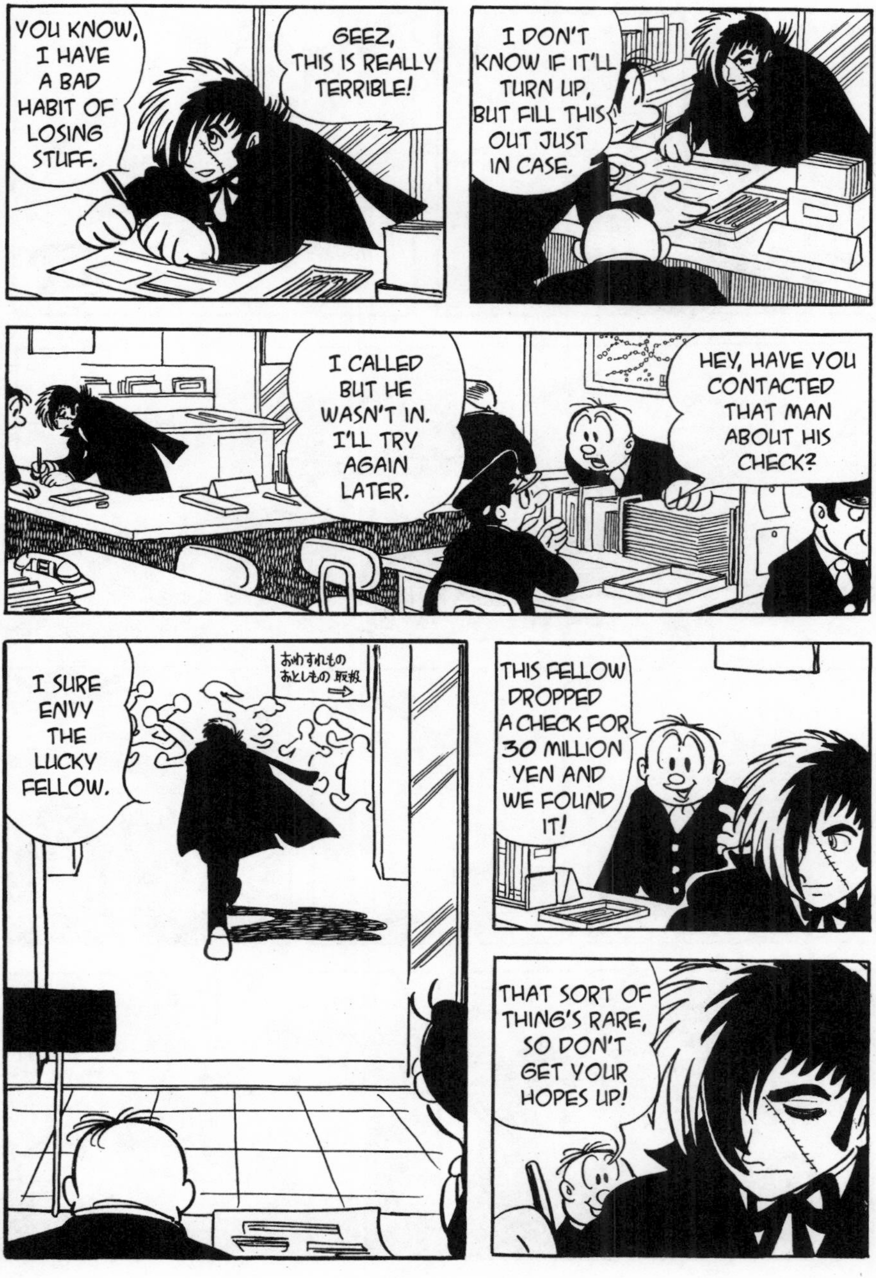
I DON'T KNOW IF IT'LL TURN UP, BUT FILL THIS OUT JUST IN CASE.
GEEZ, THIS IS REALLY TERRIBLE!
YOU KNOW, I HAVE A BAD HABIT OF LOSING STUFF.
HEY, HAVE YOU CONTACTED THAT MAN ABOUT HIS CHECK?
I CALLED BUT HE WASN'T IN. I'LL TRY AGAIN LATER.
THIS FELLOW DROPPED A CHECK FOR 30 MILLION YEN AND WE FOUND IT!
THAT SORT OF THING'S RARE, SO DON'T GET YOUR HOPES UP!
おわすれもの
おとしもの 取扱
I SURE ENVY THE LUCKY FELLOW.

BURNED DOLL

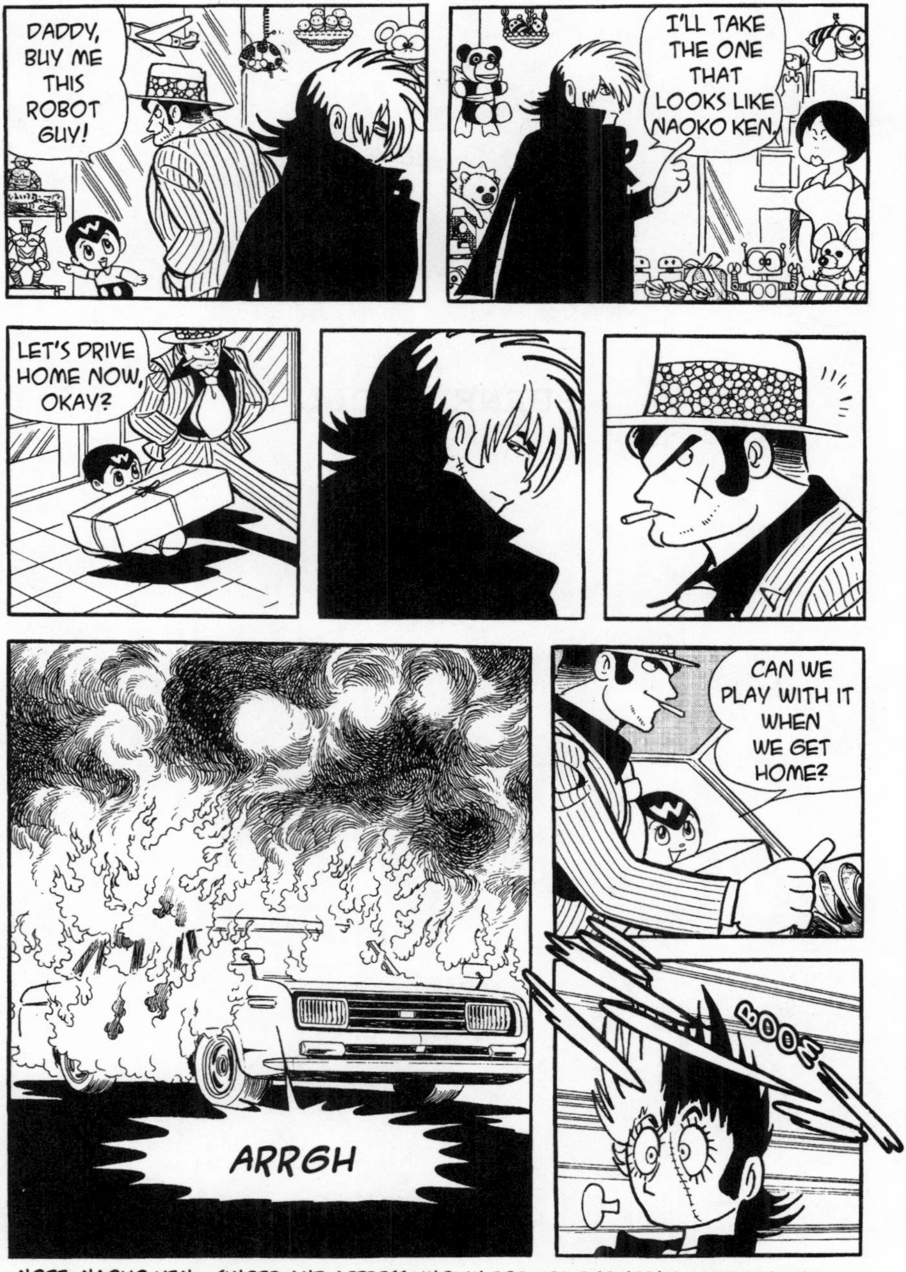
I'LL TAKE THE ONE THAT LOOKS LIKE NAOKO KEN.
DADDY, BUY ME THIS ROBOT GUY!
LET'S DRIVE HOME NOW, OKAY?
CAN WE PLAY WITH IT WHEN WE GET HOME?
BOOM
ARRGH

NOTE: NAOKO KEN = SINGER AND ACTRESS KNOWN FOR HER DISTINCTIVE FEATURES AND COMEDY ROLES

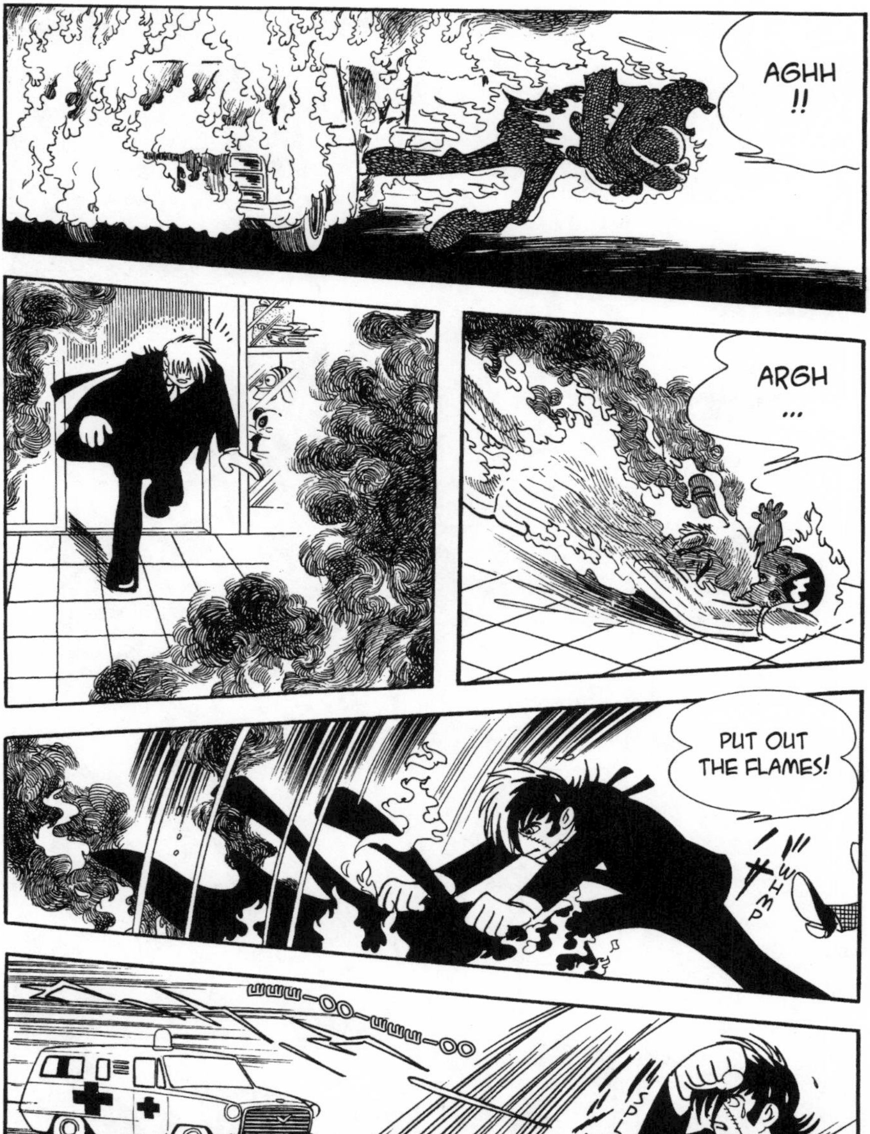
AGHH !!
ARGH ...
PUT OUT THE FLAMES!
WHIP

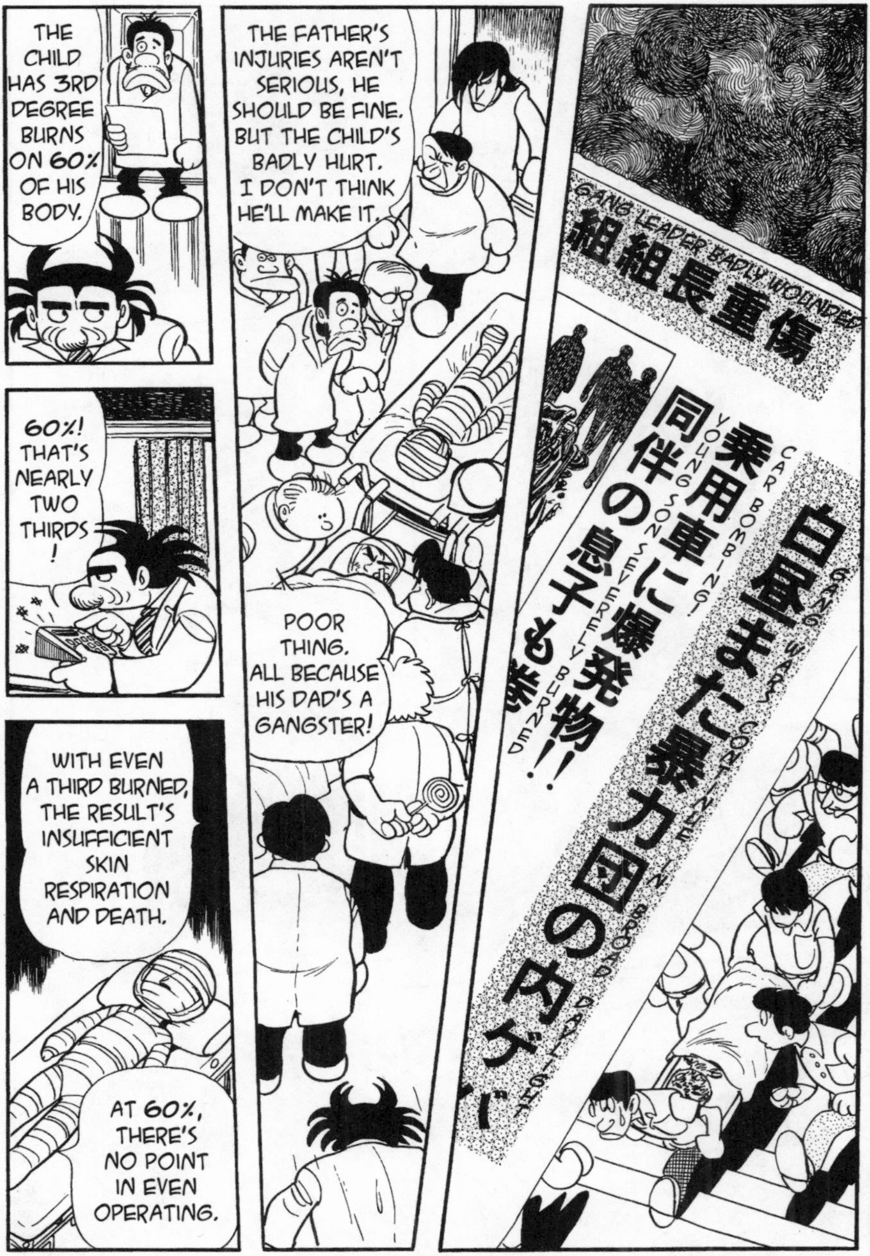
組組長重傷
GANG LEADER BADLY WOUNDED
白昼また暴力団の内ゲバ
GANG WARS CONTINUE IN BROAD DAYLIGHT
乗用車に爆発物!!
CAR BOMBING!
同伴の息子も
YOUNG SON SEVERELY BURNED
THE FATHER'S INJURIES AREN'T SERIOUS, HE SHOULD BE FINE. BUT THE CHILD'S BADLY HURT. I DON'T THINK HE'LL MAKE IT.
POOR THING. ALL BECAUSE HIS DAD'S A GANGSTER!
THE CHILD HAS 3RD DEGREE BURNS ON 60% OF HIS BODY.
60%! THAT'S NEARLY TWO THIRDS!
WITH EVEN A THIRD BURNED, THE RESULT'S INSUFFICIENT SKIN RESPIRATION AND DEATH.
AT 60%, THERE'S NO POINT IN EVEN OPERATING.

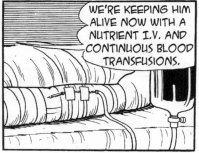

WE'RE KEEPING HIM ALIVE NOW WITH A NUTRIENT I.V. AND CONTINUOUS BLOOD TRANSFUSIONS.
HOPE-LESS.
GUESS IT'S UP TO FATE NOW.
OUR DIRECTOR'S KINDA SPINELESS...
WE'RE IN LUCK, SIR.
THERE'S A MAN WHO'S A SURGICAL GENIUS.
OVER THERE. DOCTOR BLACK JACK ...
NO, NO. HE HAS NO LICENSE!
THEY SAY HE ONLY TREATS PATIENTS WHO AGREE TO PAY RIDICULOUS SUMS OF MONEY.
THERE ARE RUMORS TO THE CONTRARY.
DR. BLACK JACK?
えー
ER...
FORGET IT.
プイ
TURN
I HAVEN'T ASKED YET...
GANGSTER FAMILY OR NOT, HE'S STILL A PATIENT.
I STEER CLEAR OF THE YAKUZA!

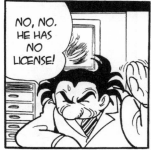

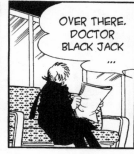

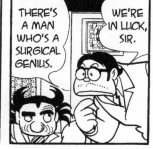

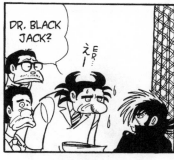

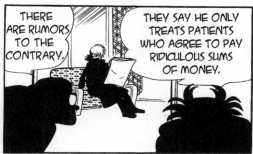

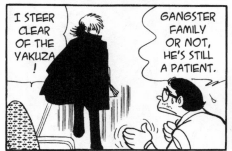

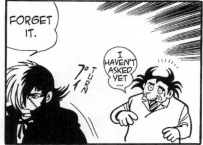

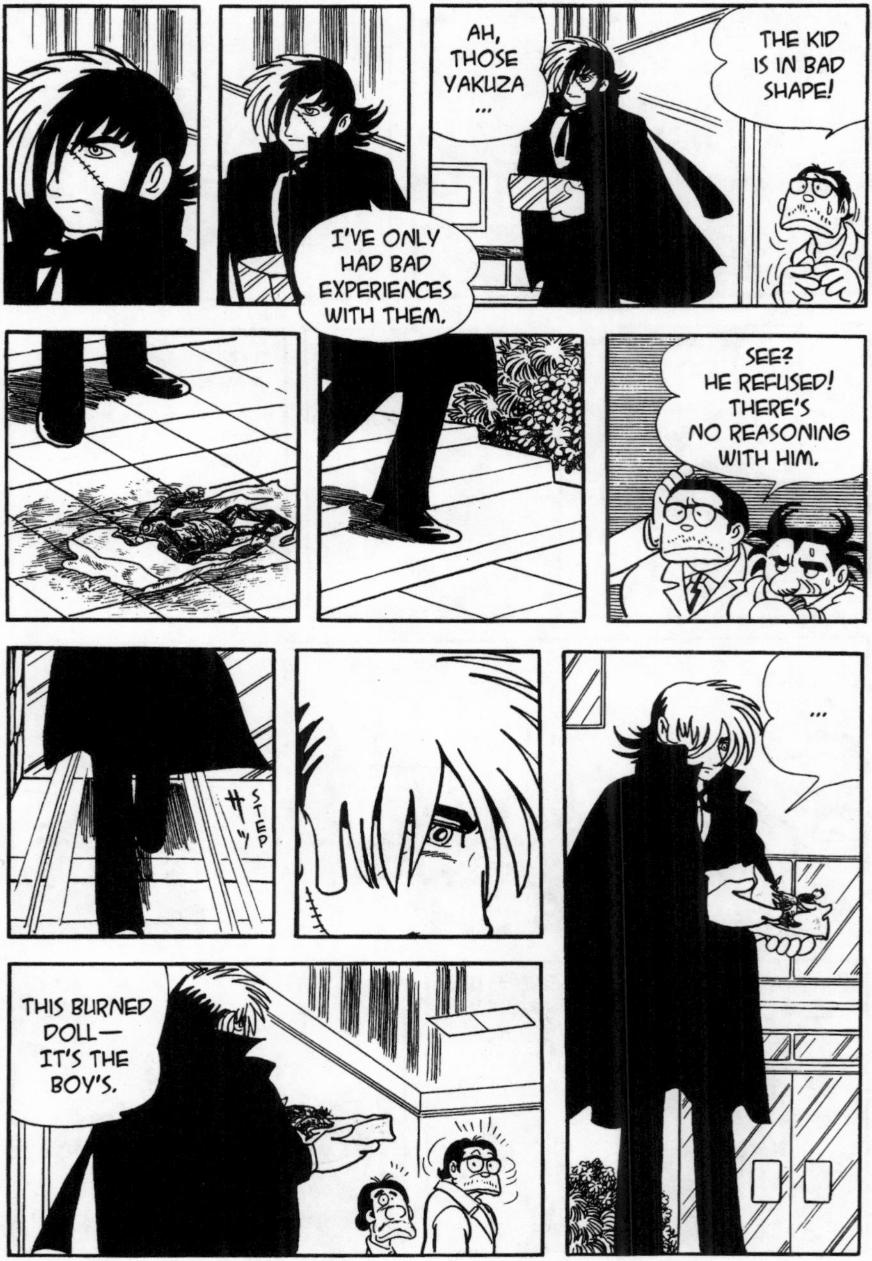
THE KID IS IN BAD SHAPE!
AH, THOSE YAKUZA ...
I'VE ONLY HAD BAD EXPERIENCES WITH THEM.
SEE? HE REFUSED! THERE'S NO REASONING WITH HIM.
...
サッ STEP
THIS BURNED DOLL— IT'S THE BOY'S.

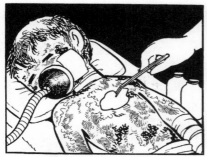

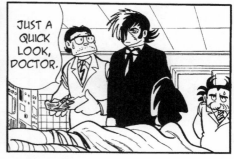

JUST A QUICK LOOK, DOCTOR.
DOC-TOR?
WILL MY BOY MAKE IT?
ONE IN TEN.
UGH
DOCTOR, PLEASE... SAVE HIM!
ARE YOU WILLING TO GIVE HIM YOUR OWN SKIN?
GLADLY! PEEL IT OFF MY WHOLE BODY IF YOU NEED TO, DOC!
EVEN IF I DO, HE MIGHT NOT MAKE IT. AND REMOVING YOUR SKIN MIGHT EARN YOU AN INFECTION.
DO YOU STILL WANT TO DO IT?
HE'S GONNA DO IT! WE'RE IN BUSINESS!

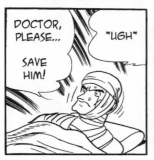

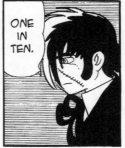

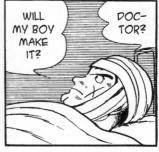

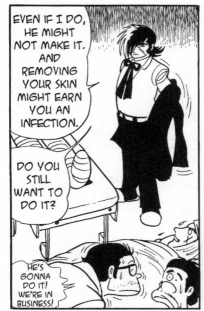

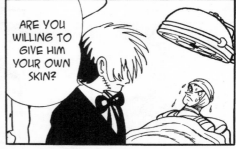

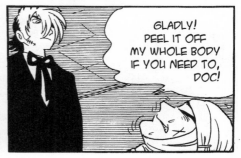

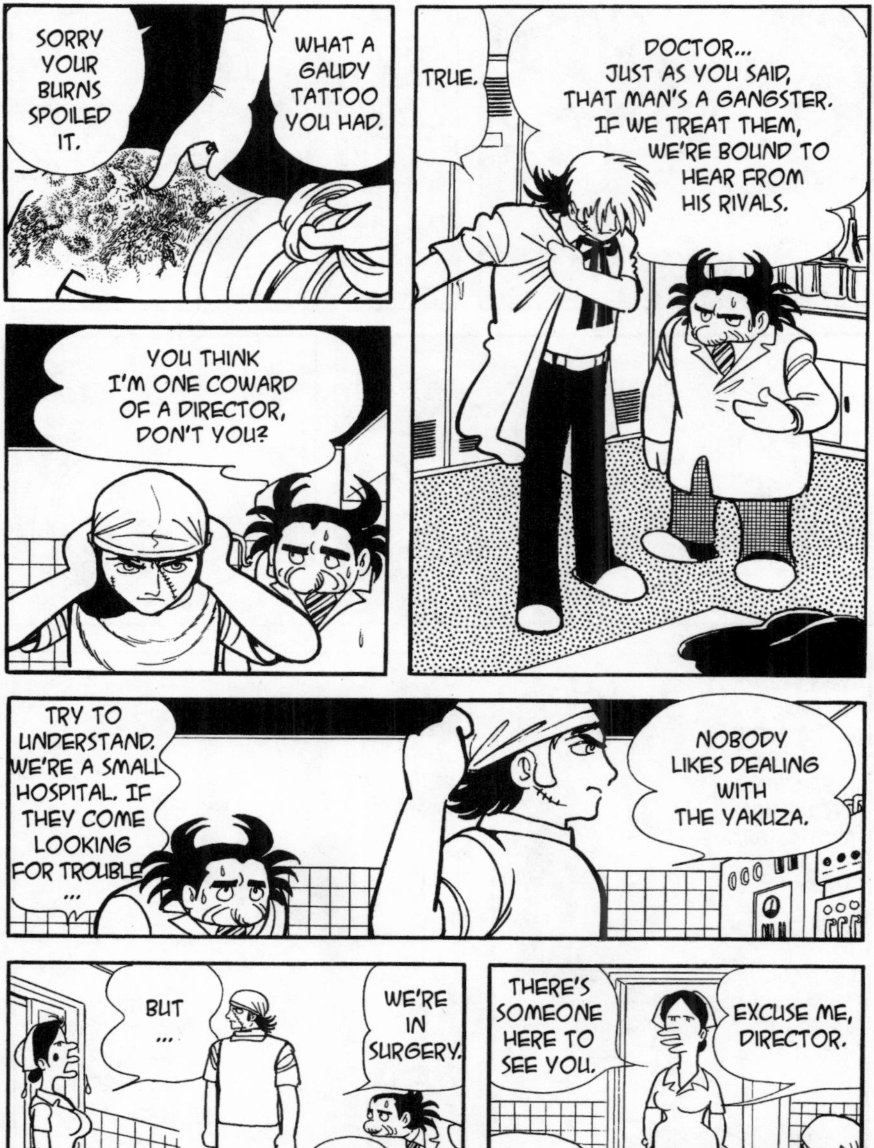
DOCTOR... JUST AS YOU SAID, THAT MAN'S A GANGSTER. IF WE TREAT THEM, WE'RE BOUND TO HEAR FROM HIS RIVALS.
TRUE.
WHAT A GAUDY TATTOO YOU HAD.
SORRY YOUR BURNS SPOILED IT.
YOU THINK I'M ONE COWARD OF A DIRECTOR, DON'T YOU?
NOBODY LIKES DEALING WITH THE YAKUZA.
TRY TO UNDERSTAND. WE'RE A SMALL HOSPITAL. IF THEY COME LOOKING FOR TROUBLE ...
EXCUSE ME, DIRECTOR.
THERE'S SOMEONE HERE TO SEE YOU.
I KNEW IT!
WE'RE IN SURGERY.
BUT ...
CAN'T THEY WAIT?

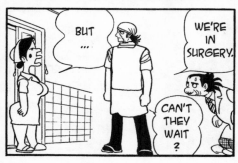

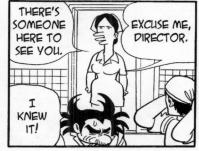

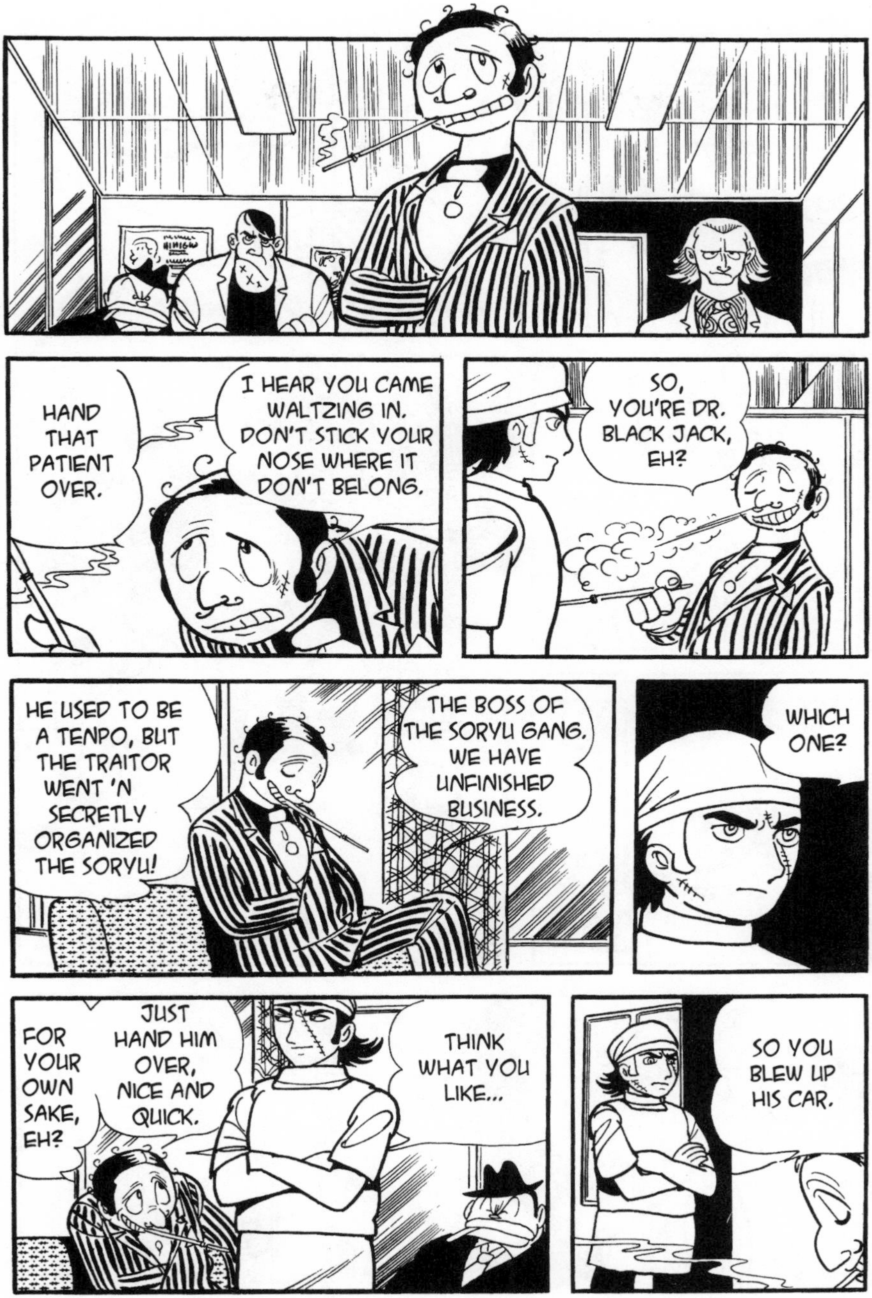
SO, YOU'RE DR. BLACK JACK, EH?
I HEAR YOU CAME WALTZING IN. DON'T STICK YOUR NOSE WHERE IT DON'T BELONG.
HAND THAT PATIENT OVER.
WHICH ONE?
THE BOSS OF THE SORYU GANG. WE HAVE UNFINISHED BUSINESS.
HE USED TO BE A TENPO, BUT THE TRAITOR WENT 'N SECRETLY ORGANIZED THE SORYU!
SO YOU BLEW UP HIS CAR.
THINK WHAT YOU LIKE...
JUST HAND HIM OVER, NICE AND QUICK.
FOR YOUR OWN SAKE, EH?

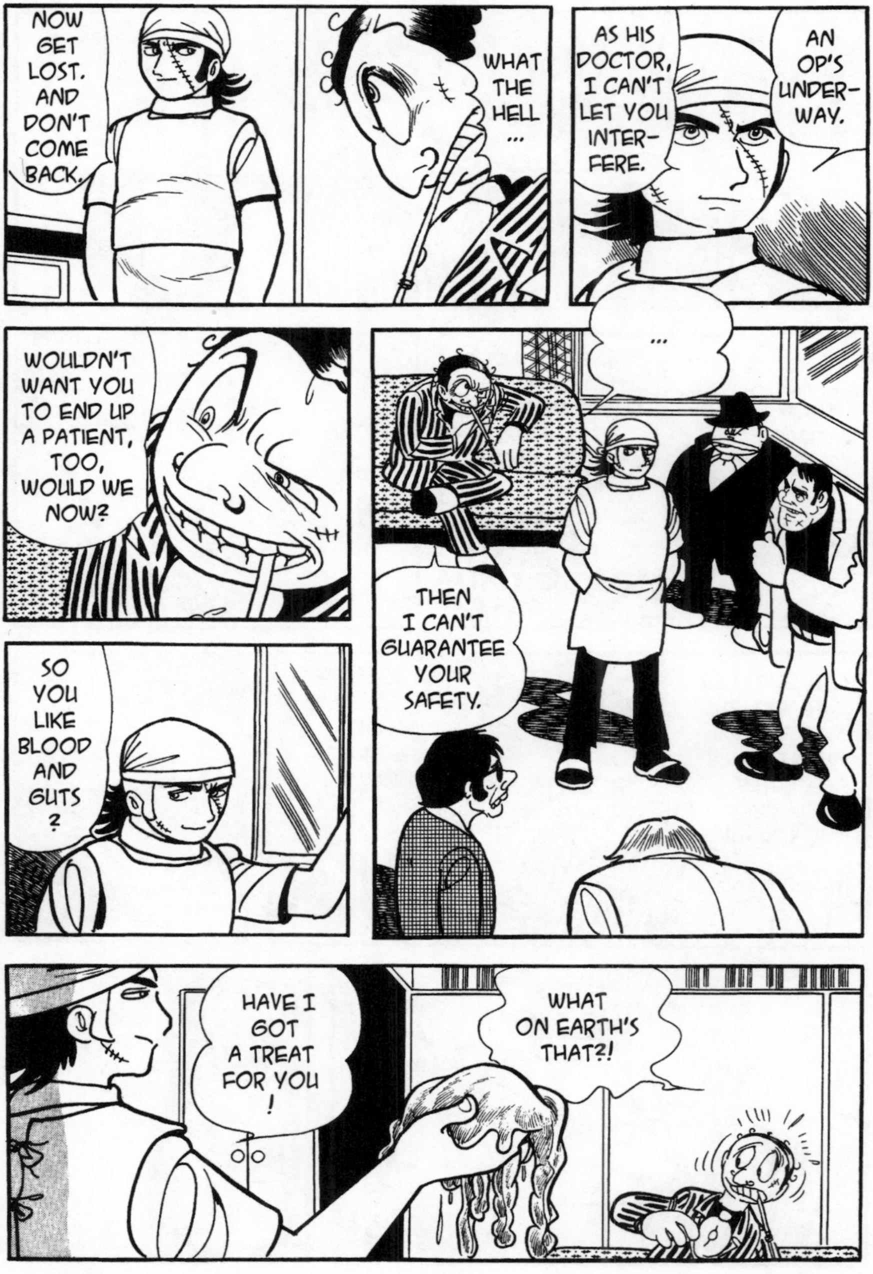
AN OP'S UNDER-WAY.
AS HIS DOCTOR, I CAN'T LET YOU INTER-FERE.
WHAT THE HELL ...
NOW GET LOST. AND DON'T COME BACK.
...
THEN I CAN'T GUARANTEE YOUR SAFETY.
WOULDN'T WANT YOU TO END UP A PATIENT, TOO, WOULD WE NOW?
SO YOU LIKE BLOOD AND GUTS?
WHAT ON EARTH'S THAT?!
HAVE I GOT A TREAT FOR YOU!

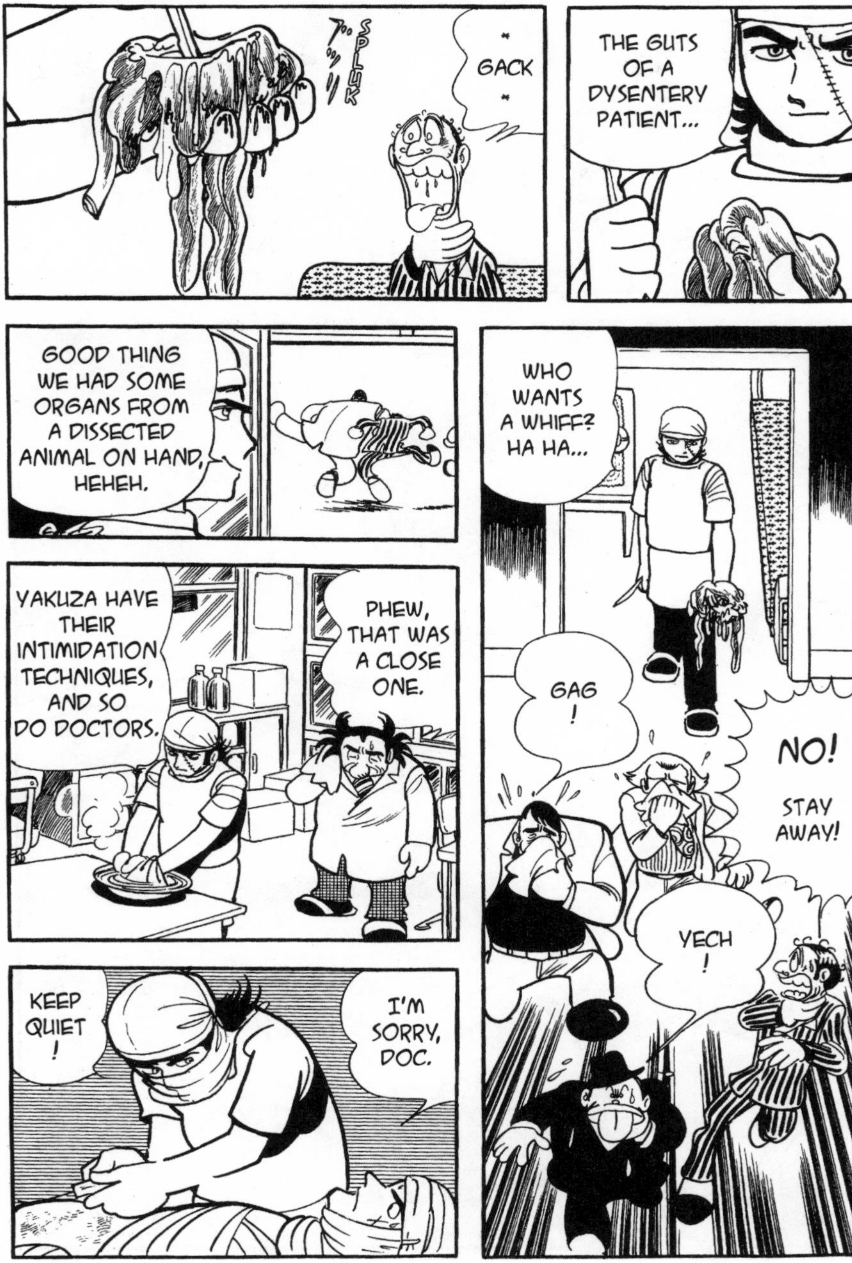
THE GUTS OF A DYSENTERY PATIENT...
* GACK *
SPLUK
WHO WANTS A WHIFF? HA HA...
NO!
STAY AWAY!
GAG!
YECH!
GOOD THING WE HAD SOME ORGANS FROM A DISSECTED ANIMAL ON HAND, HEHEH.
PHEW, THAT WAS A CLOSE ONE.
YAKUZA HAVE THEIR INTIMIDATION TECHNIQUES, AND SO DO DOCTORS.
I'M SORRY, DOC.
KEEP QUIET!

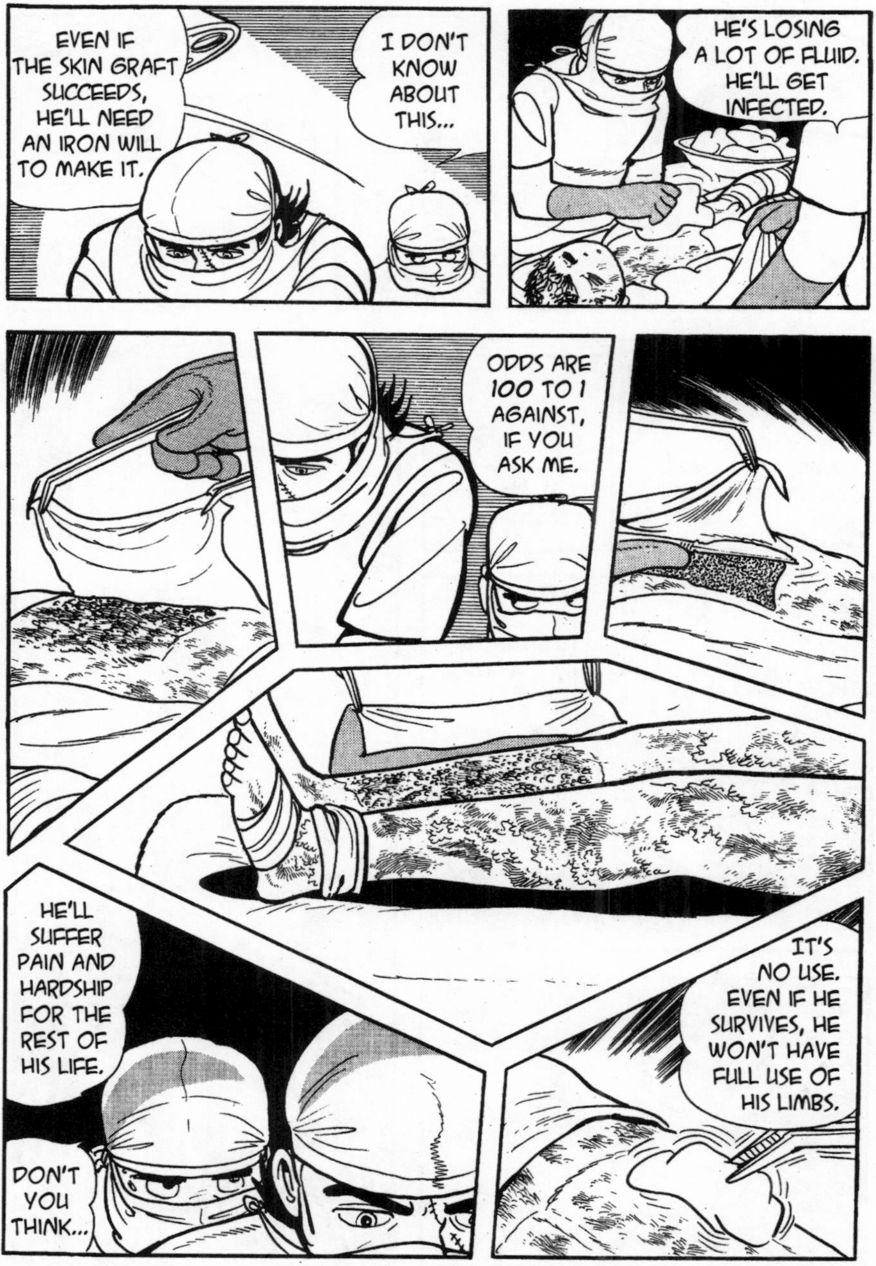
HE'S LOSING A LOT OF FLUID. HE'LL GET INFECTED.
I DON'T KNOW ABOUT THIS...
EVEN IF THE SKIN GRAFT SUCCEEDS, HE'LL NEED AN IRON WILL TO MAKE IT.
ODDS ARE 100 TO 1 AGAINST, IF YOU ASK ME.
IT'S NO USE. EVEN IF HE SURVIVES, HE WON'T HAVE FULL USE OF HIS LIMBS.
HE'LL SUFFER PAIN AND HARDSHIP FOR THE REST OF HIS LIFE.
DON'T YOU THINK...

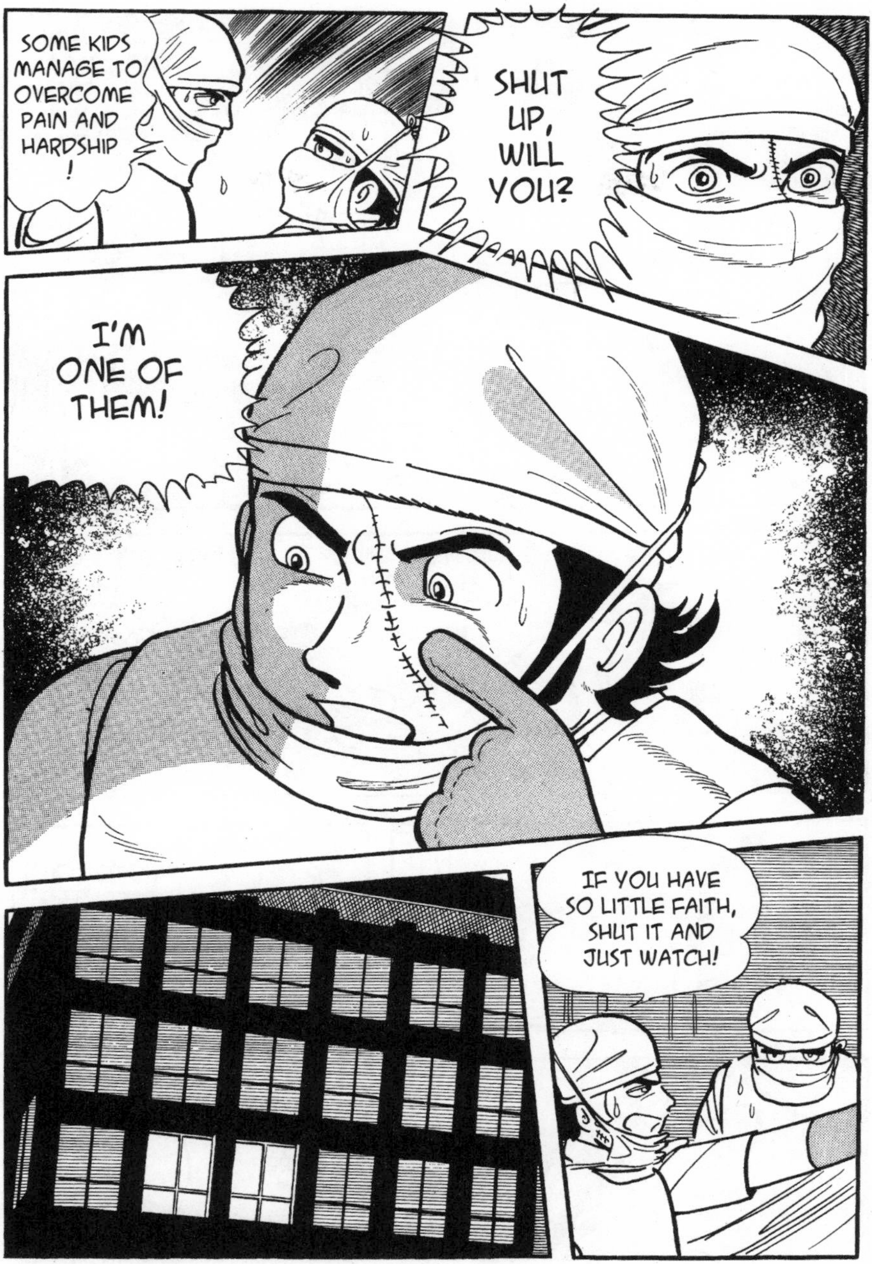
SHUT UP, WILL YOU?
SOME KIDS MANAGE TO OVERCOME PAIN AND HARDSHIP!
I'M ONE OF THEM!
IF YOU HAVE SO LITTLE FAITH, SHUT IT AND JUST WATCH!

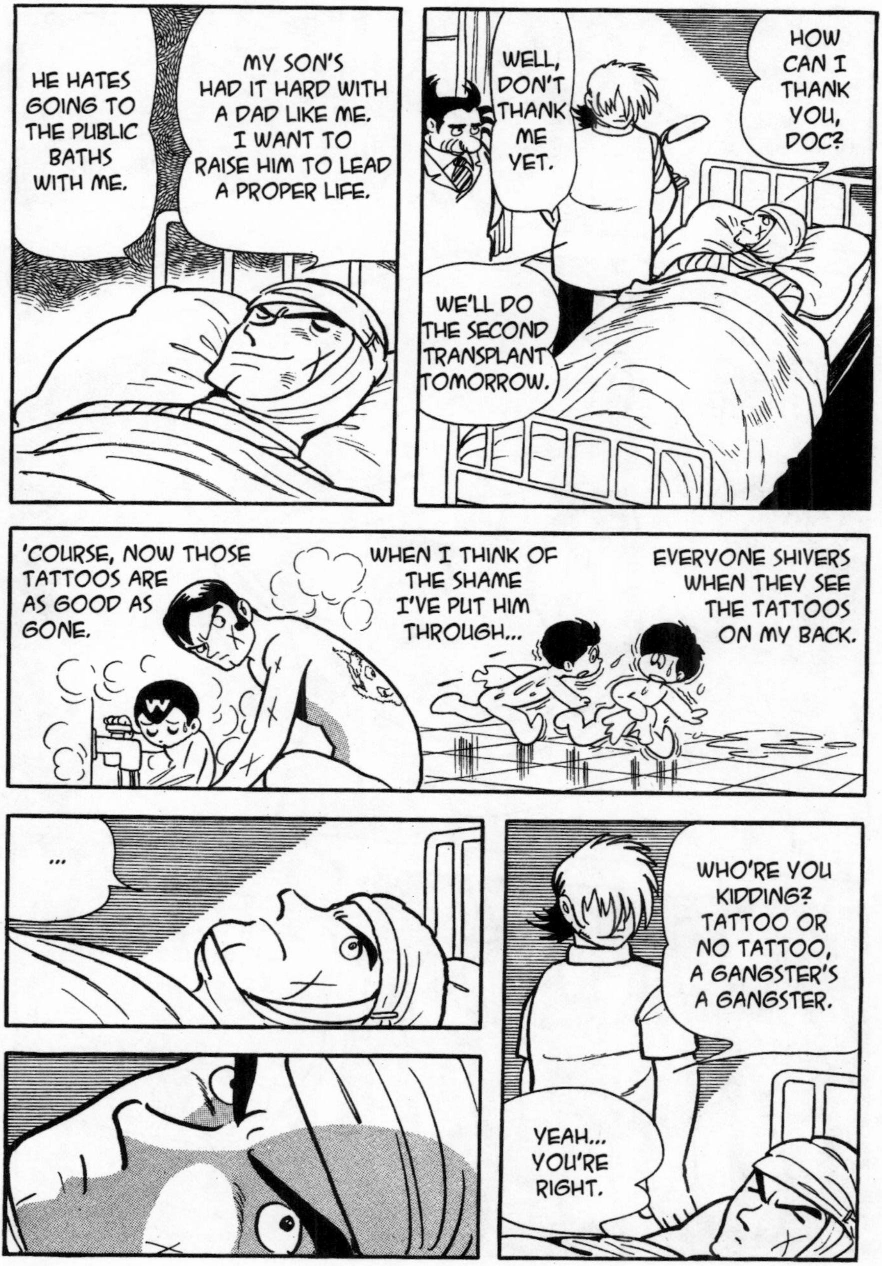
HOW CAN I THANK YOU, DOC?
WELL, DON'T THANK ME YET.
WE'LL DO THE SECOND TRANSPLANT TOMORROW.
MY SON'S HAD IT HARD WITH A DAD LIKE ME. I WANT TO RAISE HIM TO LEAD A PROPER LIFE.
HE HATES GOING TO THE PUBLIC BATHS WITH ME.
EVERYONE SHIVERS WHEN THEY SEE THE TATTOOS ON MY BACK.
WHEN I THINK OF THE SHAME I'VE PUT HIM THROUGH...
'COURSE, NOW THOSE TATTOOS ARE AS GOOD AS GONE.
WHO'RE YOU KIDDING? TATTOO OR NO TATTOO, A GANGSTER'S A GANGSTER.
YEAH... YOU'RE RIGHT.
...

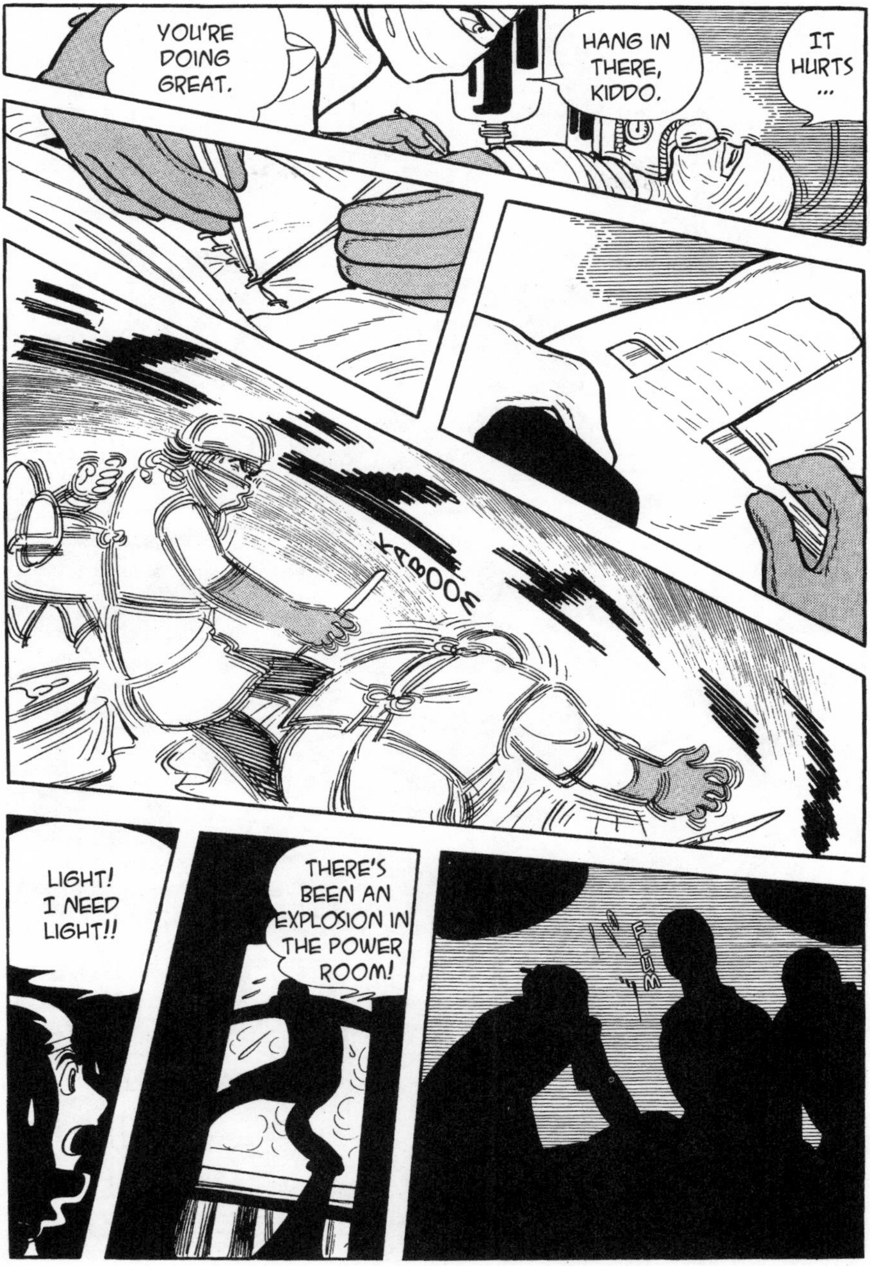
IT HURTS ...
HANG IN THERE, KIDDO.
YOU'RE DOING GREAT.
KABOOM
FLUM
THERE'S BEEN AN EXPLOSION IN THE POWER ROOM!
LIGHT! I NEED LIGHT!!

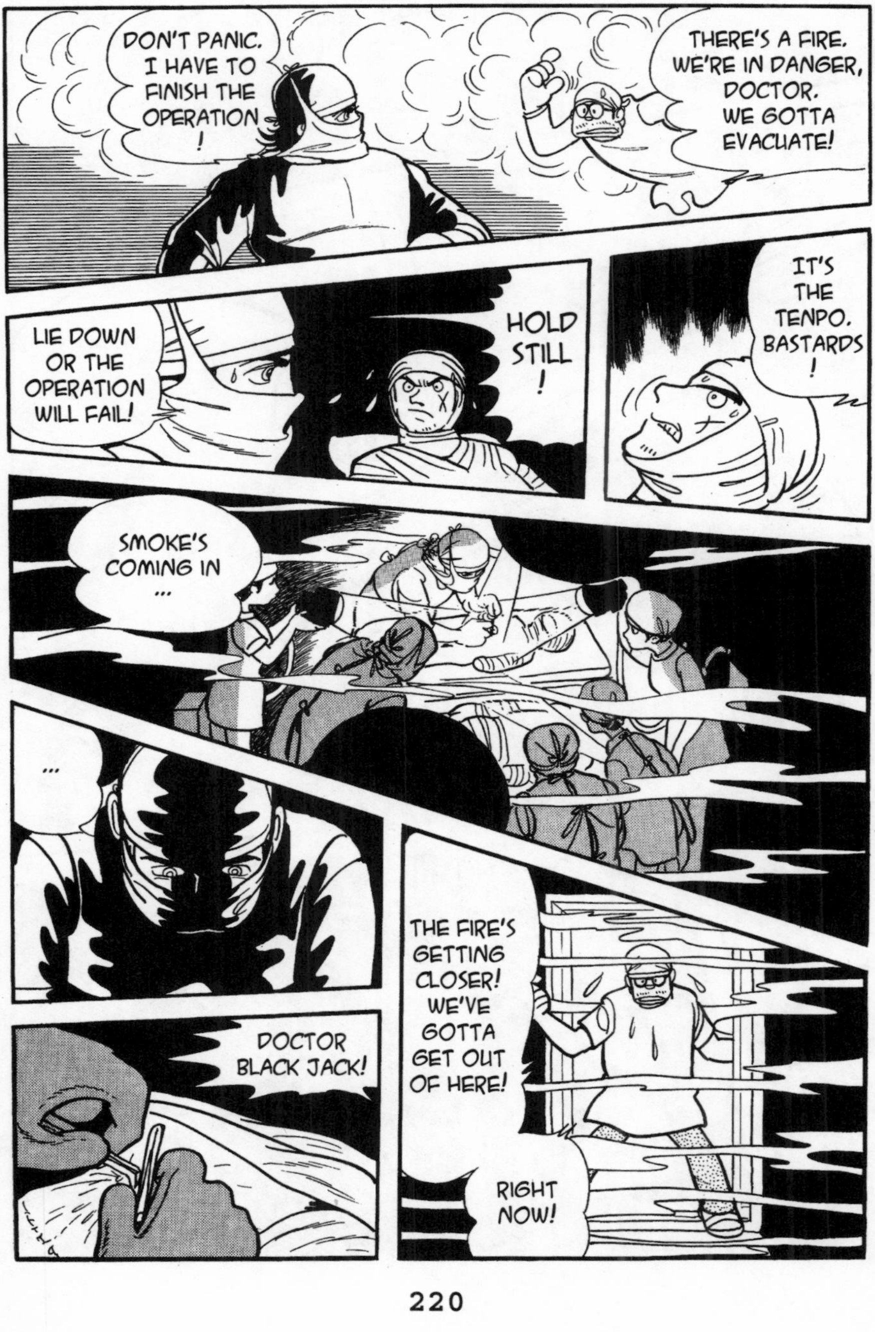
THERE'S A FIRE. WE'RE IN DANGER, DOCTOR. WE GOTTA EVACUATE!
DON'T PANIC. I HAVE TO FINISH THE OPERATION!
IT'S THE TENPO. BASTARDS!
HOLD STILL!
LIE DOWN OR THE OPERATION WILL FAIL!
SMOKE'S COMING IN ...
THE FIRE'S GETTING CLOSER! WE'VE GOTTA GET OUT OF HERE!
RIGHT NOW!
...
DOCTOR BLACK JACK!

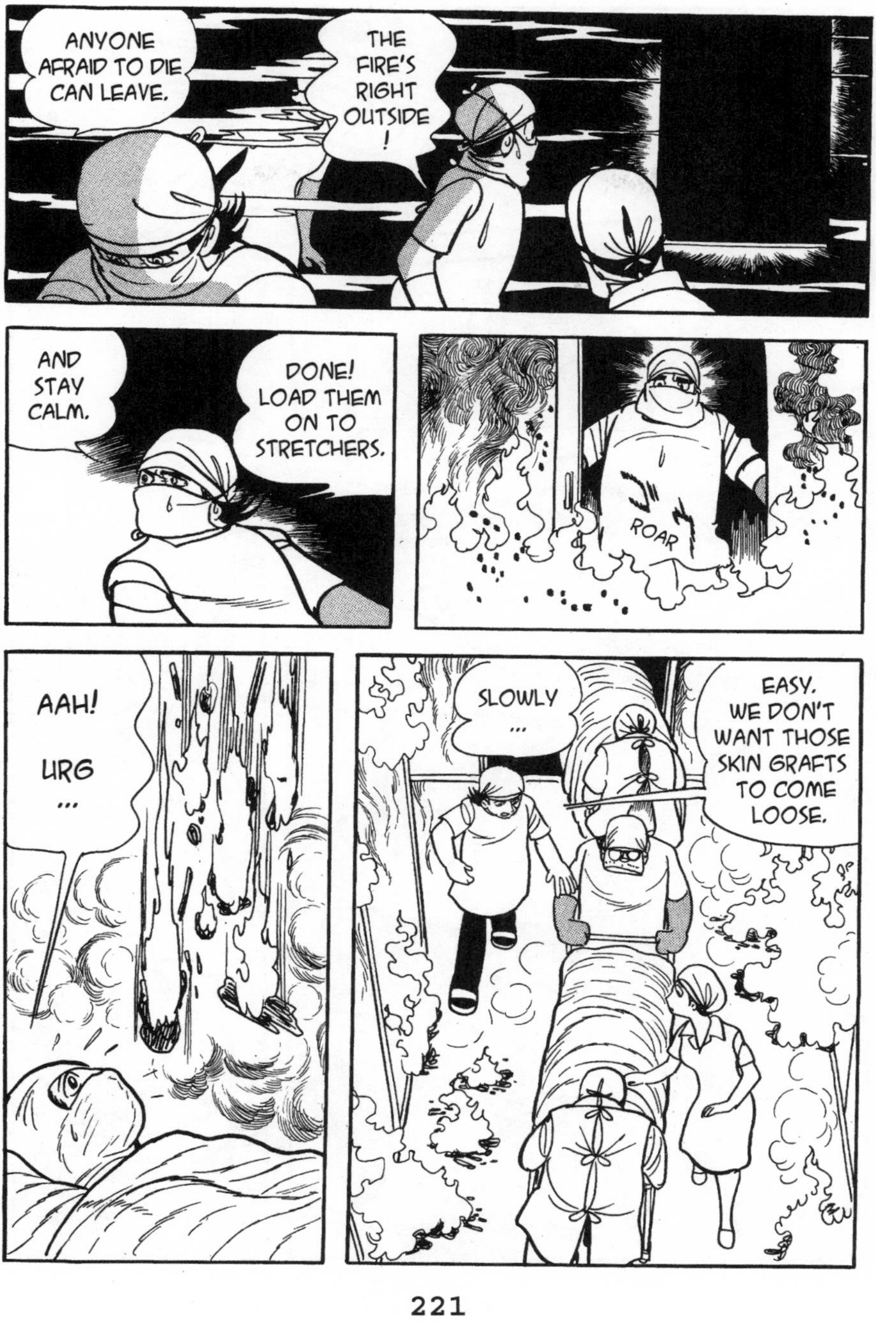
THE FIRE'S RIGHT OUTSIDE !
ANYONE AFRAID TO DIE CAN LEAVE.
ROAR
DONE! LOAD THEM ON TO STRETCHERS.
AND STAY CALM.
EASY. WE DON'T WANT THOSE SKIN GRAFTS TO COME LOOSE.
SLOWLY ...
AAH!
URG ...

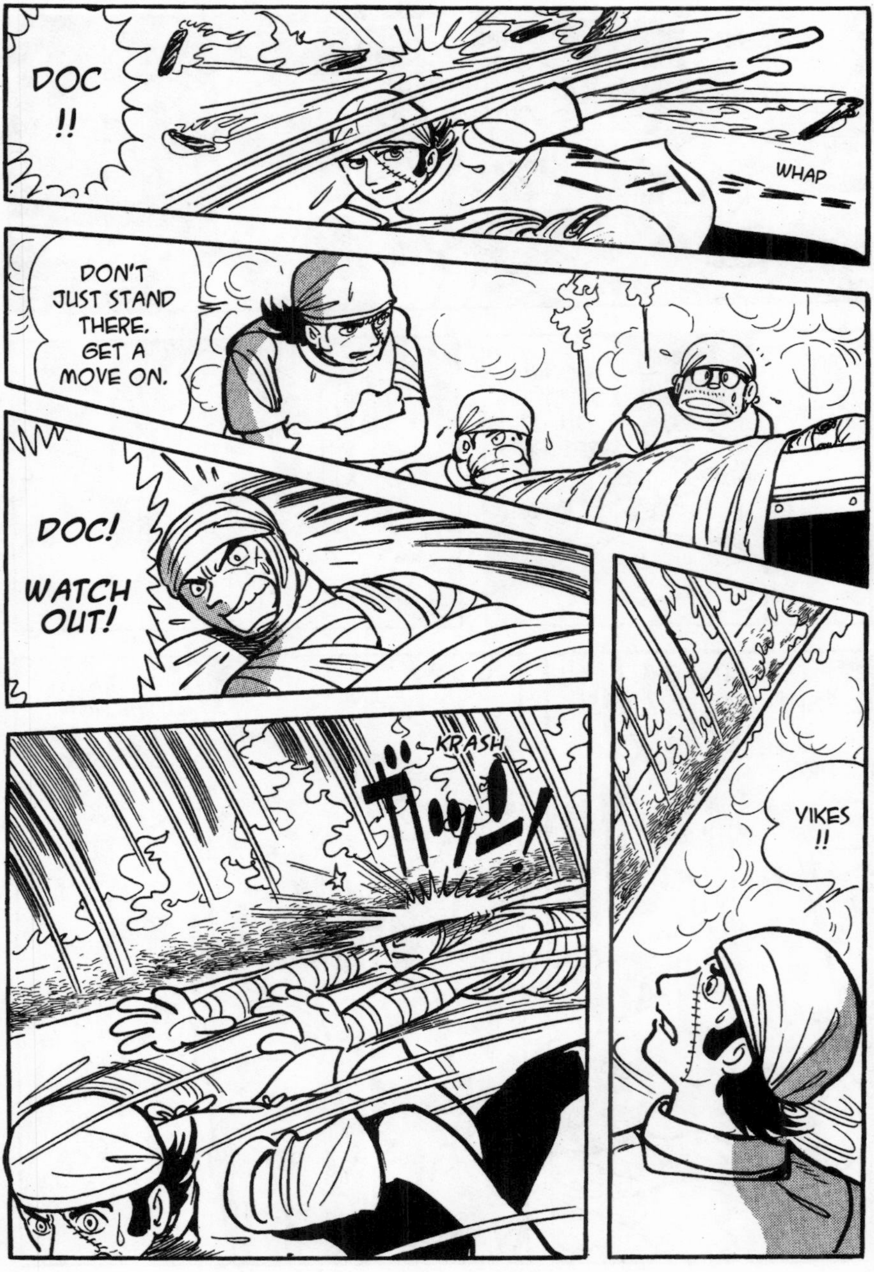
DOC !!
WHAP
DON'T JUST STAND THERE. GET A MOVE ON.
YIKES !!
DOC! WATCH OUT!
KRASH

D-DOC...
M-MY SON...
FUJIMI BATHS
富士見湯
富士見

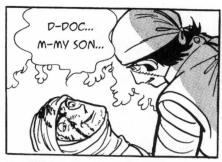

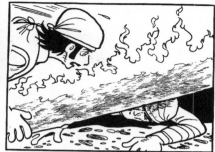

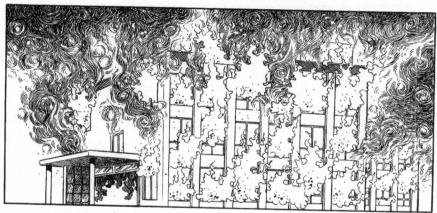

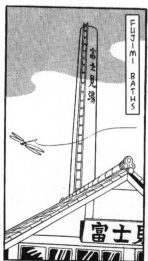

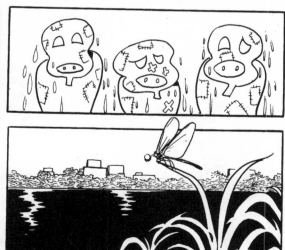

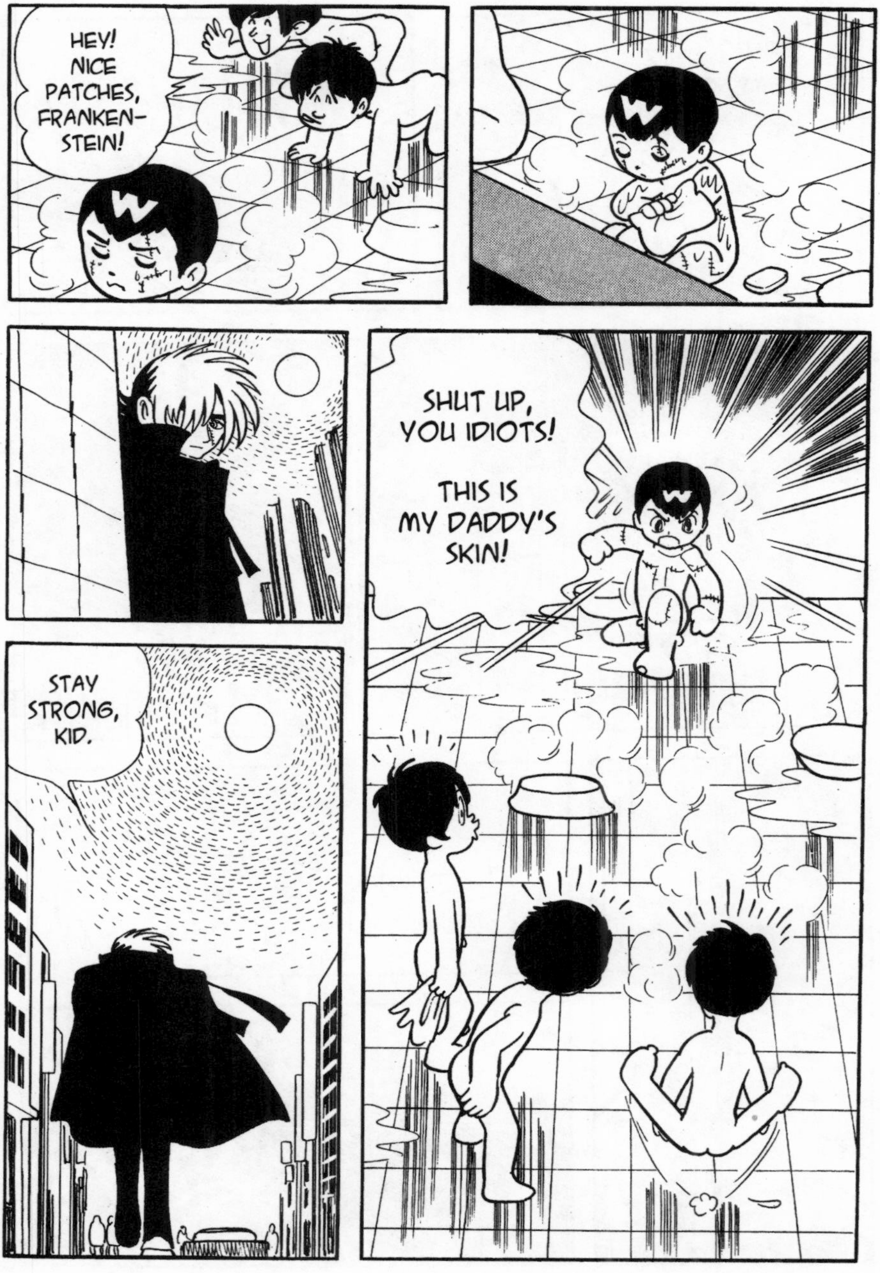
HEY! NICE PATCHES, FRANKEN-STEIN!
SHUT UP, YOU IDIOTS!
THIS IS MY DADDY'S SKIN!
STAY STRONG, KID.

THE HEART OF A GIANT

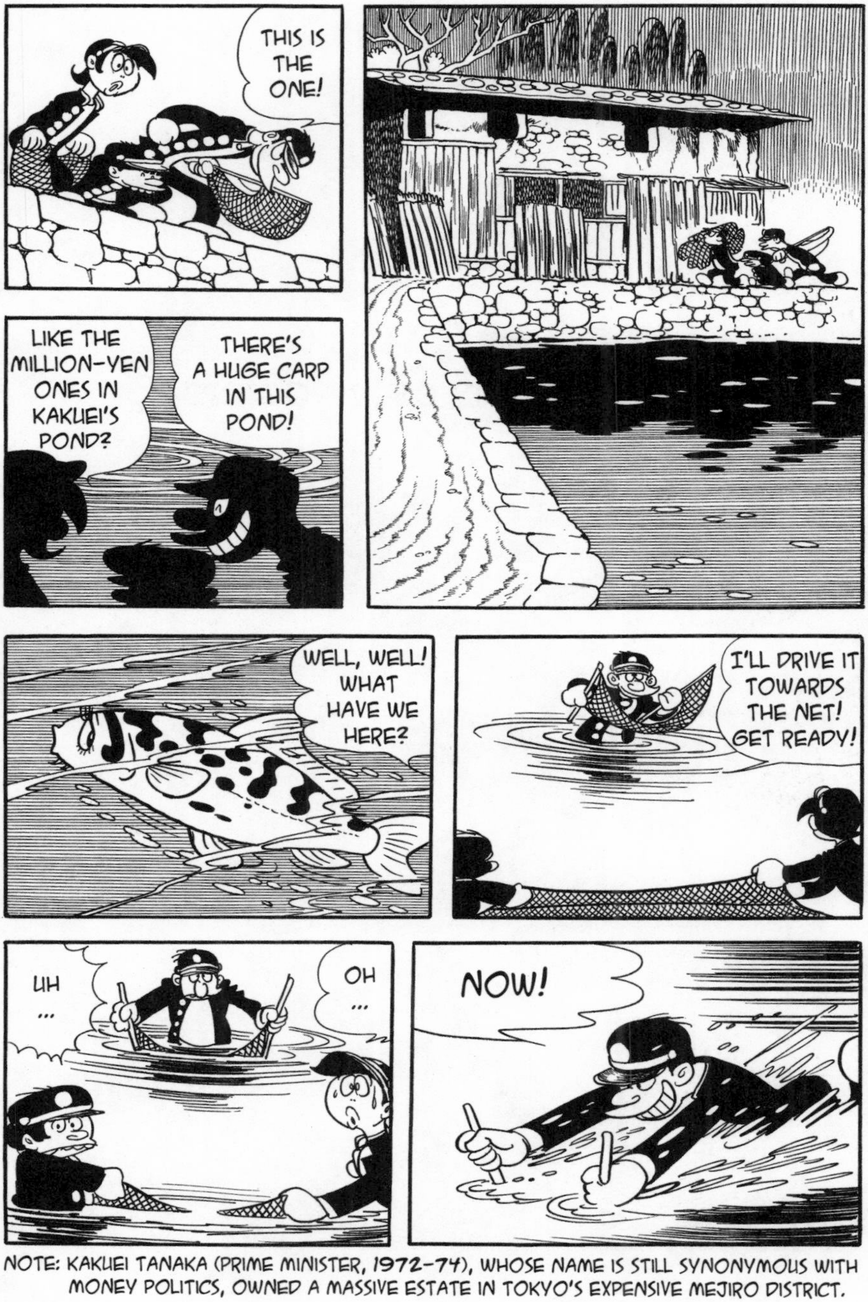
THIS IS THE ONE!
THERE'S A HUGE CARP IN THIS POND!
LIKE THE MILLION-YEN ONES IN KAKUEI'S POND?
I'LL DRIVE IT TOWARDS THE NET! GET READY!
WELL, WELL! WHAT HAVE WE HERE?
NOW!
OH ...
UH ...

NOTE: KAKUEI TANAKA (PRIME MINISTER, 1972–74), WHOSE NAME IS STILL SYNONYMOUS WITH MONEY POLITICS, OWNED A MASSIVE ESTATE IN TOKYO'S EXPENSIVE MEJIRO DISTRICT.

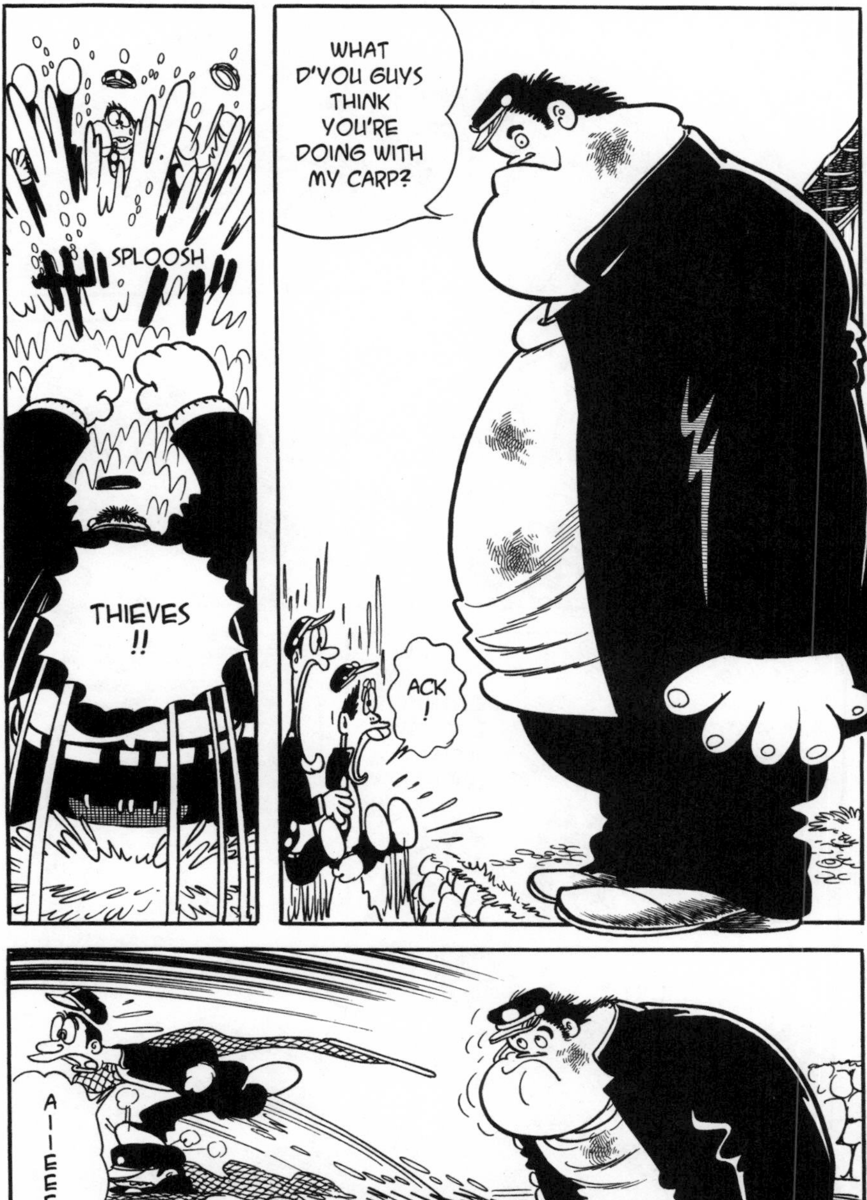
WHAT D'YOU GUYS THINK YOU'RE DOING WITH MY CARP?
ACK!
SPLOOSH
THIEVES!!
AIIEEE!

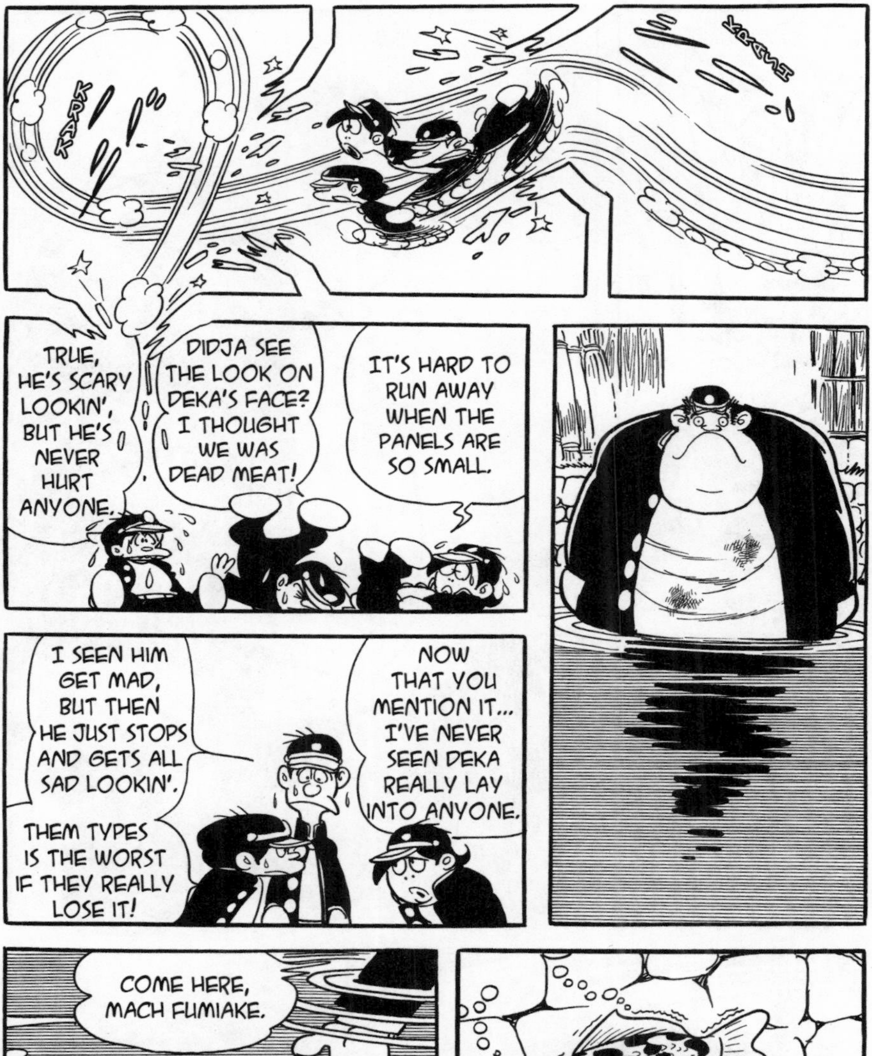
KRASH
KRAK
IT'S HARD TO RUN AWAY WHEN THE PANELS ARE SO SMALL.
DIDJA SEE THE LOOK ON DEKA'S FACE? I THOUGHT WE WAS DEAD MEAT!
TRUE, HE'S SCARY LOOKIN', BUT HE'S NEVER HURT ANYONE.
NOW THAT YOU MENTION IT... I'VE NEVER SEEN DEKA REALLY LAY INTO ANYONE.
I SEEN HIM GET MAD, BUT THEN HE JUST STOPS AND GETS ALL SAD LOOKIN'.
THEM TYPES IS THE WORST IF THEY REALLY LOSE IT!
...
COME HERE, MACH FUMIAKE.

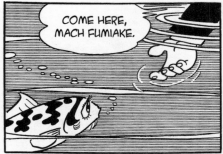

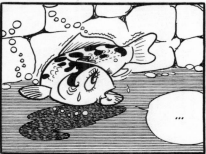

NOTE: "DEKA" MEANS *HUGE* IN JAPANESE. MACH (AS IN "SUPERSONIC") FUMIAKE, A FEMALE PRO-WRESTLER, LAUNCHED A SECOND CAREER AS A TV PERSONALITY THANKS TO HER RELATIVELY GOOD LOOKS.

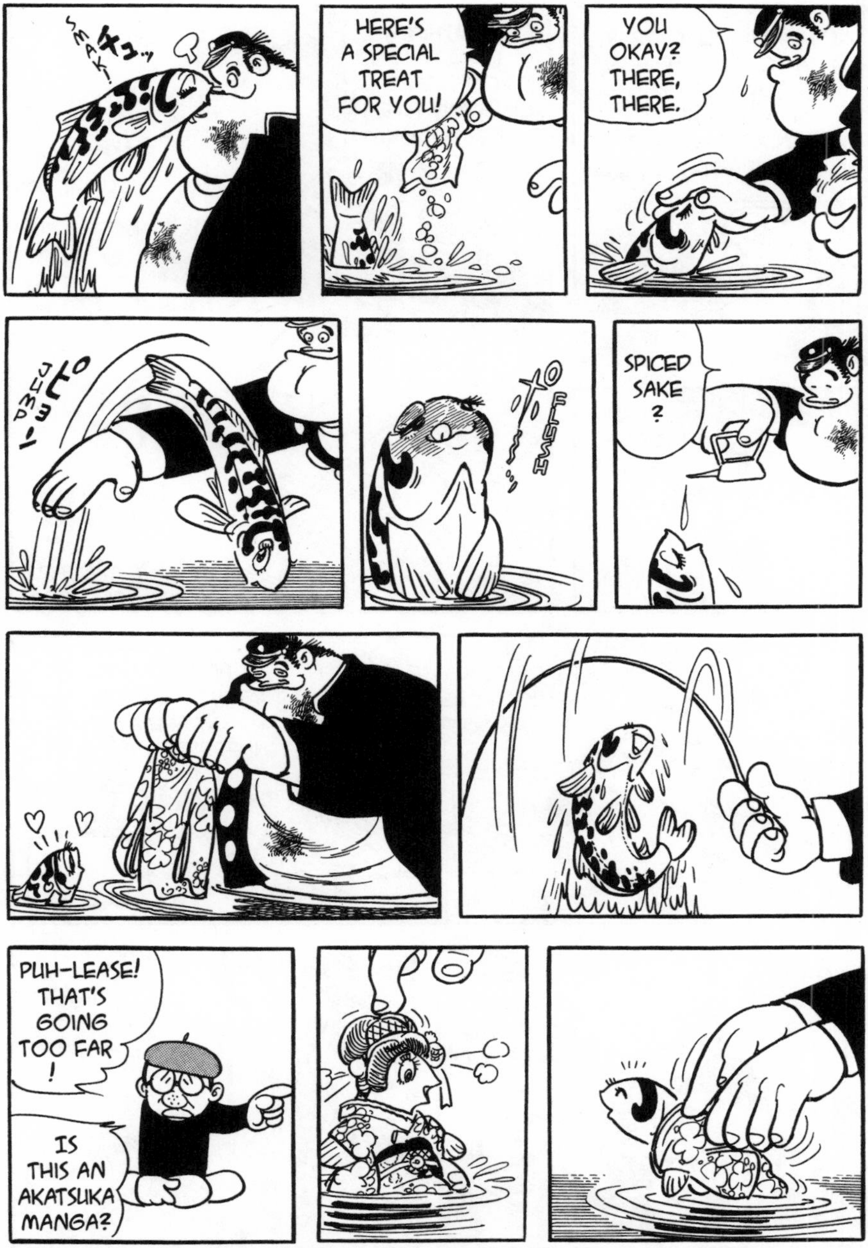
YOU OKAY? THERE, THERE.
HERE'S A SPECIAL TREAT FOR YOU!
SMAK!
SPICED SAKE ?
FLISH
JUMP!
PUH-LEASE! THAT'S GOING TOO FAR !
IS THIS AN AKATSUKA MANGA?

NOTE: FUJIO AKATSUKA = UNDISPUTED KING OF "GAG MANGA"

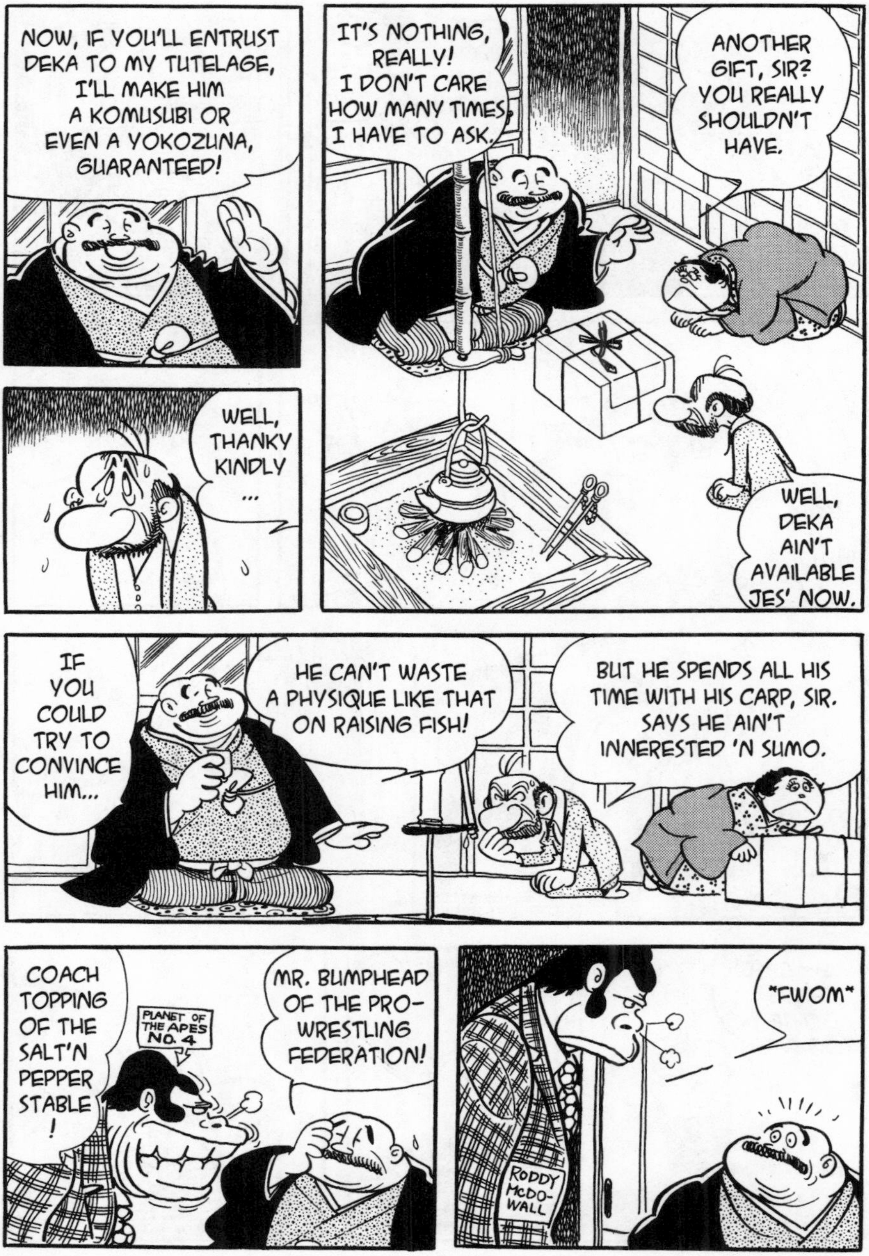
ANOTHER GIFT, SIR? YOU REALLY SHOULDN'T HAVE.
IT'S NOTHING, REALLY! I DON'T CARE HOW MANY TIMES I HAVE TO ASK.
WELL, DEKA AIN'T AVAILABLE JES' NOW.
NOW, IF YOU'LL ENTRUST DEKA TO MY TUTELAGE, I'LL MAKE HIM A KOMUSUBI OR EVEN A YOKOZUNA, GUARANTEED!
WELL, THANKY KINDLY ...
BUT HE SPENDS ALL HIS TIME WITH HIS CARP, SIR. SAYS HE AIN'T INNERESTED 'N SUMO.
HE CAN'T WASTE A PHYSIQUE LIKE THAT ON RAISING FISH!
IF YOU COULD TRY TO CONVINCE HIM...
FWOM
RODDY McDOWALL
MR. BUMPHEAD OF THE PRO-WRESTLING FEDERATION!
PLANET OF THE APES NO. 4
COACH TOPPING OF THE SALT'N PEPPER STABLE!

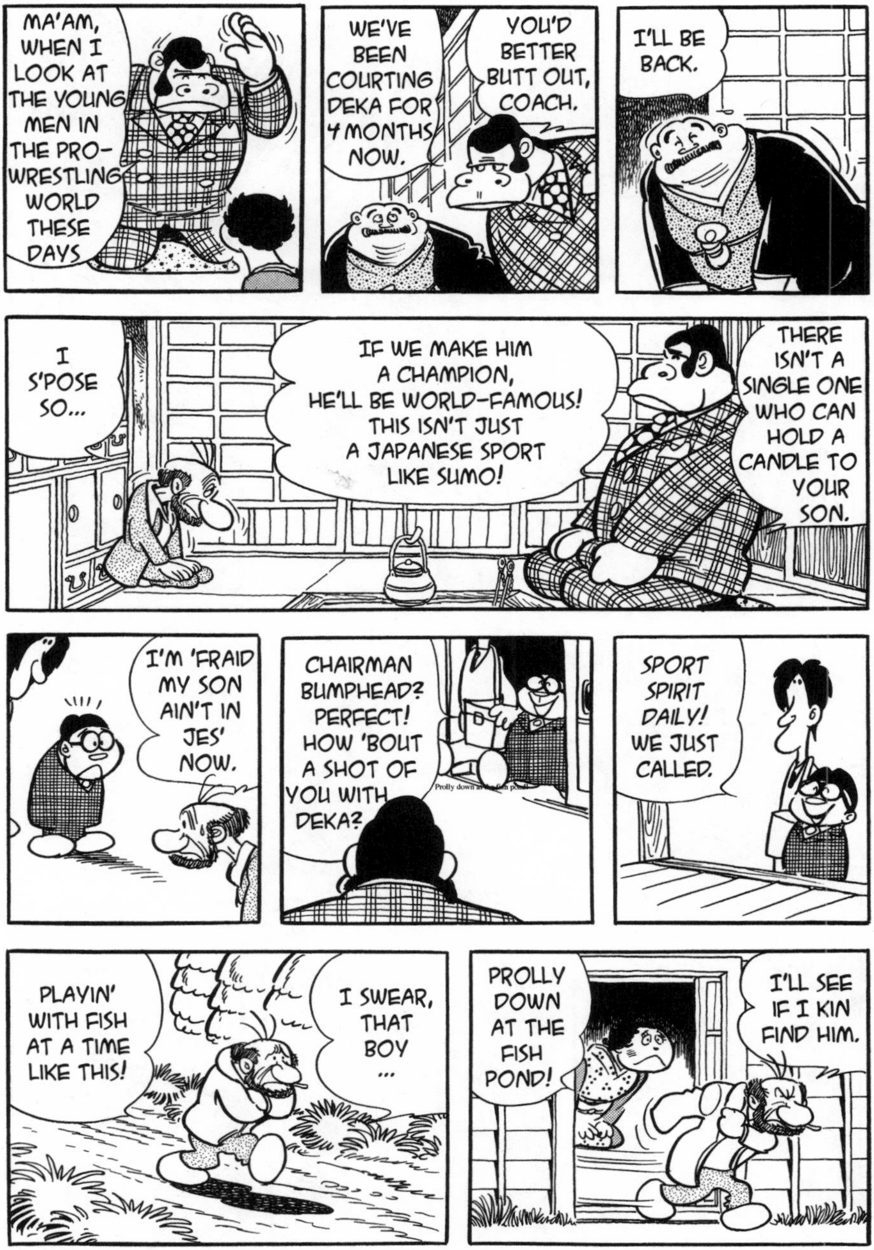
I'LL BE BACK.
YOU'D BETTER BUTT OUT, COACH.
WE'VE BEEN COURTING DEKA FOR 4 MONTHS NOW.
MA'AM, WHEN I LOOK AT THE YOUNG MEN IN THE PRO-WRESTLING WORLD THESE DAYS
THERE ISN'T A SINGLE ONE WHO CAN HOLD A CANDLE TO YOUR SON.
IF WE MAKE HIM A CHAMPION, HE'LL BE WORLD-FAMOUS! THIS ISN'T JUST A JAPANESE SPORT LIKE SUMO!
I S'POSE SO...
SPORT SPIRIT DAILY! WE JUST CALLED.
CHAIRMAN BUMPHEAD? PERFECT! HOW 'BOUT A SHOT OF YOU WITH DEKA?
I'M 'FRAID MY SON AIN'T IN JES' NOW.
I'LL SEE IF I KIN FIND HIM.
PROLLY DOWN AT THE FISH POND!
I SWEAR, THAT BOY ...
PLAYIN' WITH FISH AT A TIME LIKE THIS!

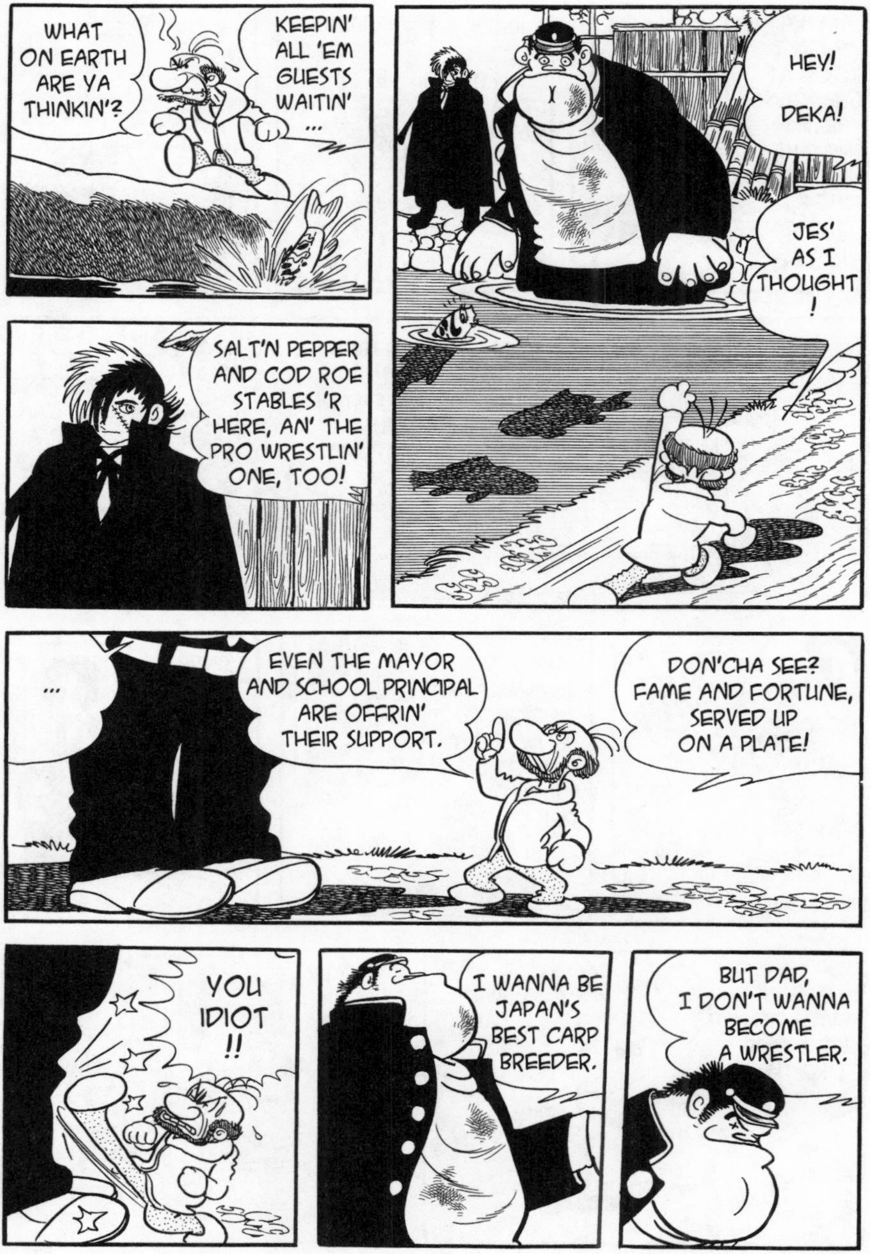
HEY!
DEKA!
JES' AS I THOUGHT !
KEEPIN' ALL 'EM GUESTS WAITIN' ...
WHAT ON EARTH ARE YA THINKIN'?
SALT'N PEPPER AND COD ROE STABLES 'R HERE, AN' THE PRO WRESTLIN' ONE, TOO!
DON'CHA SEE? FAME AND FORTUNE, SERVED UP ON A PLATE!
EVEN THE MAYOR AND SCHOOL PRINCIPAL ARE OFFRIN' THEIR SUPPORT.
...
BUT DAD, I DON'T WANNA BECOME A WRESTLER.
I WANNA BE JAPAN'S BEST CARP BREEDER.
YOU IDIOT !!

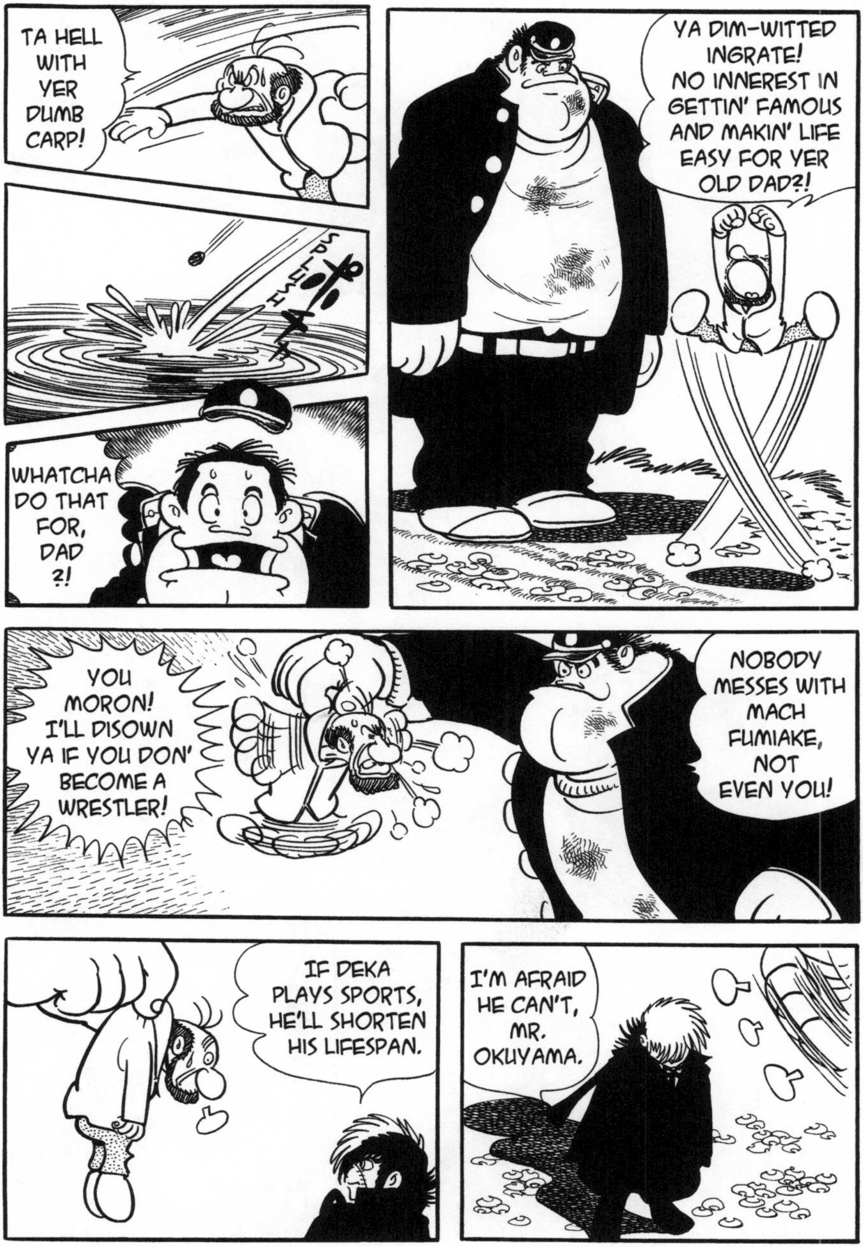
YA DIM-WITTED INGRATE! NO INNEREST IN GETTIN' FAMOUS AND MAKIN' LIFE EASY FOR YER OLD DAD?!
TA HELL WITH YER DUMB CARP!
SPLASH
WHATCHA DO THAT FOR, DAD ?!
NOBODY MESSES WITH MACH FUMIAKE, NOT EVEN YOU!
YOU MORON! I'LL DISOWN YA IF YOU DON' BECOME A WRESTLER!
I'M AFRAID HE CAN'T, MR. OKUYAMA.
IF DEKA PLAYS SPORTS, HE'LL SHORTEN HIS LIFESPAN.

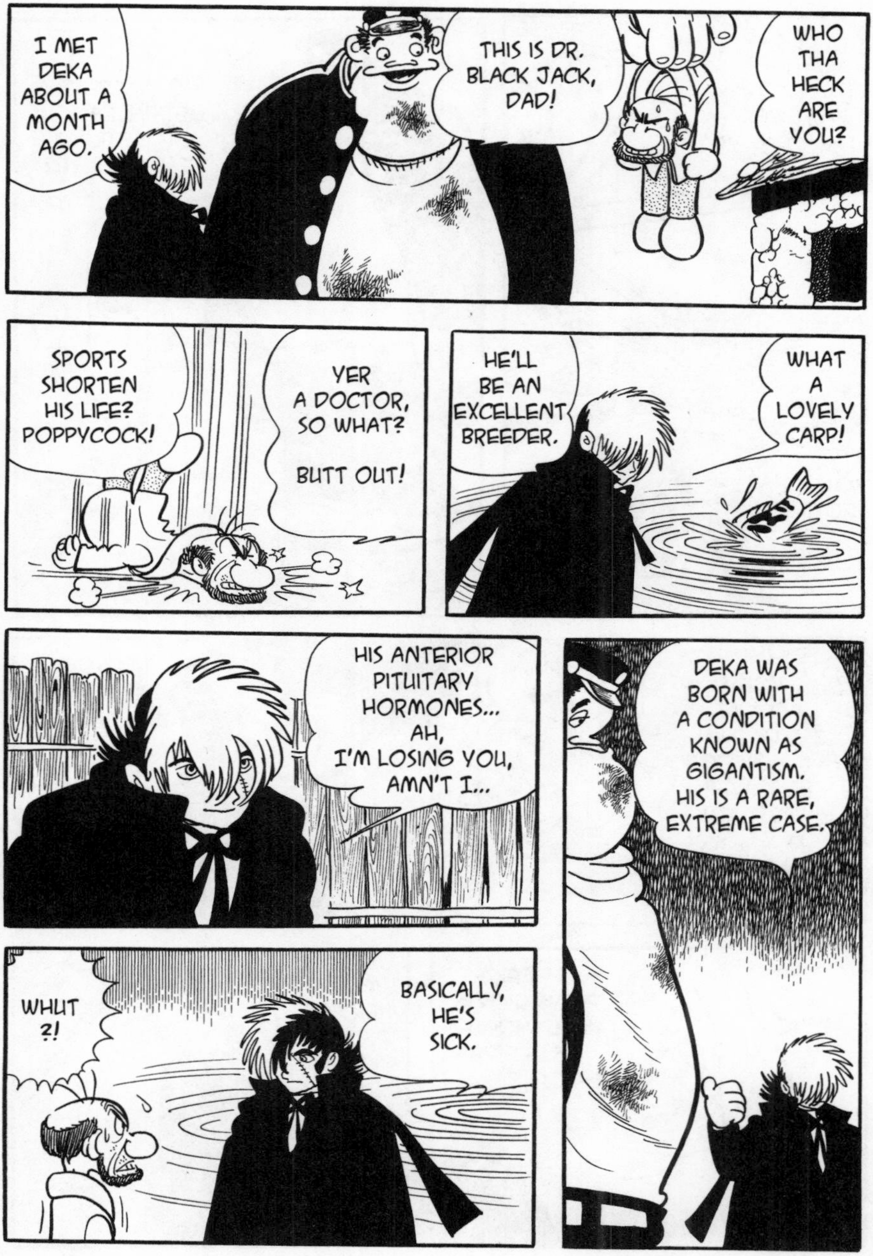
WHO THA HECK ARE YOU?
THIS IS DR. BLACK JACK, DAD!
I MET DEKA ABOUT A MONTH AGO.
WHAT A LOVELY CARP!
HE'LL BE AN EXCELLENT BREEDER.
YER A DOCTOR, SO WHAT? BUTT OUT!
SPORTS SHORTEN HIS LIFE? POPPYCOCK!
DEKA WAS BORN WITH A CONDITION KNOWN AS GIGANTISM. HIS IS A RARE, EXTREME CASE.
HIS ANTERIOR PITUITARY HORMONES... AH, I'M LOSING YOU, AMN'T I...
BASICALLY, HE'S SICK.
WHUT ?!

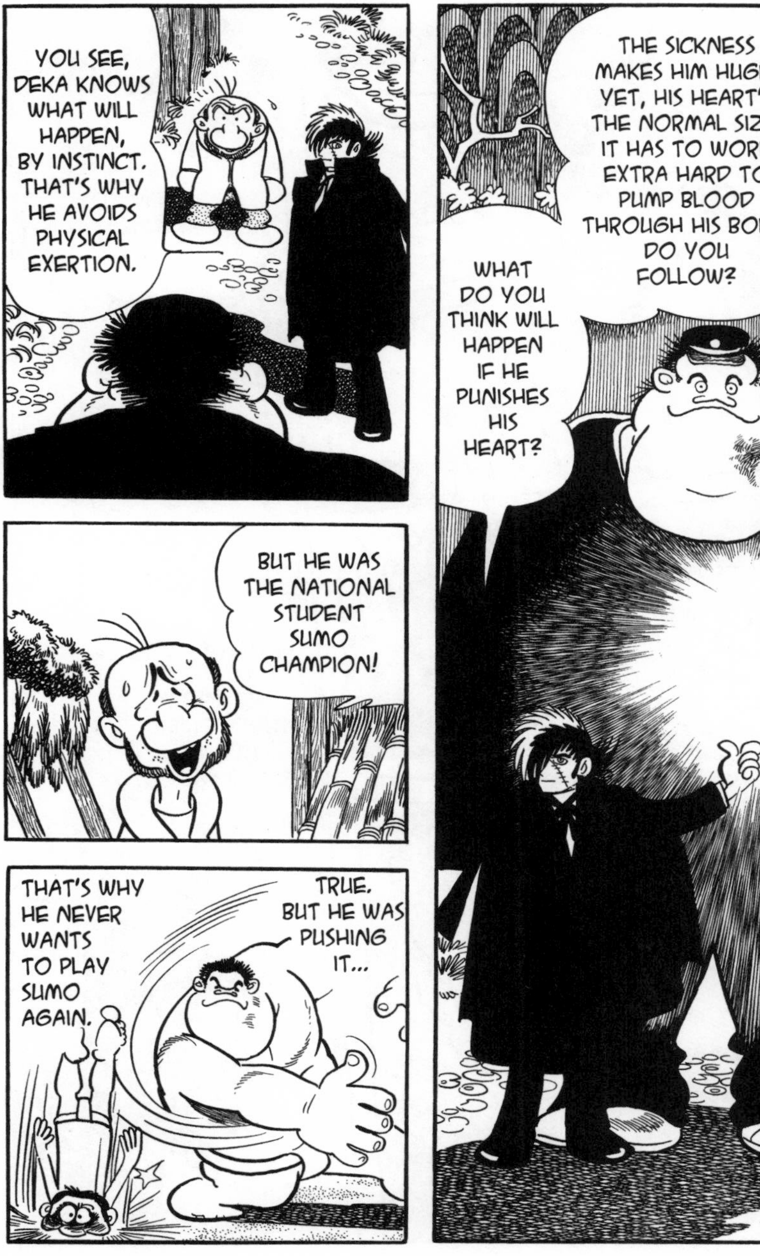
THE SICKNESS MAKES HIM HUGE. YET, HIS HEART'S THE NORMAL SIZE. IT HAS TO WORK EXTRA HARD TO PUMP BLOOD THROUGH HIS BODY. DO YOU FOLLOW?
WHAT DO YOU THINK WILL HAPPEN IF HE PUNISHES HIS HEART?
YOU SEE, DEKA KNOWS WHAT WILL HAPPEN, BY INSTINCT. THAT'S WHY HE AVOIDS PHYSICAL EXERTION.
BUT HE WAS THE NATIONAL STUDENT SUMO CHAMPION!
TRUE. BUT HE WAS PUSHING IT...
THAT'S WHY HE NEVER WANTS TO PLAY SUMO AGAIN.

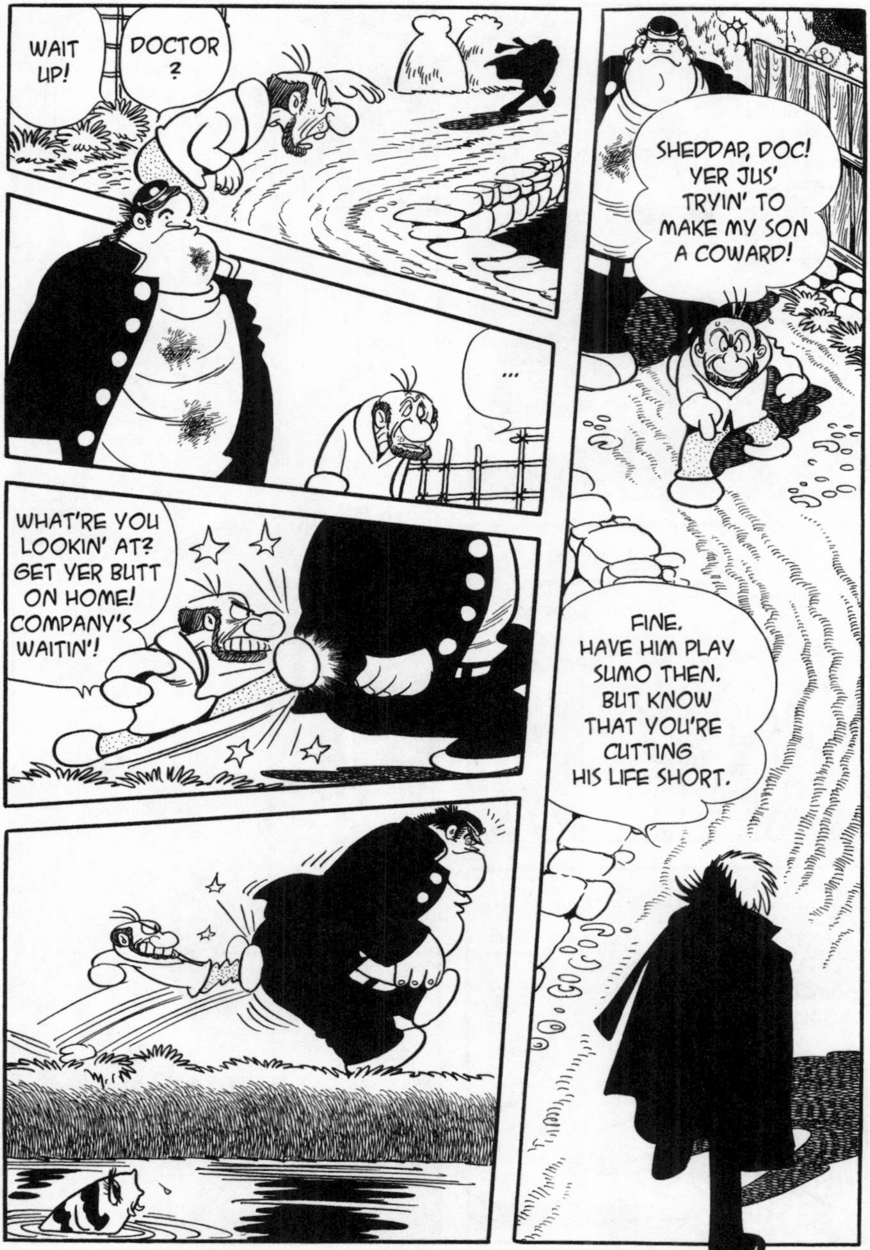
SHEDDAP, DOC! YER JUS' TRYIN' TO MAKE MY SON A COWARD!
FINE. HAVE HIM PLAY SUMO THEN. BUT KNOW THAT YOU'RE CUTTING HIS LIFE SHORT.
DOCTOR ?
WAIT UP!
...
WHAT'RE YOU LOOKIN' AT? GET YER BUTT ON HOME! COMPANY'S WAITIN'!

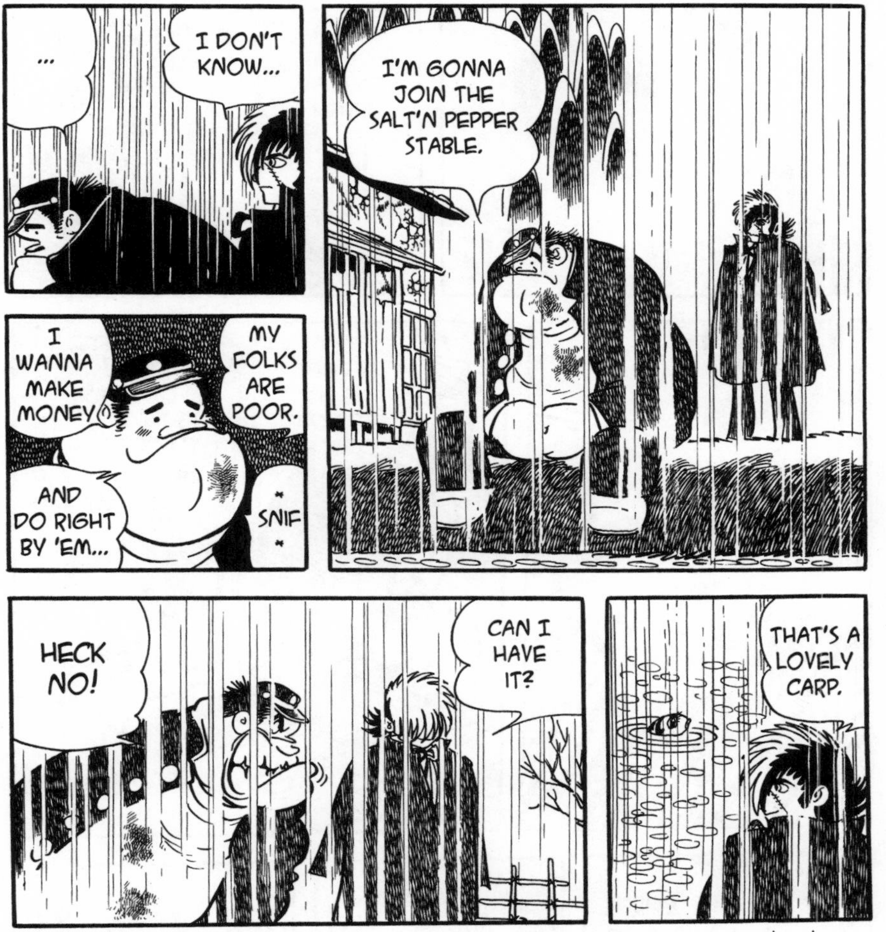
I'M GONNA JOIN THE SALT'N PEPPER STABLE.
I DON'T KNOW...
...
MY FOLKS ARE POOR.
I WANNA MAKE MONEY
AND DO RIGHT BY 'EM...
SNIF
THAT'S A LOVELY CARP.
CAN I HAVE IT?
HECK NO!
SHE'S MY FISH!
YOU SURE LOVE THAT THING.
A FISH FETISH, HEH.
SINCE YOU'RE GOING TO DIE ANYWAY, WHY NOT GIVE IT TO ME?

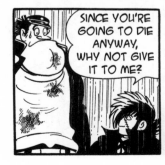

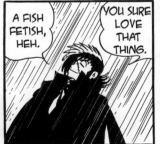

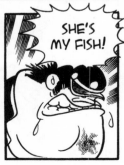

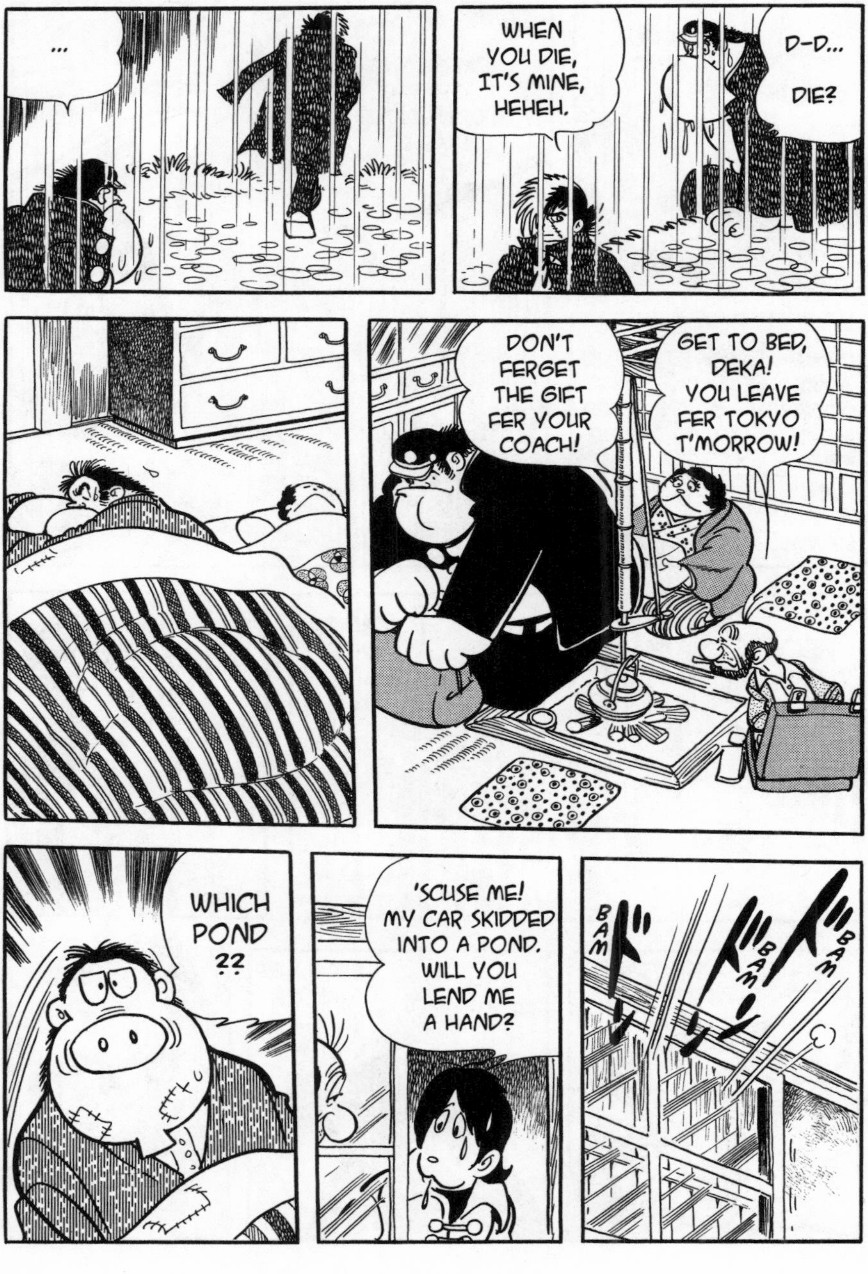
D-D...
DIE?
WHEN YOU DIE, IT'S MINE, HEHEH.
...
GET TO BED, DEKA! YOU LEAVE FER TOKYO T'MORROW!
DON'T FERGET THE GIFT FER YOUR COACH!
BAM
BAM
BAM
BAM
'SCUSE ME! MY CAR SKIDDED INTO A POND. WILL YOU LEND ME A HAND?
WHICH POND ??

NO...
NOT MY CARP POND !!
YOU BASTARD!!
OIL... THERE'S OIL IN MY POND!

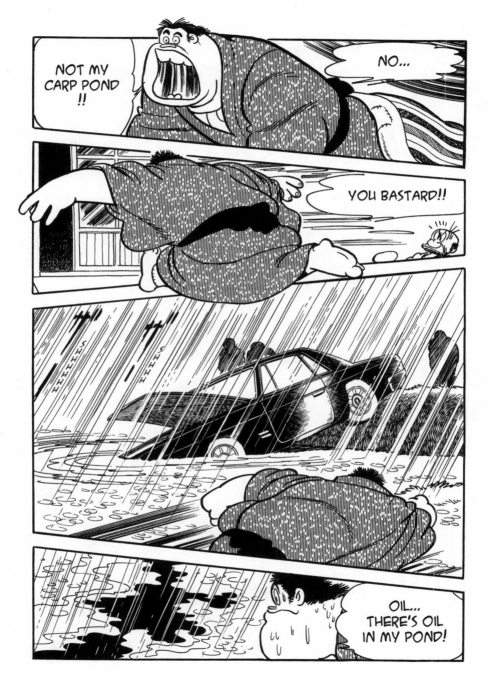

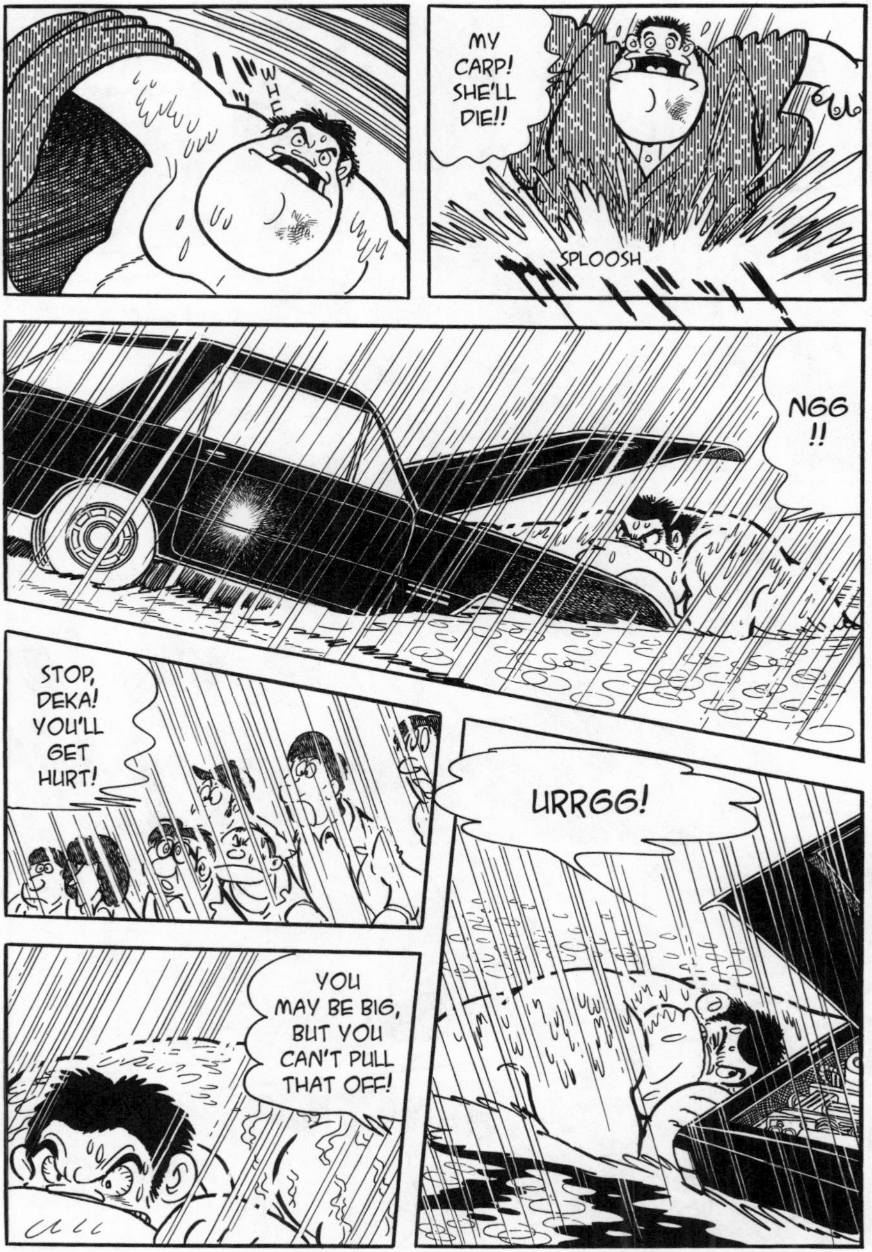
MY CARP! SHE'LL DIE!!
SPLOOSH
WHE
NGG !!
URRGG!
STOP, DEKA! YOU'LL GET HURT!
YOU MAY BE BIG, BUT YOU CAN'T PULL THAT OFF!

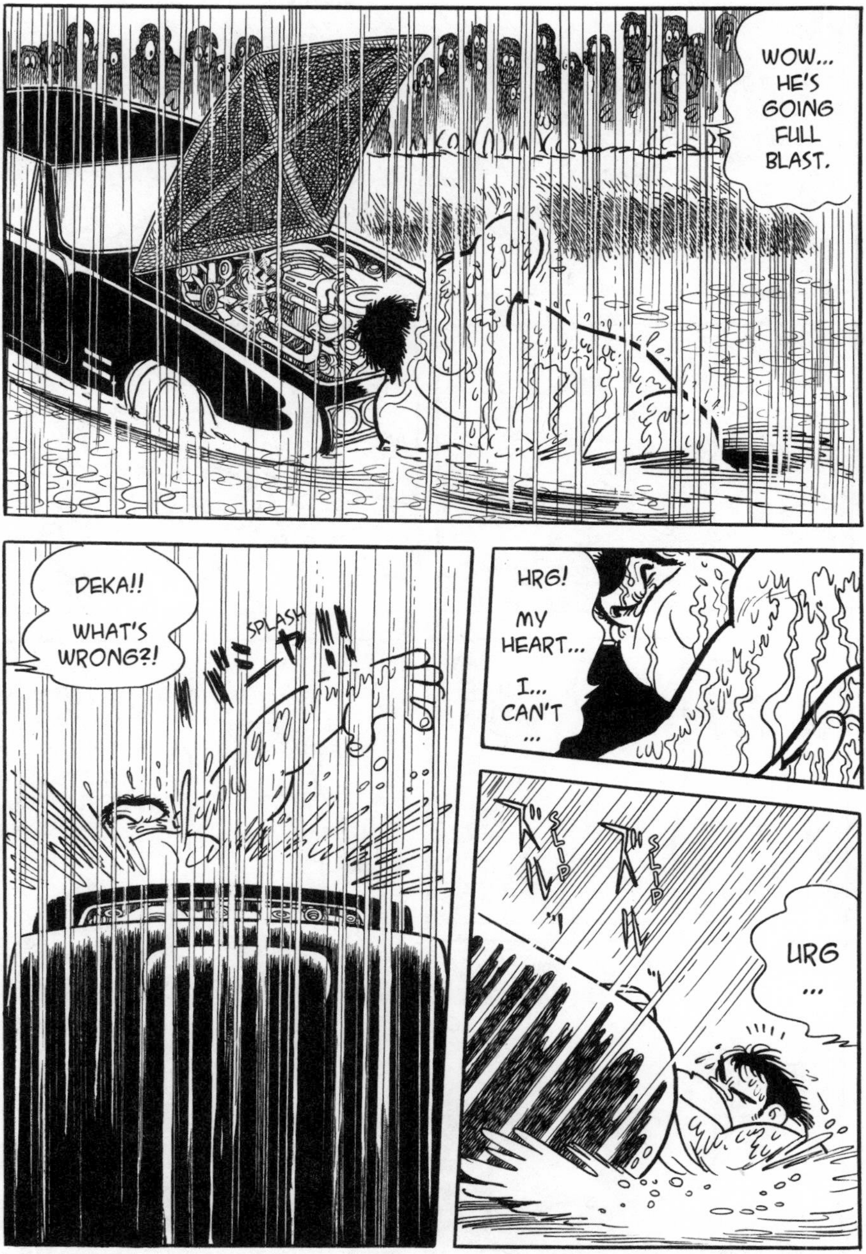

WOW... HE'S GOING FULL BLAST.
HRG!
MY HEART...
I... CAN'T ...
SLIP
SLIP
URG ...
DEKA!!
WHAT'S WRONG?!
SPLASH

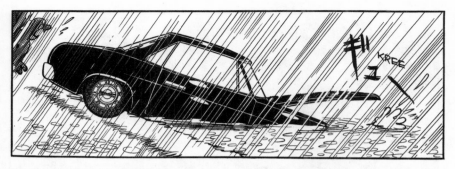

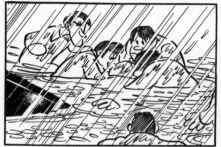

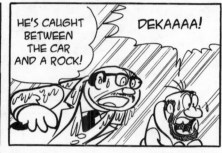

ギュー
KREE
DEKAAAA!
HE'S CAUGHT BETWEEN THE CAR AND A ROCK!
HIS HEART COULDN'T TAKE IT. JUST AS I TOLD YOU, MR. OKUYAMA.
YOU CAN EITHER LET HIM DIE...
OR I CAN AMPUTATE HIS LEGS TO SAVE HIS LIFE.
I HOPE YOU OPT FOR THE LATTER.

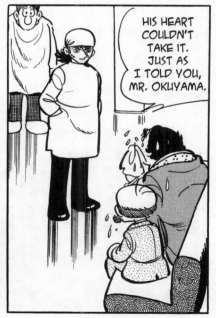

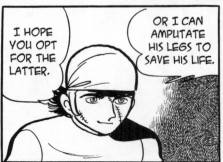

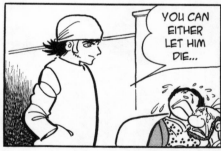

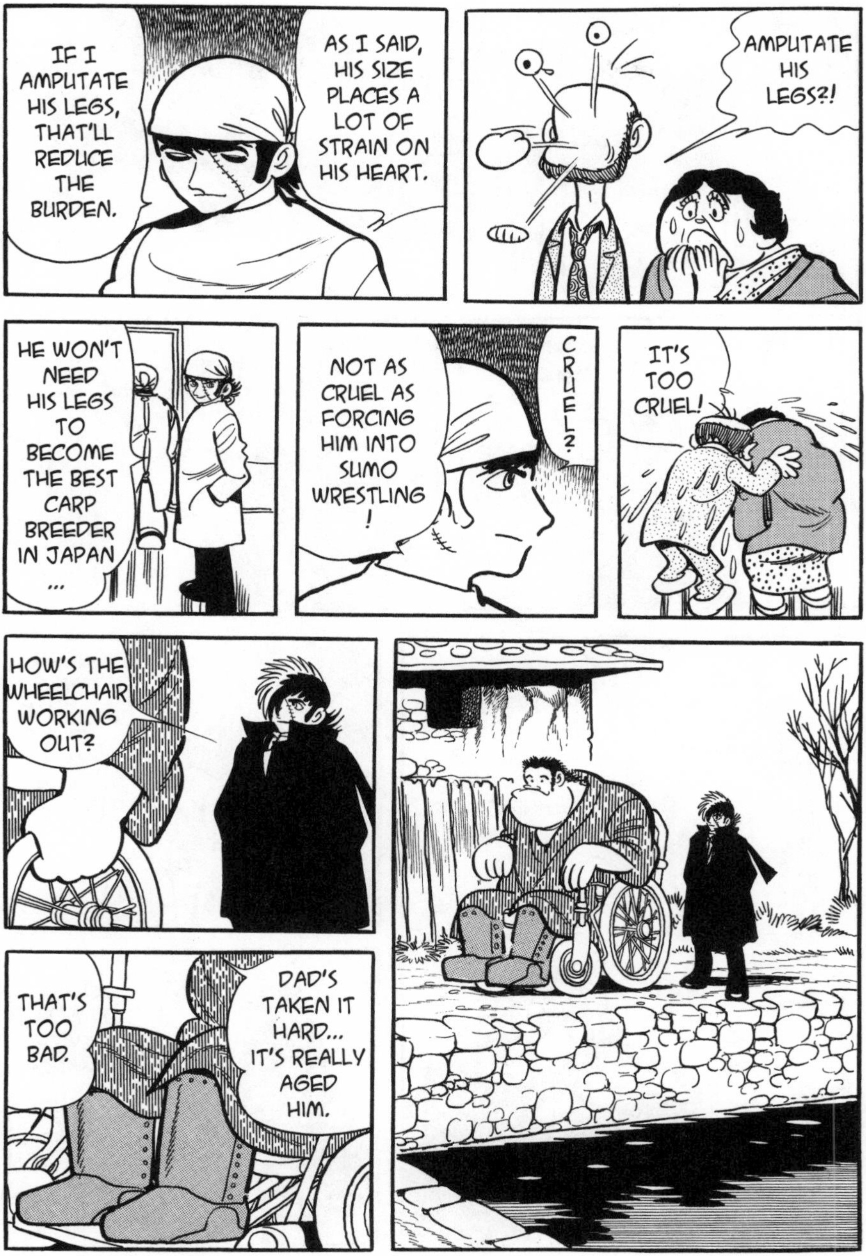
AMPUTATE HIS LEGS?!
AS I SAID, HIS SIZE PLACES A LOT OF STRAIN ON HIS HEART.
IF I AMPUTATE HIS LEGS, THAT'LL REDUCE THE BURDEN.
IT'S TOO CRUEL!
CRUEL?
NOT AS CRUEL AS FORCING HIM INTO SUMO WRESTLING!
HE WON'T NEED HIS LEGS TO BECOME THE BEST CARP BREEDER IN JAPAN ...
HOW'S THE WHEELCHAIR WORKING OUT?
DAD'S TAKEN IT HARD... IT'S REALLY AGED HIM.
THAT'S TOO BAD.

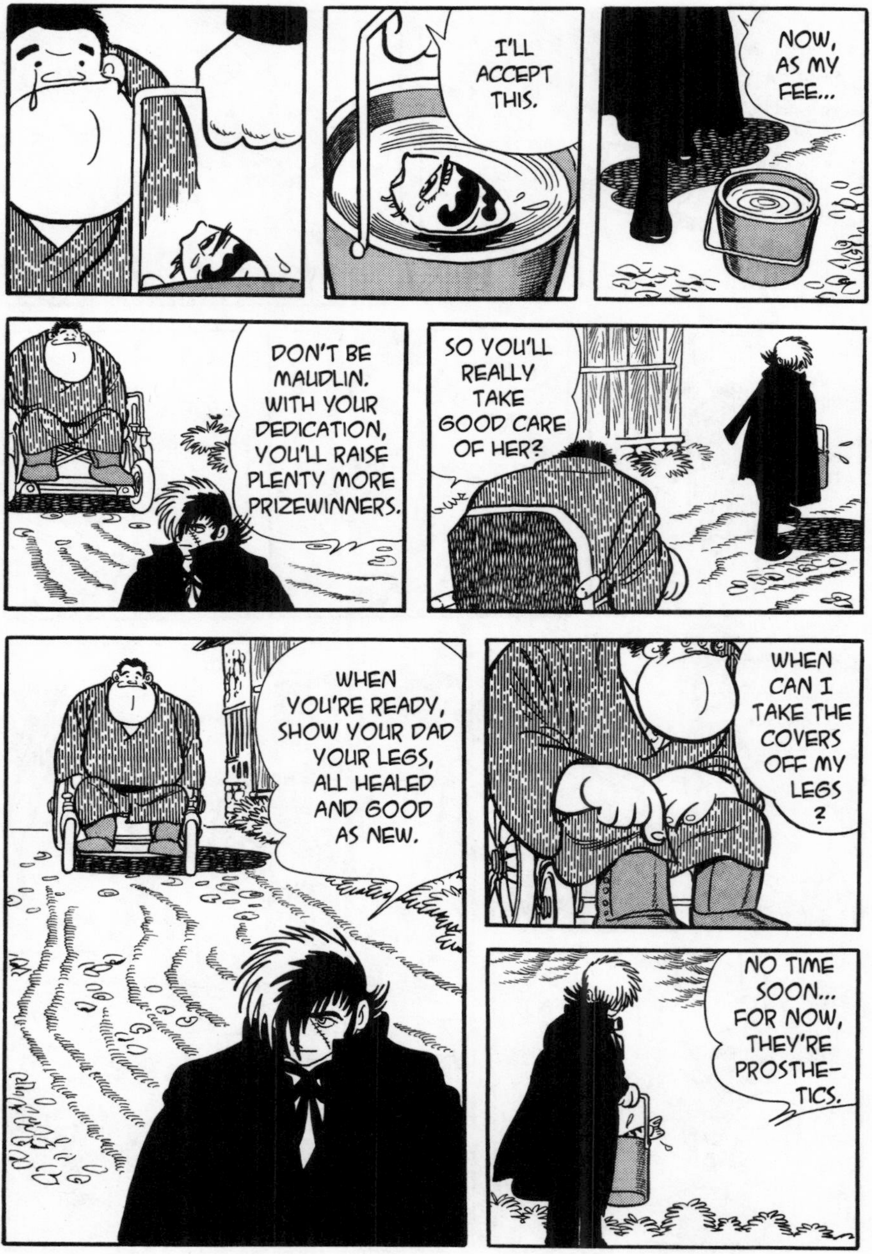
NOW, AS MY FEE...
I'LL ACCEPT THIS.
SO YOU'LL REALLY TAKE GOOD CARE OF HER?
DON'T BE MAUDLIN. WITH YOUR DEDICATION, YOU'LL RAISE PLENTY MORE PRIZEWINNERS.
WHEN CAN I TAKE THE COVERS OFF MY LEGS ?
NO TIME SOON... FOR NOW, THEY'RE PROSTHE-TICS.
WHEN YOU'RE READY, SHOW YOUR DAD YOUR LEGS, ALL HEALED AND GOOD AS NEW.

GAS

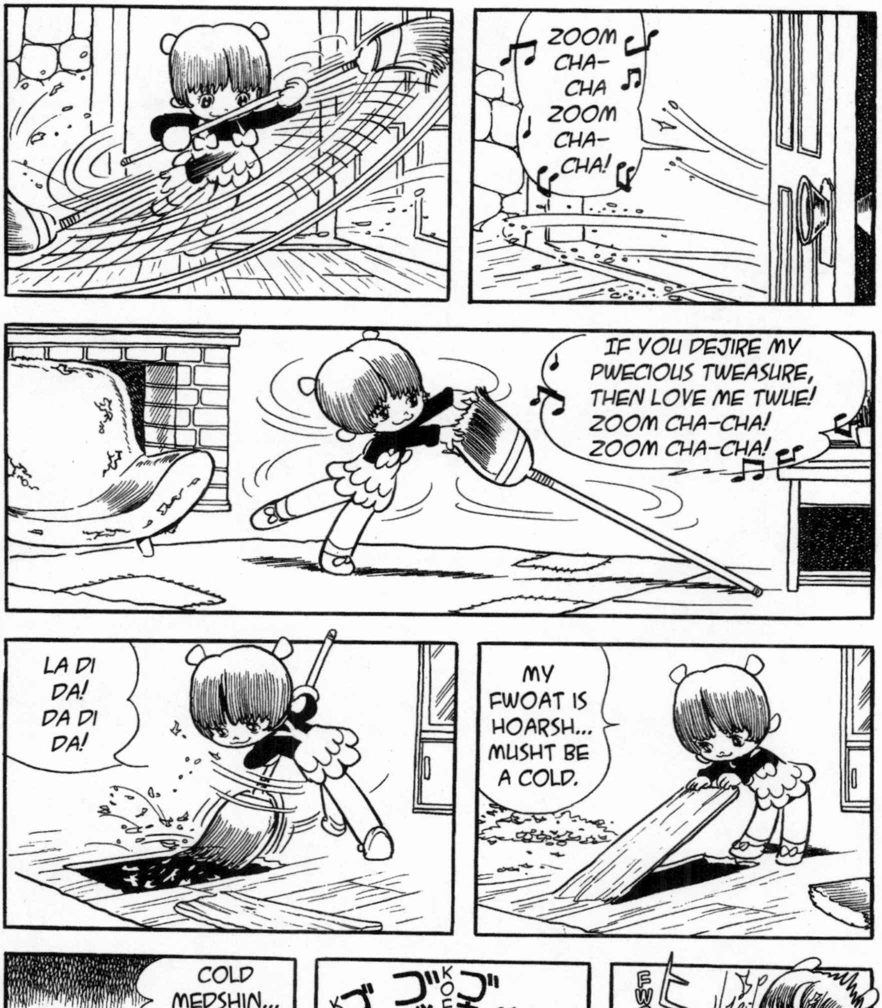
ZOOM CHA-CHA ZOOM CHA-CHA!
IF YOU DEJIRE MY PWECIOUS TWEASURE, THEN LOVE ME TWUE! ZOOM CHA-CHA! ZOOM CHA-CHA!
MY FWOAT IS HOARSH... MUSHT BE A COLD.
LA DI DA! DA DI DA!
ヒュー
FWOOO
ゴホ
KOFF
ゴッホ
KOFF
ゴホ
COLD MEDSHIN... FOUND IT!

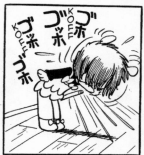

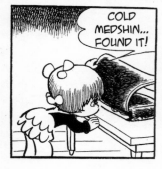

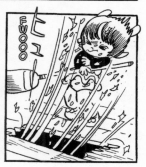

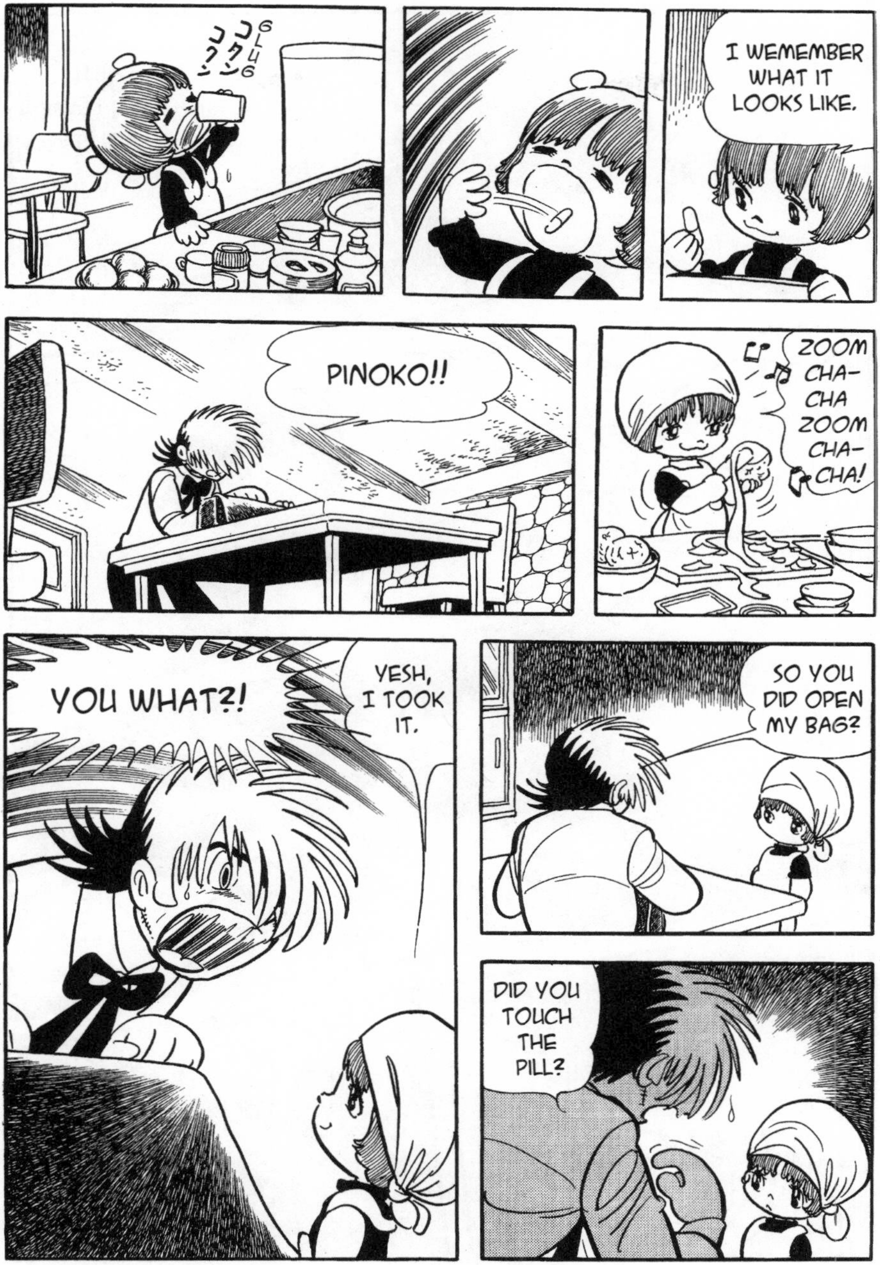
I WEMEMBER WHAT IT LOOKS LIKE.
GLUG
コクン コクン
ZOOM CHA-CHA ZOOM CHA-CHA!
PINOKO!!
SO YOU DID OPEN MY BAG?
DID YOU TOUCH THE PILL?
YESH, I TOOK IT.
YOU WHAT?!

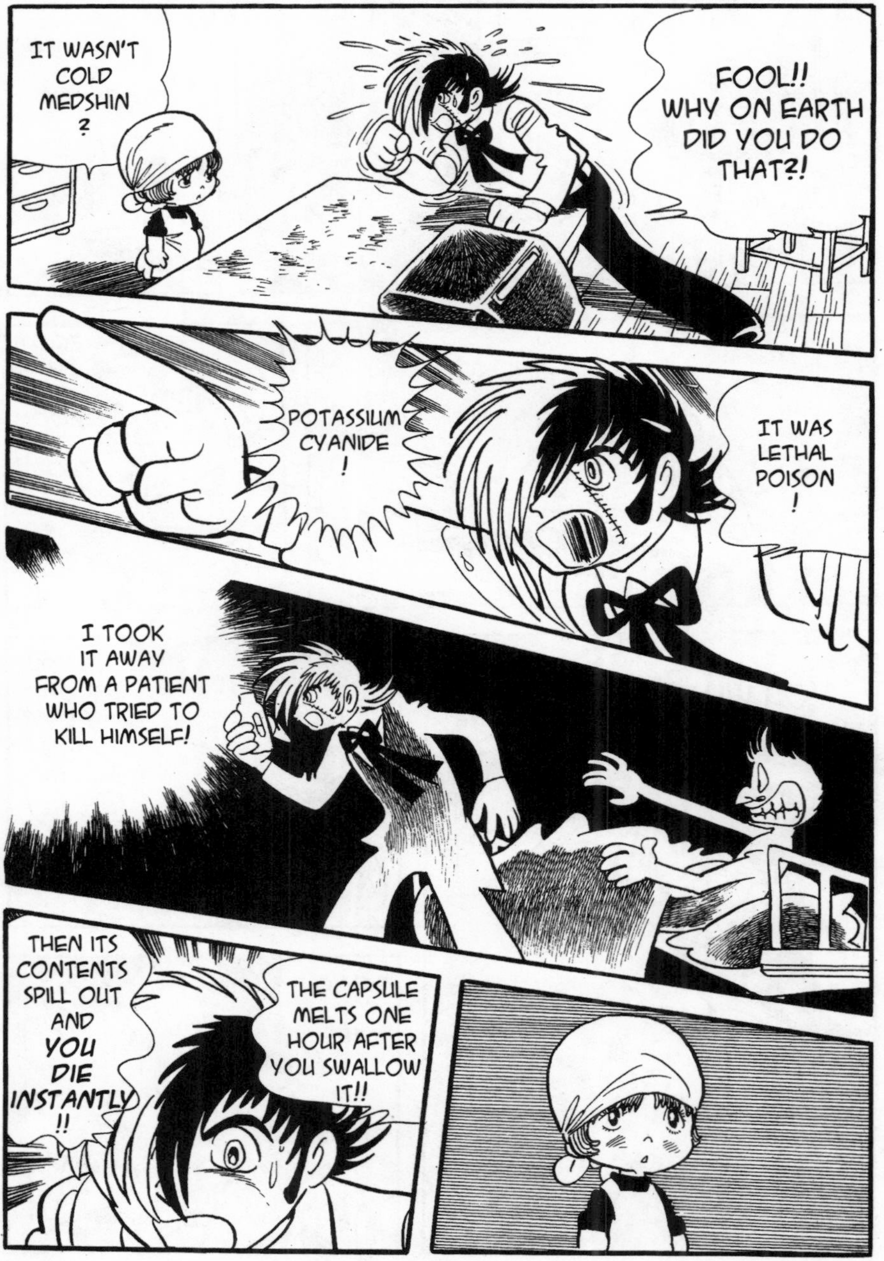
FOOL!! WHY ON EARTH DID YOU DO THAT?!
IT WASN'T COLD MEDSHIN ?
IT WAS LETHAL POISON !
POTASSIUM CYANIDE !
I TOOK IT AWAY FROM A PATIENT WHO TRIED TO KILL HIMSELF!
THE CAPSULE MELTS ONE HOUR AFTER YOU SWALLOW IT!!
THEN ITS CONTENTS SPILL OUT AND YOU DIE INSTANTLY !!

PINOKO'S GONNA DIE?
HOW LONG AGO DID YOU TAKE IT ?
BEFORE COOKING SHUPPER, 'BOUT HALF AN HOUR AGO?
PINOKO!! YOU DON'T GET IT, DO YOU?
YOU'RE GOING TO DIE IN THIRTY MINUTES !!
WAAAAA
WAAAH

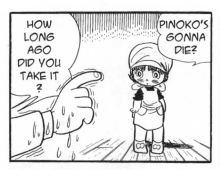

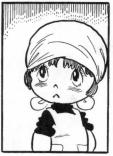

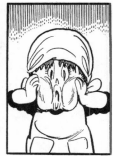

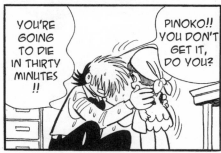

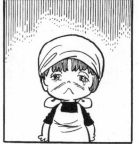

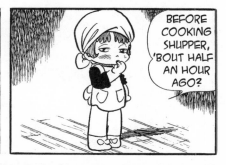

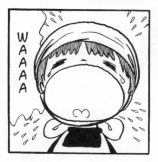

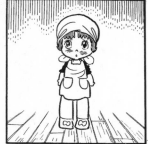

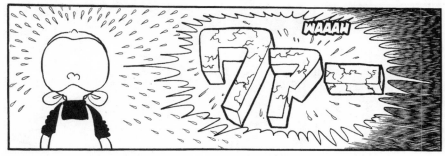

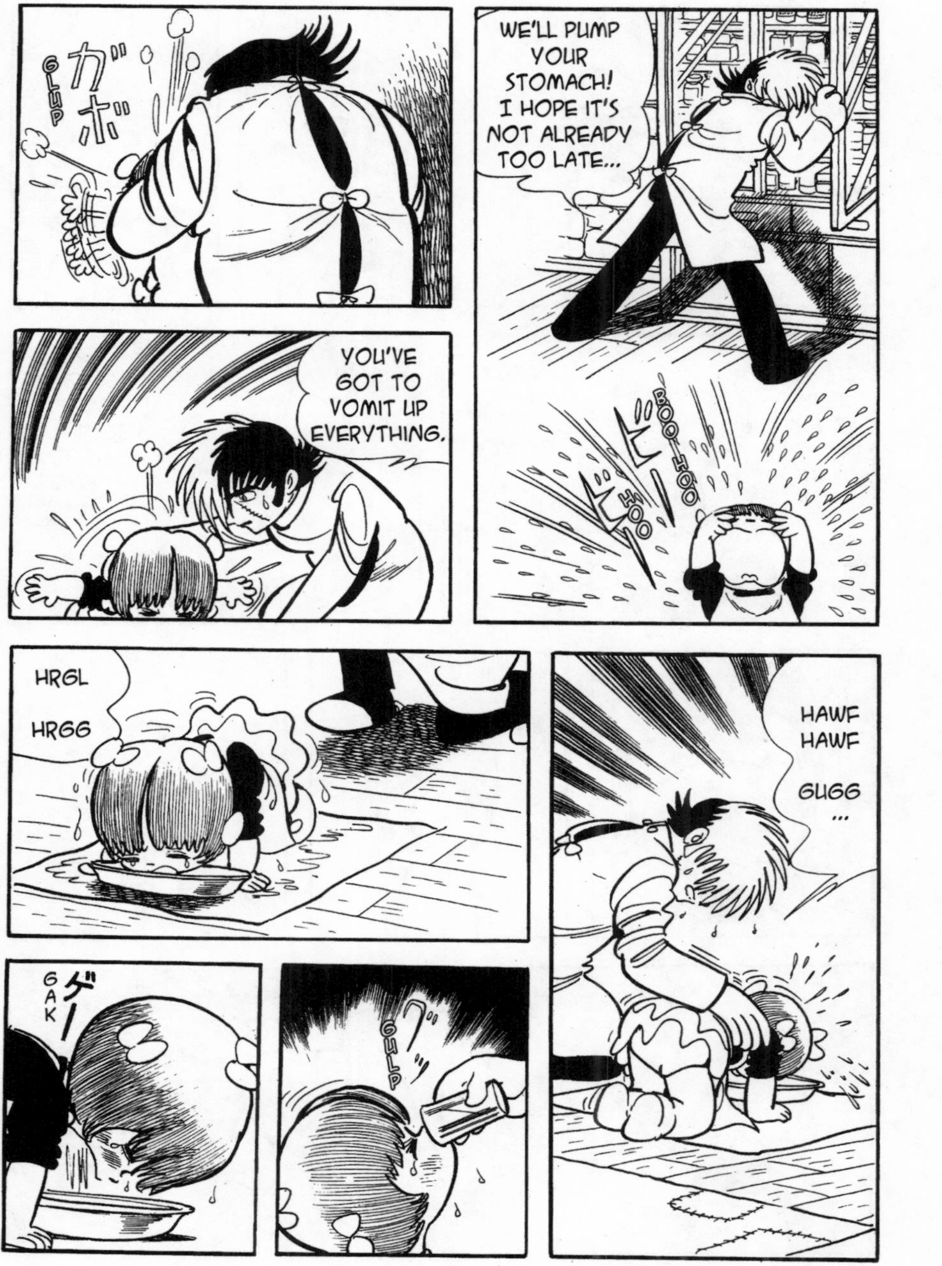
WE'LL PUMP YOUR STOMACH! I HOPE IT'S NOT ALREADY TOO LATE...
BOO-HOO
HOO HOO
ガボ
GLUP
YOU'VE GOT TO VOMIT UP EVERYTHING.
HAWF HAWF
GUGG ...
HRGL
HRGG
GULP
ゲー
GAK

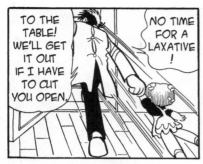

DARN! NOTHING ...
IT'S ALREADY SLIPPED THROUGH YOUR STOMACH!
NO TIME FOR A LAXATIVE!
TO THE TABLE! WE'LL GET IT OUT IF I HAVE TO CUT YOU OPEN.
HOW IS PINOKO GONNA DIE? WILL IT HURT?
POTASSIUM CYANIDE CAUSES INSTANT DEATH. YOUR BODY SEIZES UP, AND IT'S OVER.
I'LL TAKE AN X-RAY TO FIND THE PILL!

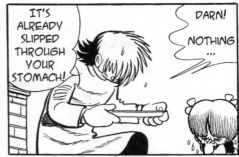

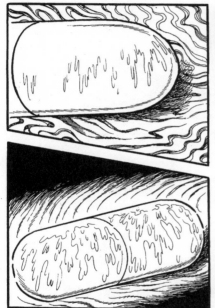

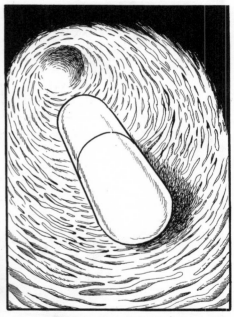

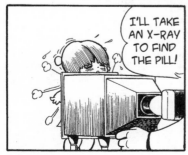

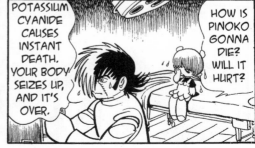

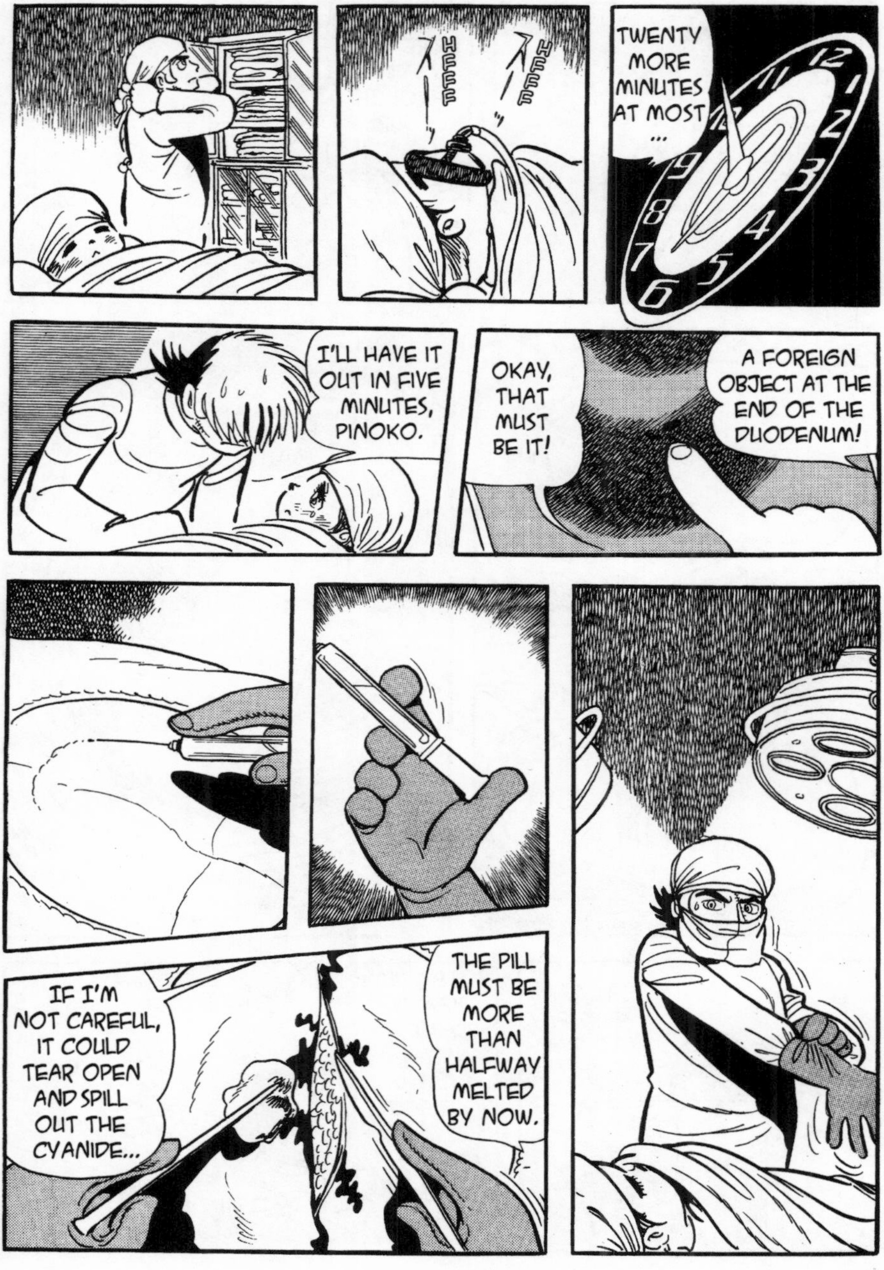
TWENTY MORE MINUTES AT MOST ...
HEFFF
HEFFF
A FOREIGN OBJECT AT THE END OF THE DUODENUM!
OKAY, THAT MUST BE IT!
I'LL HAVE IT OUT IN FIVE MINUTES, PINOKO.
THE PILL MUST BE MORE THAN HALFWAY MELTED BY NOW.
IF I'M NOT CAREFUL, IT COULD TEAR OPEN AND SPILL OUT THE CYANIDE...

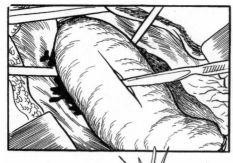

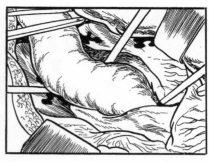

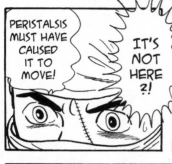

NOT HERE ...
NOT HERE !
IT'S NOT HERE ?!
PERISTALSIS MUST HAVE CAUSED IT TO MOVE!
THIS ISN'T LIKE ME. I'VE GOTTA CALM DOWN, RELAX.
IT MUST BE IN THE SMALL INTESTINE ...
I'D BETTER CLOSE UP THE DUODENUM AND INCISE LOWER.
I'VE ONLY MADE SUCH AN AMATEURISH BLUNDER A FEW TIMES IN MY CAREER...
SHK
SHK

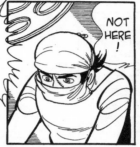

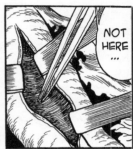

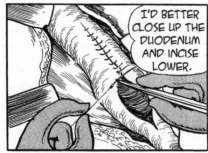

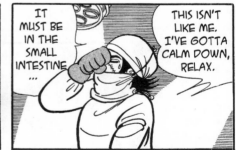

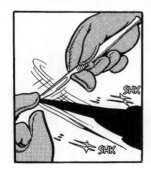

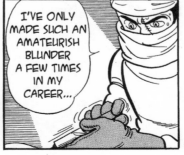

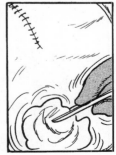

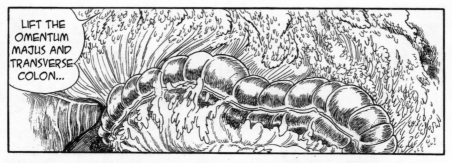

LIFT THE OMENTUM MAJUS AND TRANSVERSE COLON...
AND LOCATE THE LIGAMENT OF TREITZ AT THE ENTRANCE TO THE JEJUNUM!
IT EXTENDS THROUGH THE UPPER-LEFT PORTION OF THE PERITONEAL CAVITY...
BECOMING THE ILEUM. FOOD IS DIGESTED AND ABSORBED AS IT MAKES A JOURNEY SEVERAL METERS LONG...
THE CAPSULE IS IN THERE SOMEWHERE—MELTING AWAY!

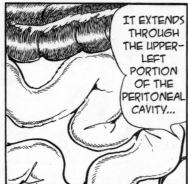

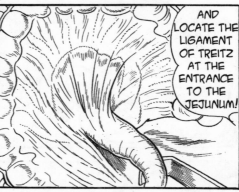

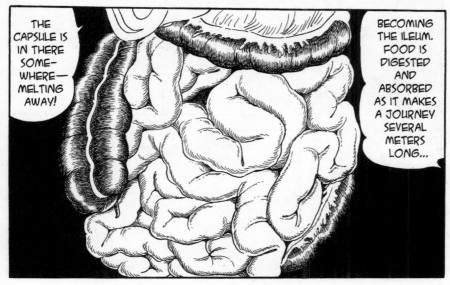

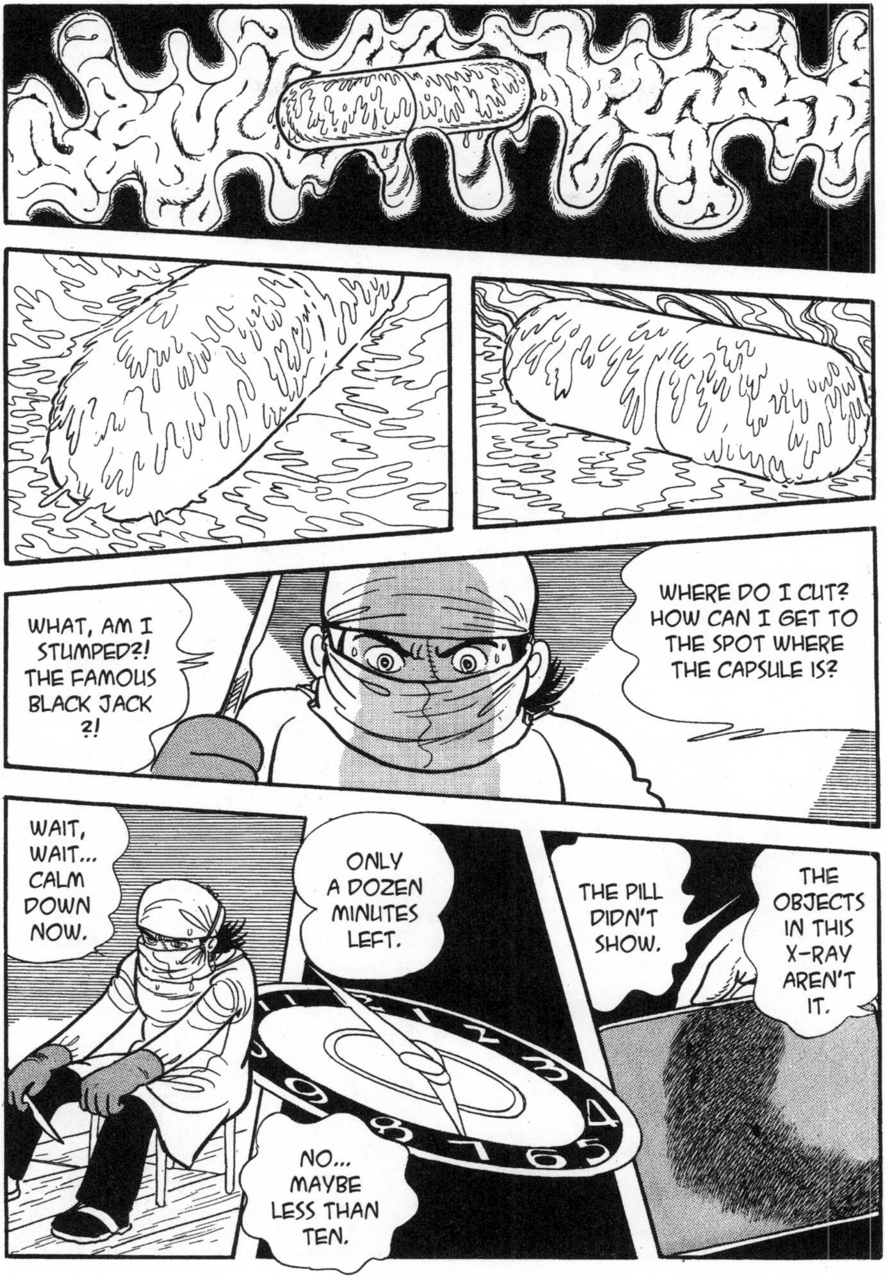
WHERE DO I CUT? HOW CAN I GET TO THE SPOT WHERE THE CAPSULE IS?
WHAT, AM I STUMPED?! THE FAMOUS BLACK JACK ?!
THE OBJECTS IN THIS X-RAY AREN'T IT.
THE PILL DIDN'T SHOW.
WAIT, WAIT... CALM DOWN NOW.
ONLY A DOZEN MINUTES LEFT.
NO... MAYBE LESS THAN TEN.

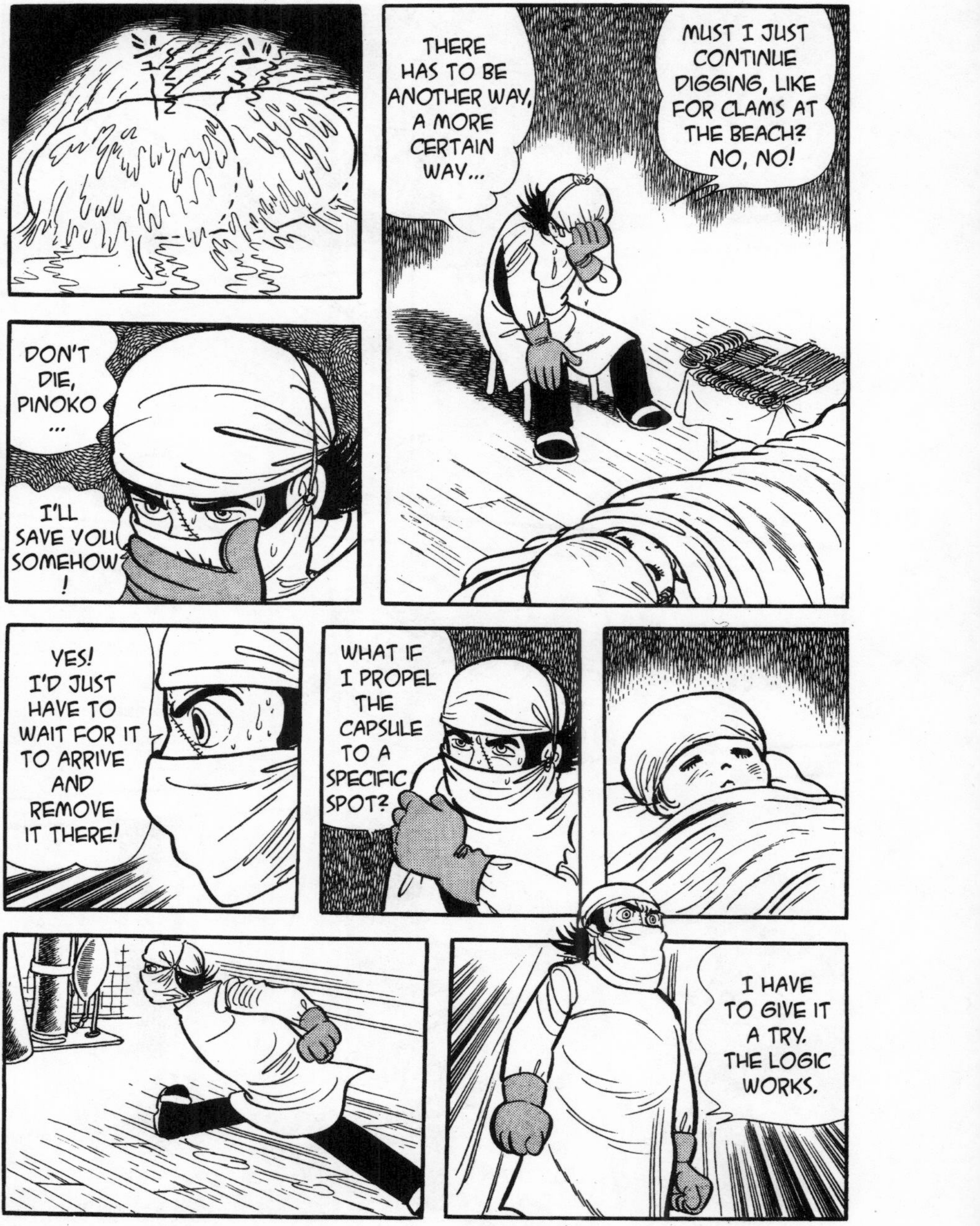
MUST I JUST CONTINUE DIGGING, LIKE FOR CLAMS AT THE BEACH? NO, NO!
THERE HAS TO BE ANOTHER WAY, A MORE CERTAIN WAY...
DON'T DIE, PINOKO ...
I'LL SAVE YOU SOMEHOW!
WHAT IF I PROPEL THE CAPSULE TO A SPECIFIC SPOT?
YES! I'D JUST HAVE TO WAIT FOR IT TO ARRIVE AND REMOVE IT THERE!
I HAVE TO GIVE IT A TRY. THE LOGIC WORKS.

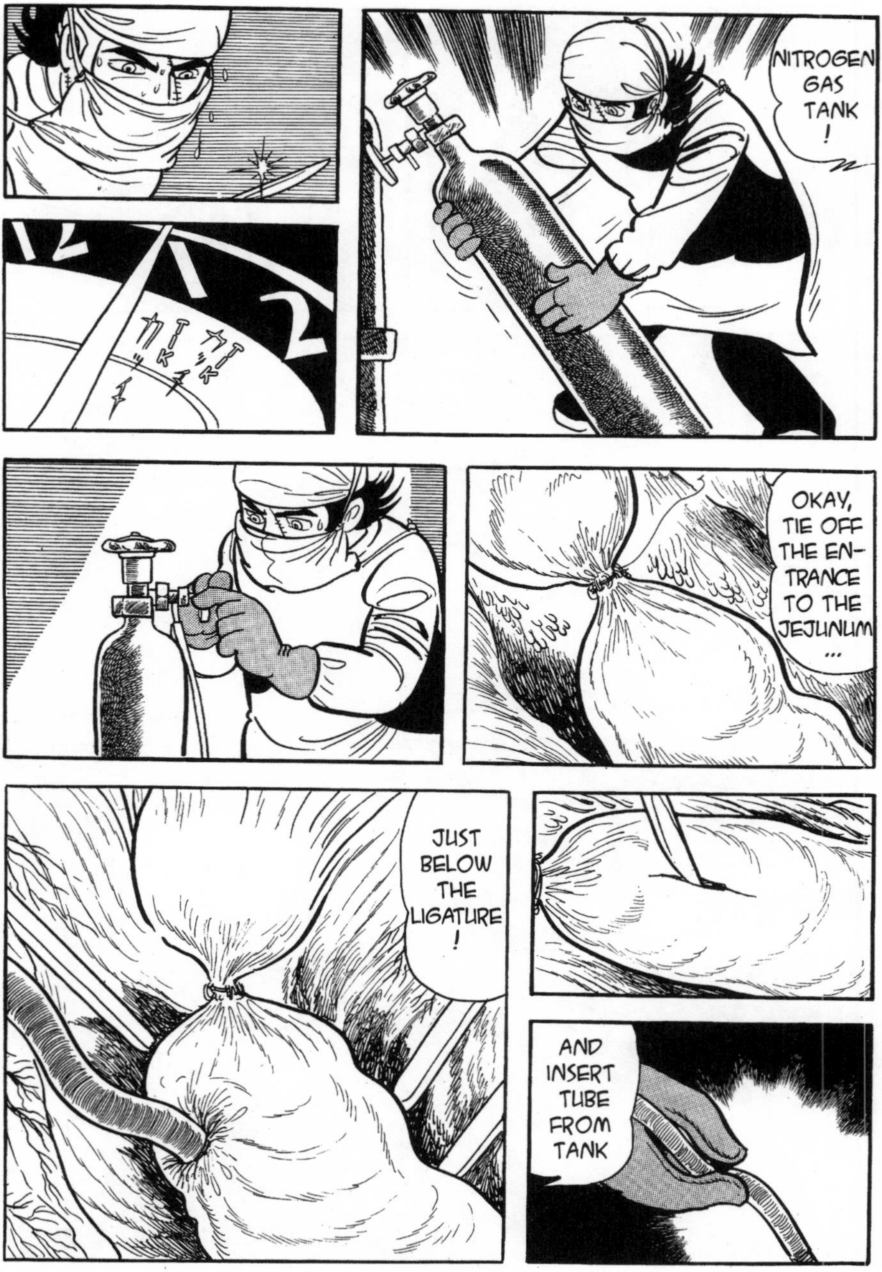
NITROGEN GAS TANK !
TIK
TIK
OKAY, TIE OFF THE EN- TRANCE TO THE JEJUNUM ...
AND INSERT TUBE FROM TANK
JUST BELOW THE LIGATURE !

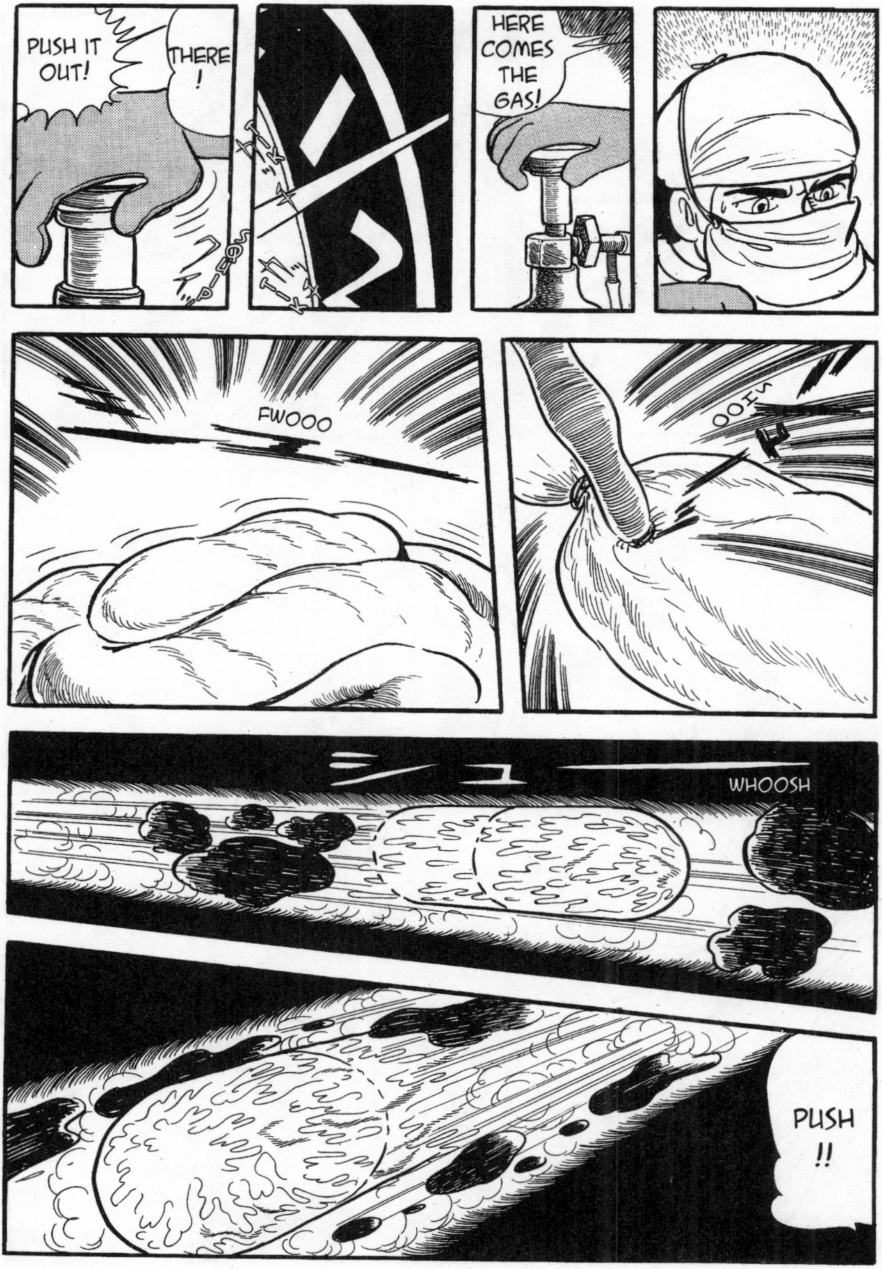
HERE COMES THE GAS!
THERE!
PUSH IT OUT!
FWOOO
WHOOSH
PUSH !!

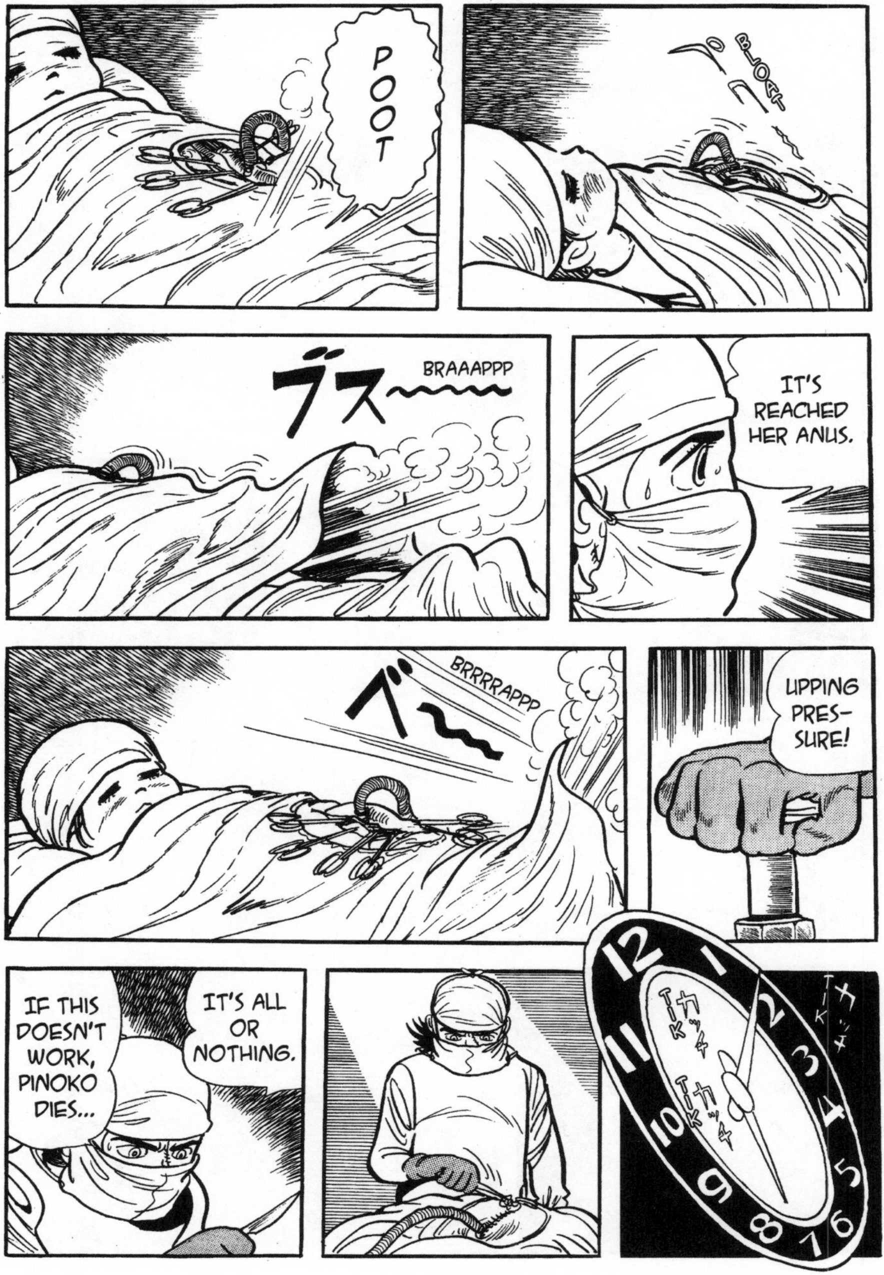
BLOOF
POOT
IT'S REACHED HER ANUS.
ブス～
BRAAAPPP
UPPING PRES-SURE!
ベ～
BRRRRAPPP
TIK
TIK
TIK
IT'S ALL OR NOTHING.
IF THIS DOESN'T WORK, PINOKO DIES...

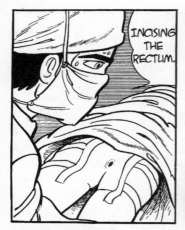

INCISING THE RECTUM.

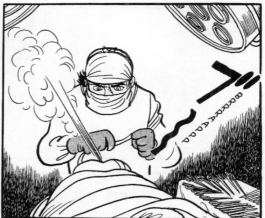

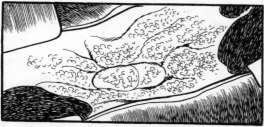

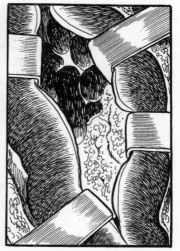

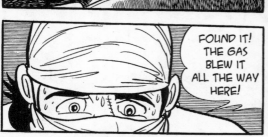

FOUND IT! THE GAS BLEW IT ALL THE WAY HERE!

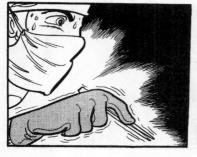

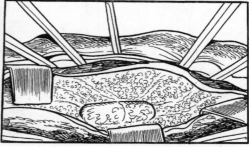

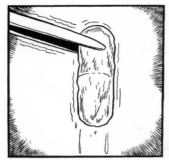

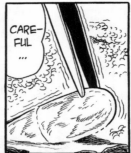

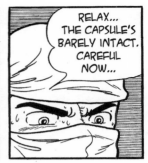

RELAX... THE CAPSULE'S BARELY INTACT. CAREFUL NOW...
CARE-FUL ...
ボロリ
SPILL
OHH !
フー
PHEW
ブー
BRAPPP

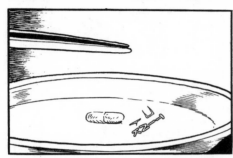

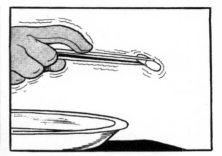

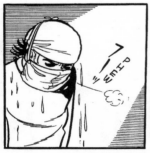

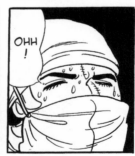

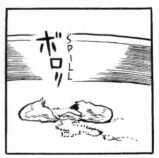

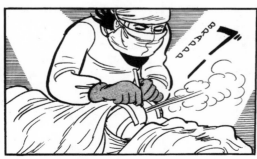

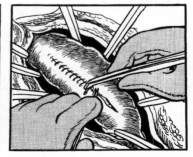

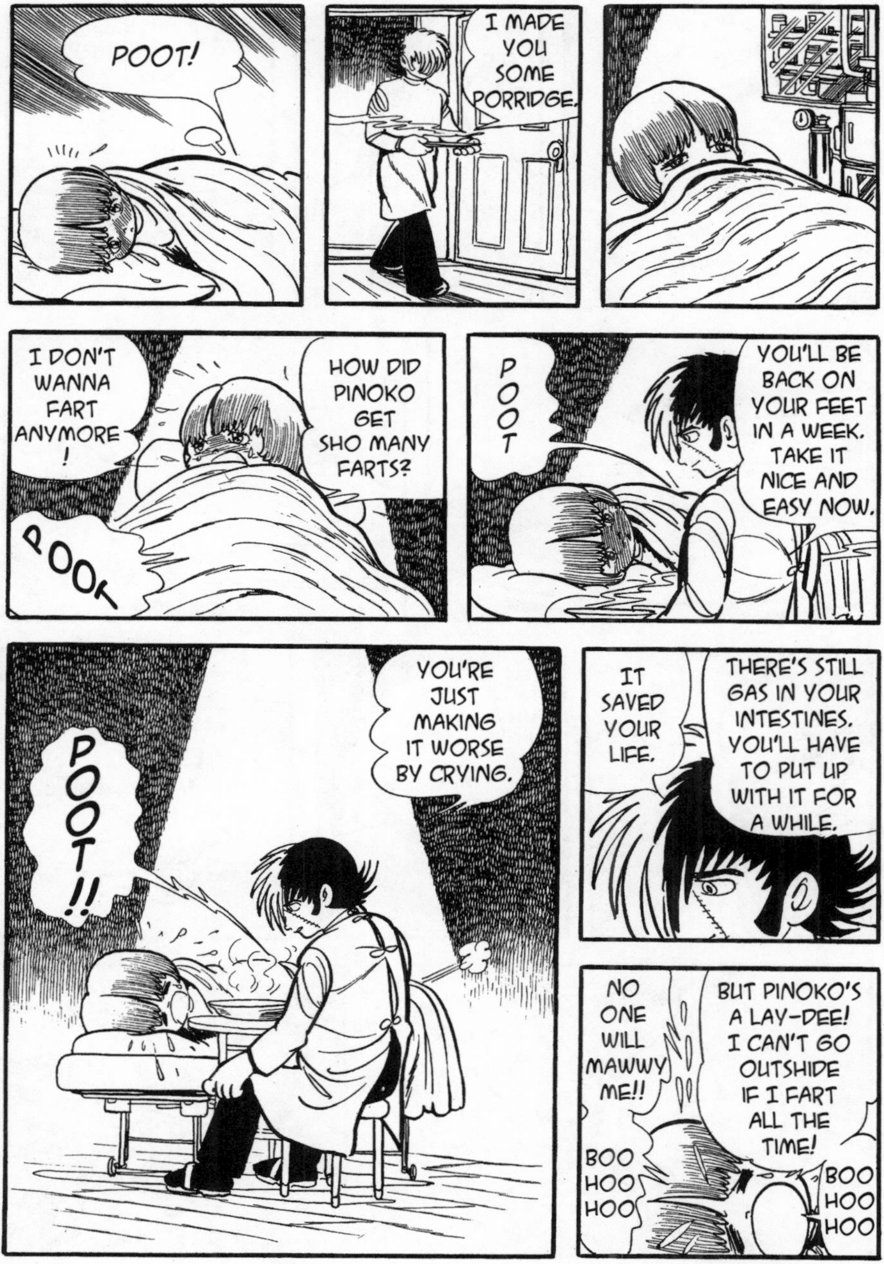
I MADE YOU SOME PORRIDGE.
POOT!
YOU'LL BE BACK ON YOUR FEET IN A WEEK. TAKE IT NICE AND EASY NOW.
POOT
HOW DID PINOKO GET SHO MANY FARTS?
I DON'T WANNA FART ANYMORE!
POOT
THERE'S STILL GAS IN YOUR INTESTINES. YOU'LL HAVE TO PUT UP WITH IT FOR A WHILE.
IT SAVED YOUR LIFE.
BUT PINOKO'S A LAY-DEE! I CAN'T GO OUTSHIDE IF I FART ALL THE TIME!
NO ONE WILL MAWWY ME!!
BOO HOO HOO
BOO HOO HOO
YOU'RE JUST MAKING IT WORSE BY CRYING.
POOT!!

FROM AFAR

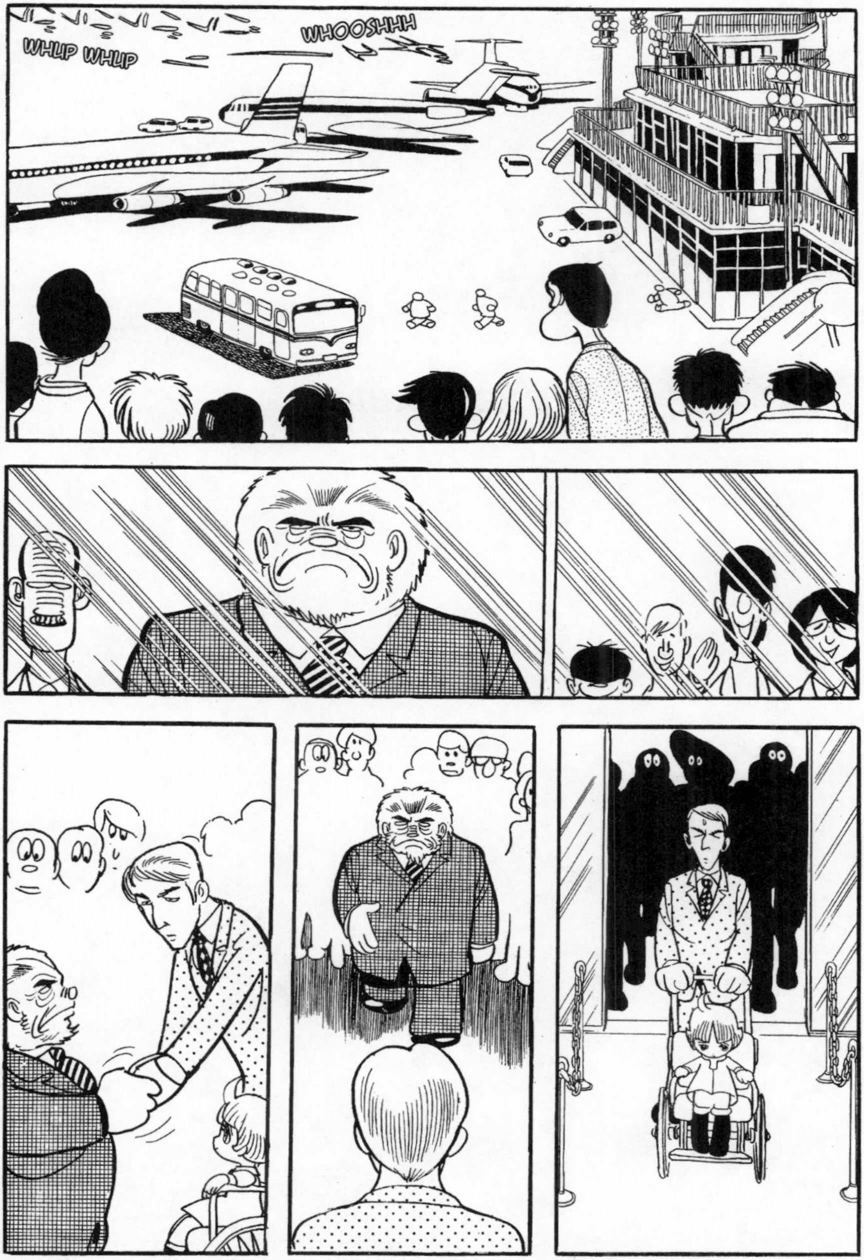
WHOOSHHH
WHUP WHUP

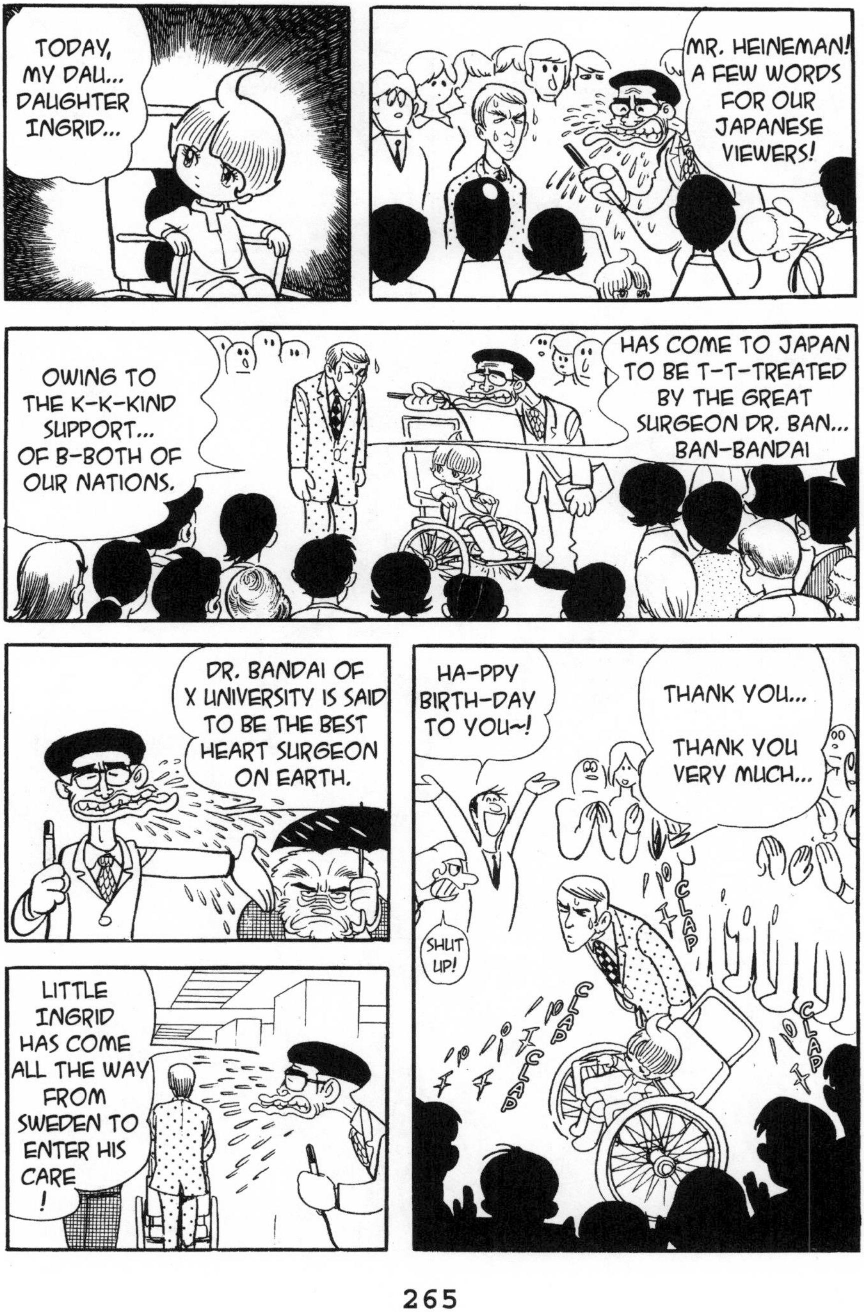

MR. HEINEMAN! A FEW WORDS FOR OUR JAPANESE VIEWERS!
TODAY, MY DAU... DAUGHTER INGRID...
HAS COME TO JAPAN TO BE T-T-TREATED BY THE GREAT SURGEON DR. BAN... BAN-BANDAI
OWING TO THE K-K-KIND SUPPORT... OF B-BOTH OF OUR NATIONS.
THANK YOU... THANK YOU VERY MUCH...
HA-PPY BIRTH-DAY TO YOU~!
CLAP
SHUT UP!
CLAP
CLAP
CLAP
DR. BANDAI OF X UNIVERSITY IS SAID TO BE THE BEST HEART SURGEON ON EARTH.
LITTLE INGRID HAS COME ALL THE WAY FROM SWEDEN TO ENTER HIS CARE!

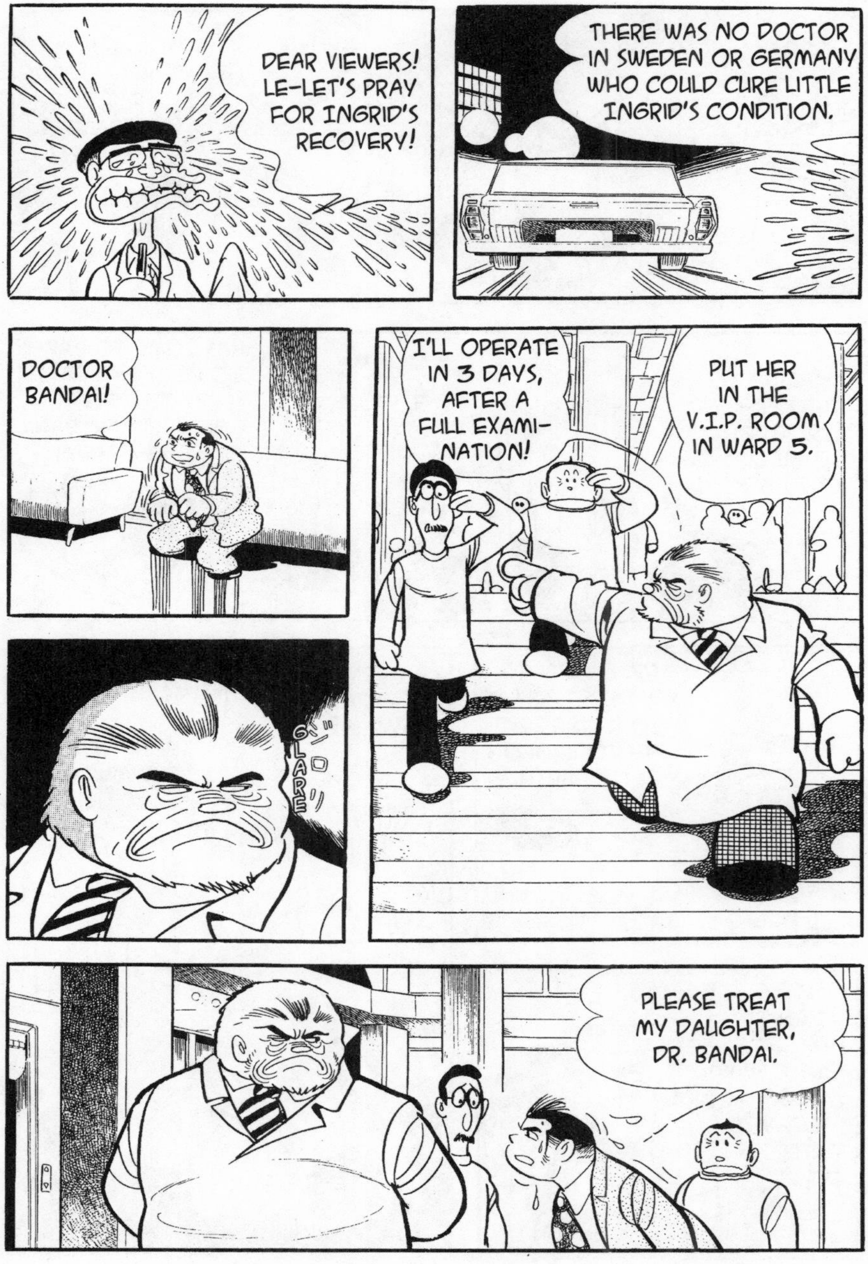
THERE WAS NO DOCTOR IN SWEDEN OR GERMANY WHO COULD CURE LITTLE INGRID'S CONDITION.
DEAR VIEWERS! LE-LET'S PRAY FOR INGRID'S RECOVERY!
PUT HER IN THE V.I.P. ROOM IN WARD 5.
I'LL OPERATE IN 3 DAYS, AFTER A FULL EXAMI-NATION!
DOCTOR BANDAI!
GLARE
PLEASE TREAT MY DAUGHTER, DR. BANDAI.

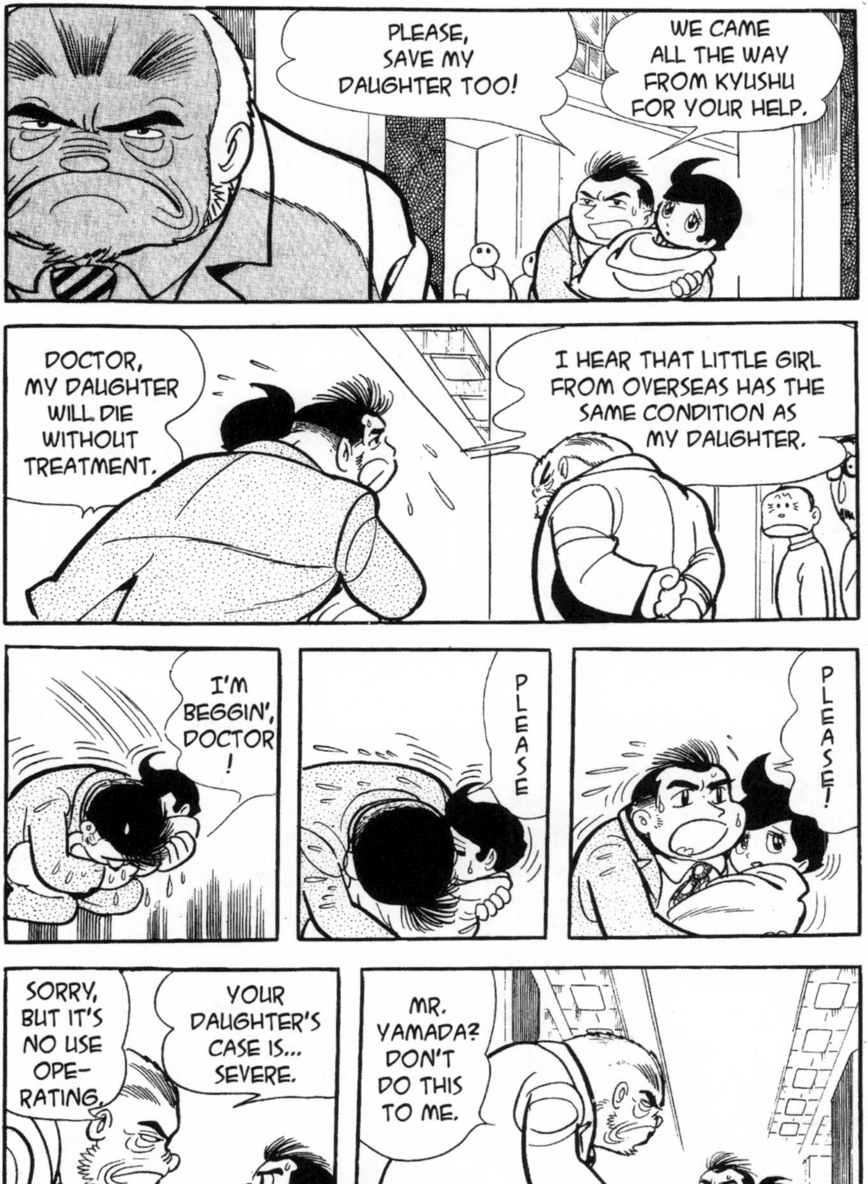
WE CAME ALL THE WAY FROM KYUSHU FOR YOUR HELP.
PLEASE, SAVE MY DAUGHTER TOO!
I HEAR THAT LITTLE GIRL FROM OVERSEAS HAS THE SAME CONDITION AS MY DAUGHTER.
DOCTOR, MY DAUGHTER WILL DIE WITHOUT TREATMENT.
PLEASE!
PLEASE
I'M BEGGIN', DOCTOR!
MR. YAMADA? DON'T DO THIS TO ME.
YOUR DAUGHTER'S CASE IS... SEVERE.
SORRY, BUT IT'S NO USE OPE-RATING.

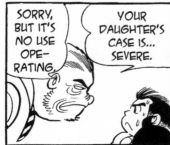

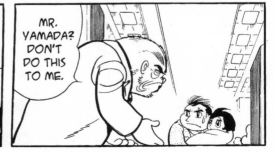

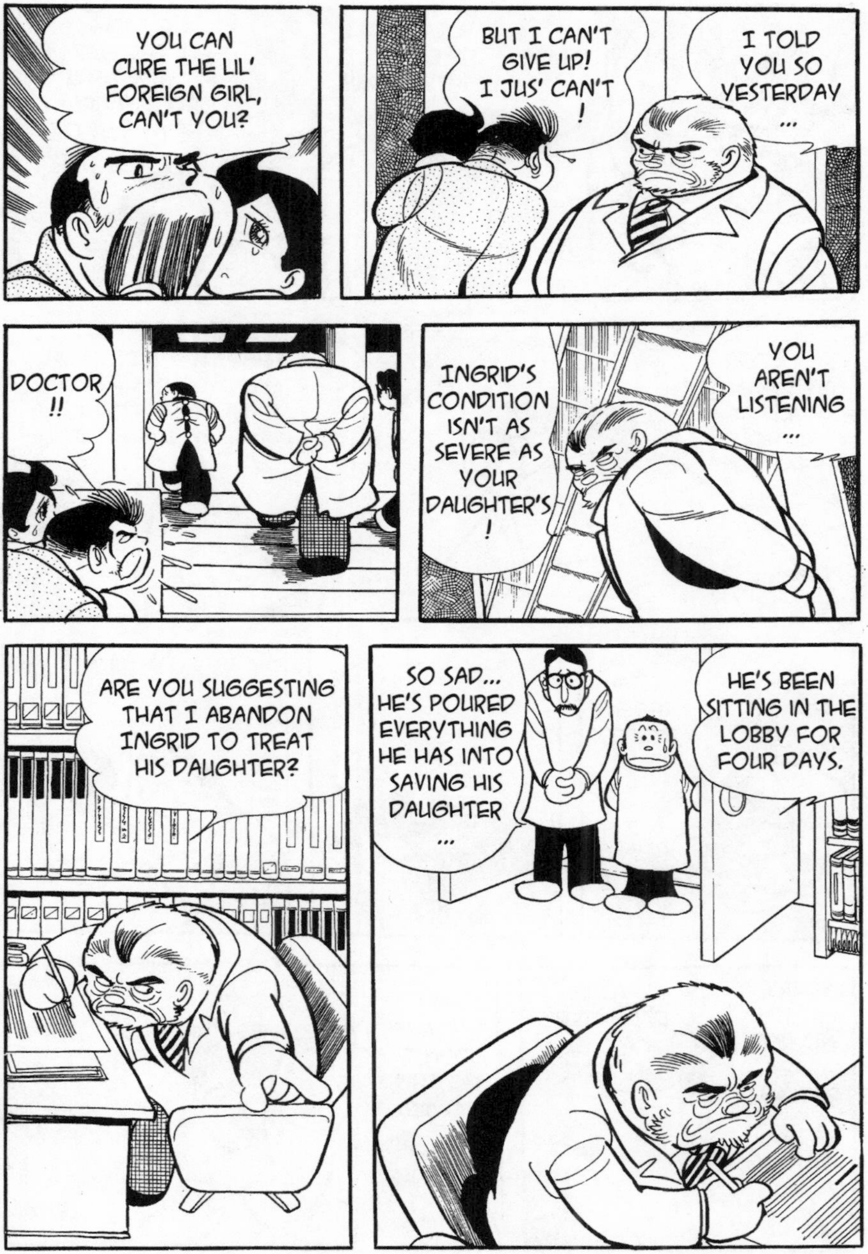
I TOLD YOU SO YESTERDAY ...
BUT I CAN'T GIVE UP! I JUS' CAN'T !
YOU CAN CURE THE LIL' FOREIGN GIRL, CAN'T YOU?
YOU AREN'T LISTENING ...
INGRID'S CONDITION ISN'T AS SEVERE AS YOUR DAUGHTER'S !
DOCTOR !!
HE'S BEEN SITTING IN THE LOBBY FOR FOUR DAYS.
SO SAD... HE'S POURED EVERYTHING HE HAS INTO SAVING HIS DAUGHTER ...
ARE YOU SUGGESTING THAT I ABANDON INGRID TO TREAT HIS DAUGHTER?

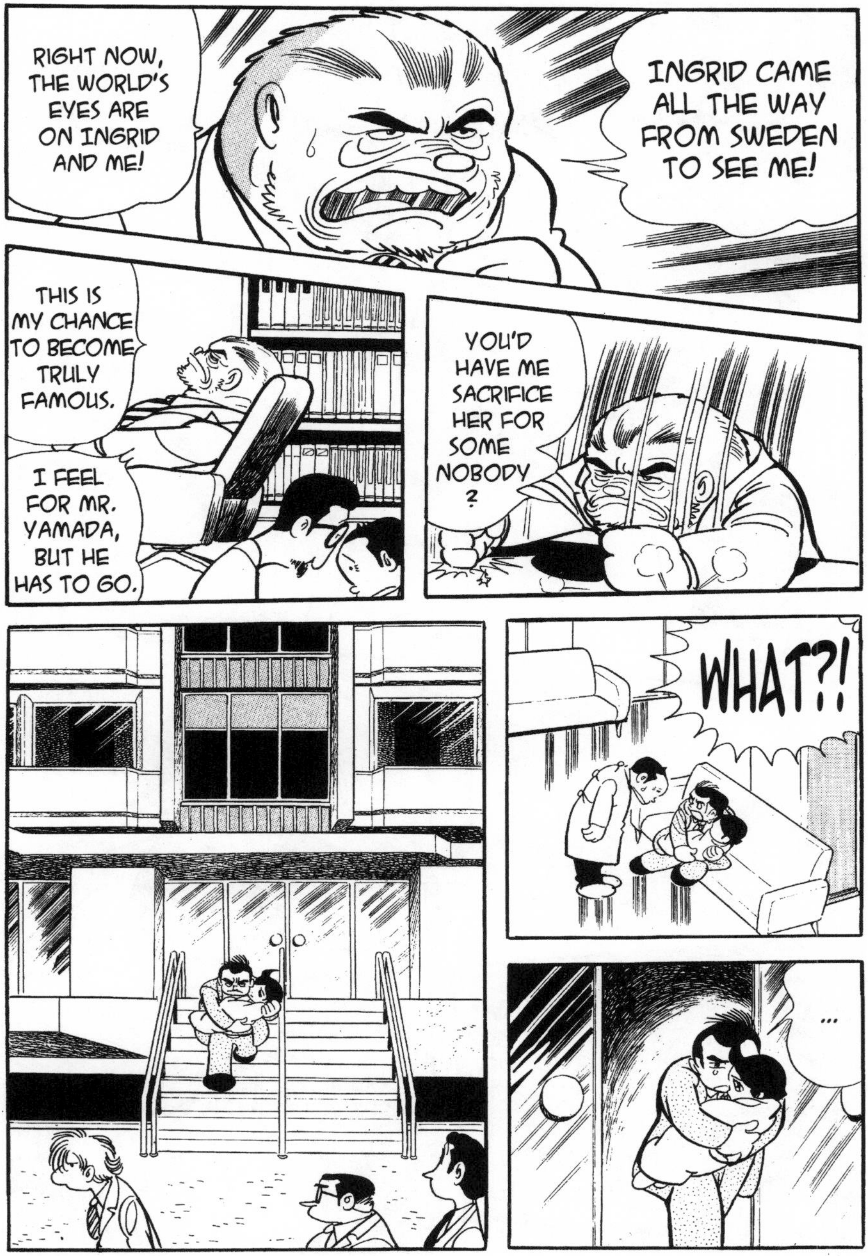
INGRID CAME ALL THE WAY FROM SWEDEN TO SEE ME!
RIGHT NOW, THE WORLD'S EYES ARE ON INGRID AND ME!
YOU'D HAVE ME SACRIFICE HER FOR SOME NOBODY?
THIS IS MY CHANCE TO BECOME TRULY FAMOUS.
I FEEL FOR MR. YAMADA, BUT HE HAS TO GO.
WHAT?!
...

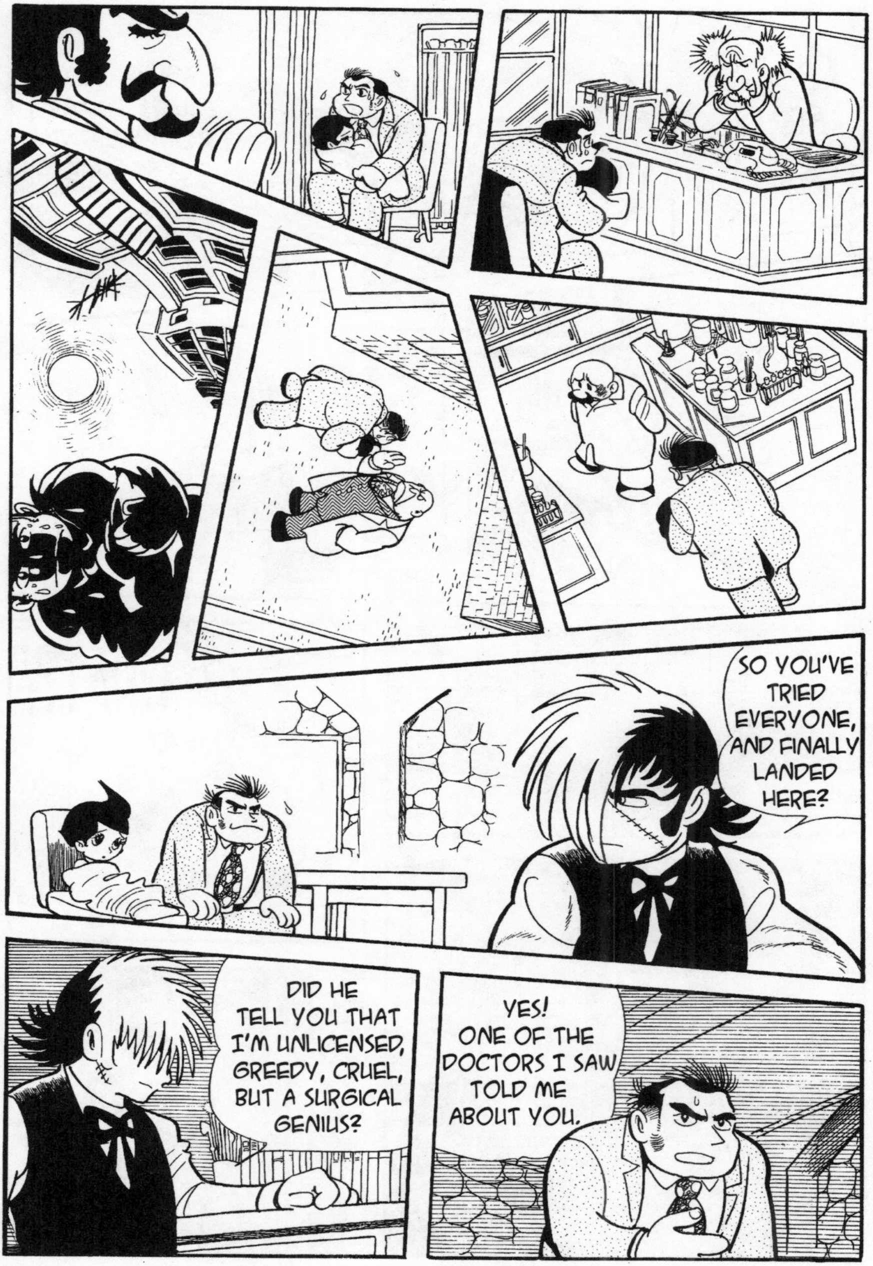
SO YOU'VE TRIED EVERYONE, AND FINALLY LANDED HERE?
YES! ONE OF THE DOCTORS I SAW TOLD ME ABOUT YOU.
DID HE TELL YOU THAT I'M UNLICENSED, GREEDY, CRUEL, BUT A SURGICAL GENIUS?

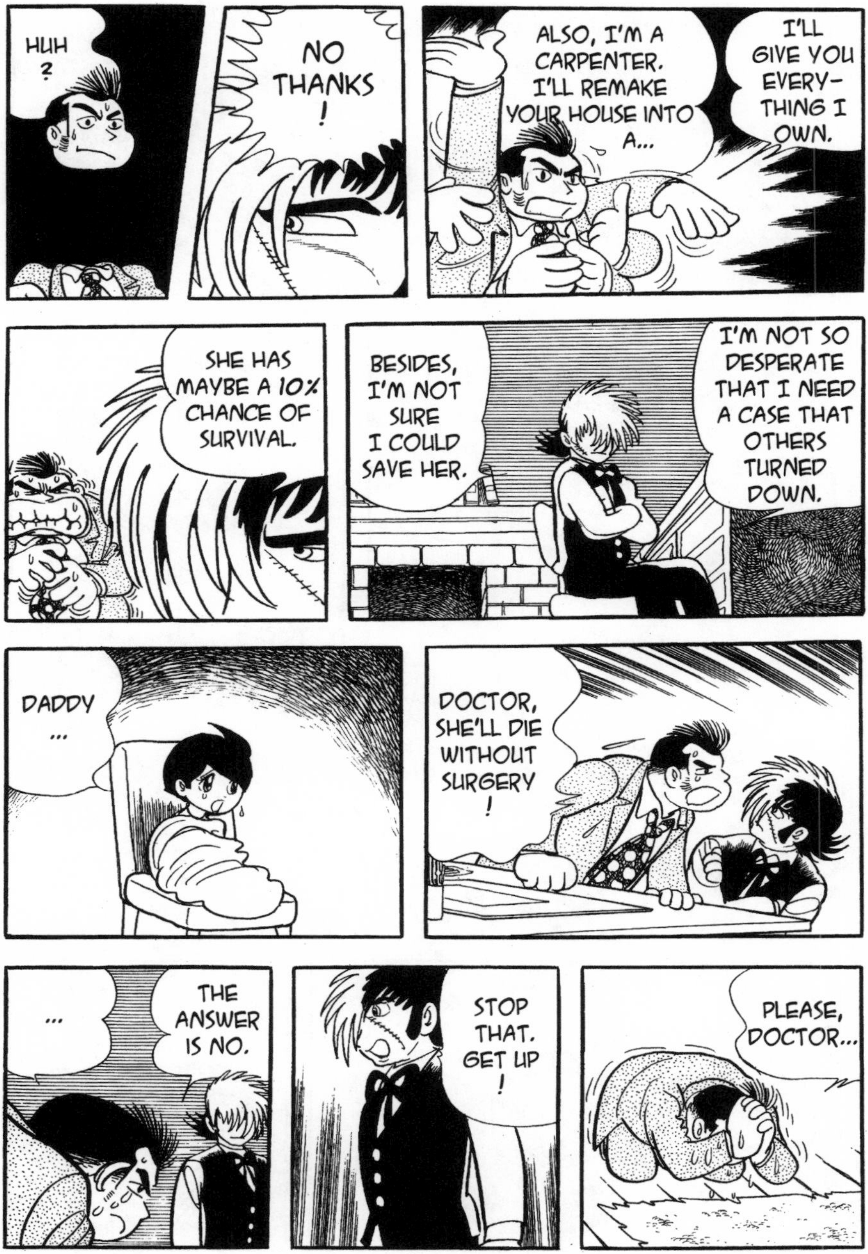
I'LL GIVE YOU EVERY-THING I OWN.
ALSO, I'M A CARPENTER. I'LL REMAKE YOUR HOUSE INTO A...
NO THANKS!
HUH?
I'M NOT SO DESPERATE THAT I NEED A CASE THAT OTHERS TURNED DOWN.
BESIDES, I'M NOT SURE I COULD SAVE HER.
SHE HAS MAYBE A 10% CHANCE OF SURVIVAL.
DOCTOR, SHE'LL DIE WITHOUT SURGERY!
DADDY...
PLEASE, DOCTOR...
STOP THAT. GET UP!
THE ANSWER IS NO.
...

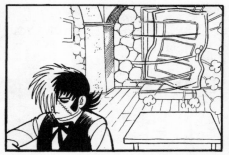

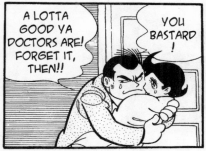

YOU BASTARD!
A LOTTA GOOD YA DOCTORS ARE! FORGET IT, THEN!!
LITTLE INGRID SUFFERS FROM A CONDITION CALLED "CARDIAC SEPTAL DEFECT WITH CALCIFICATION OF THE MITRAL AND AORTIC VALVES," WHICH REQUIRES EXTREMELY DIFFICULT SURGERY.
QUIT SPITTING, THIS IS A HOSPITAL!
YES. I HAVE PERFORMED THIS OPERATION SUCCESSFULLY 9 TIMES.
IF THERE'S ANOTHER DOCTOR WHO THINKS HE CAN PULL IT OFF, I'D LIKE TO MEET HIM!
HAR HAR HAR
MODERN TECHNOLOGY HAS HELPED, YES?
IT'S TRUE, TECHNOLOGY PLAYS A ROLE. THERE'S THE HEART-LUNG MACHINE.
BUT ULTIMATELY, IT BOILS DOWN TO SKILL— A GREAT DOCTOR'S SKILL!

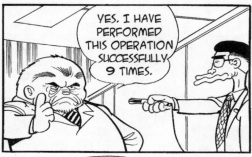

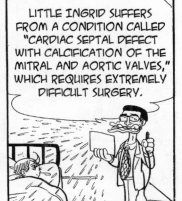

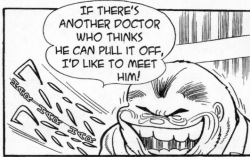

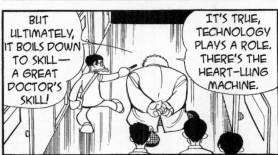

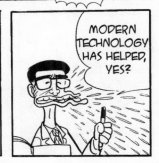

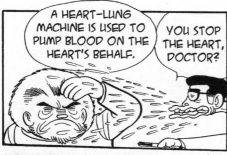

HEART SURGERY MUST BE UNIQUE, WHAT WITH THE BLOOD FLOWING IN AND OUT.
CORRECT. THAT'S WHY WE STOP THE BLOOD FLOW FOR THE DURATION.
YOU STOP THE HEART, DOCTOR?
A HEART-LUNG MACHINE IS USED TO PUMP BLOOD ON THE HEART'S BEHALF.
LET'S GET A SHOT OF THE APPARATUS FOR OUR VIEWERS!
THAT'S IT. THAT'S THE ARTIFICIAL LUNG.
NOW YOU'RE SEEING A ROLLER-STYLE ARTIFICIAL HEART.
WHAT'S YOUR PROGNOSIS, DOCTOR?
IF I WEREN'T SURE, I'D HAVE DECLINED.

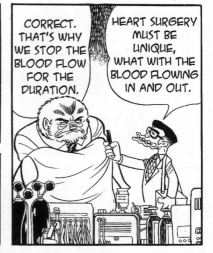

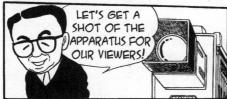

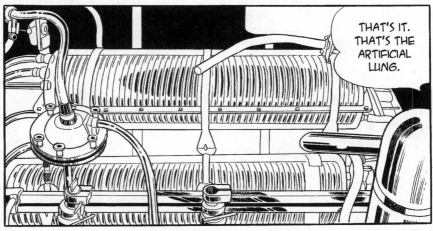

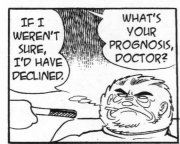

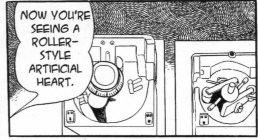

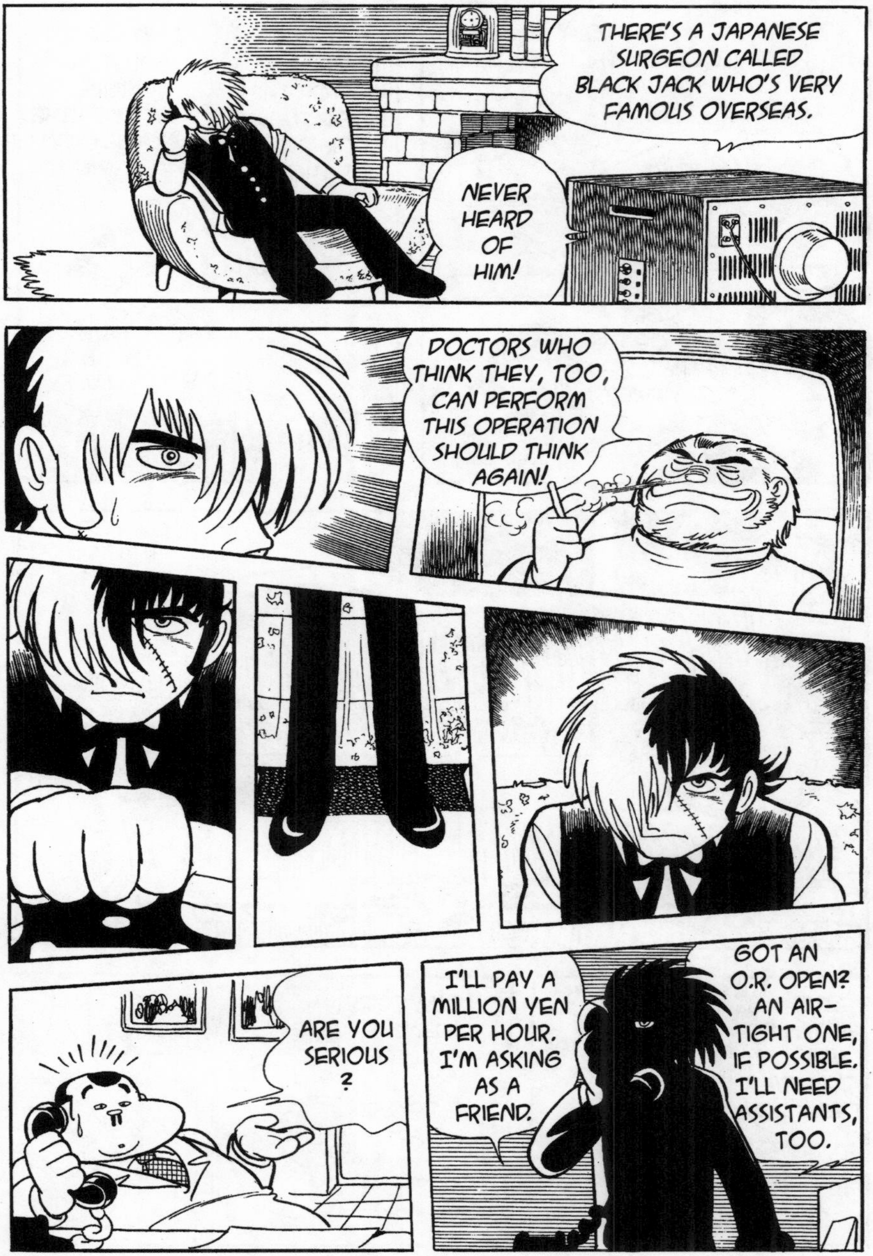
THERE'S A JAPANESE SURGEON CALLED BLACK JACK WHO'S VERY FAMOUS OVERSEAS.
NEVER HEARD OF HIM!
DOCTORS WHO THINK THEY, TOO, CAN PERFORM THIS OPERATION SHOULD THINK AGAIN!
GOT AN O.R. OPEN? AN AIR-TIGHT ONE, IF POSSIBLE. I'LL NEED ASSISTANTS, TOO.
I'LL PAY A MILLION YEN PER HOUR. I'M ASKING AS A FRIEND.
ARE YOU SERIOUS ?

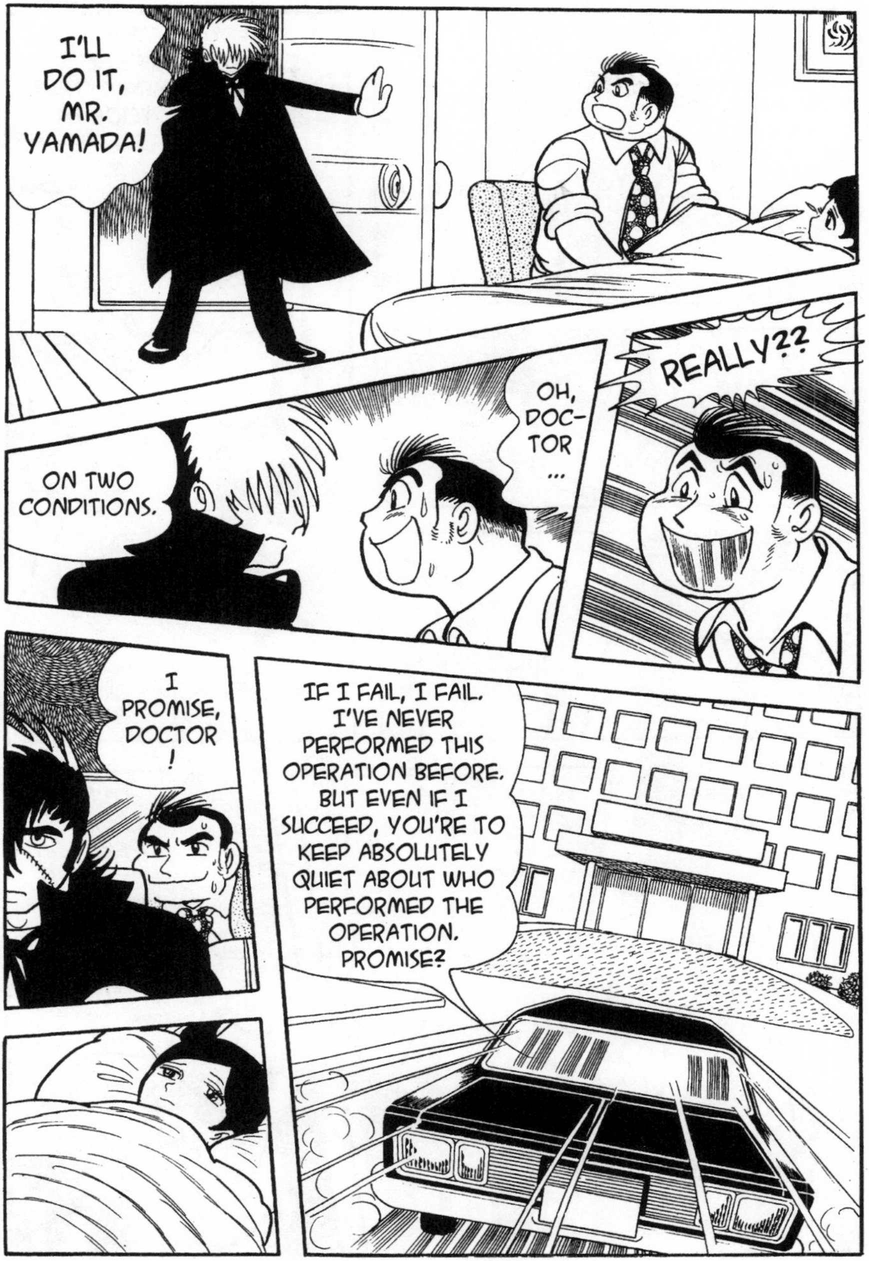
I'LL DO IT, MR. YAMADA!
REALLY??
OH, DOCTOR ...
ON TWO CONDITIONS.
IF I FAIL, I FAIL. I'VE NEVER PERFORMED THIS OPERATION BEFORE. BUT EVEN IF I SUCCEED, YOU'RE TO KEEP ABSOLUTELY QUIET ABOUT WHO PERFORMED THE OPERATION. PROMISE?
I PROMISE, DOCTOR!

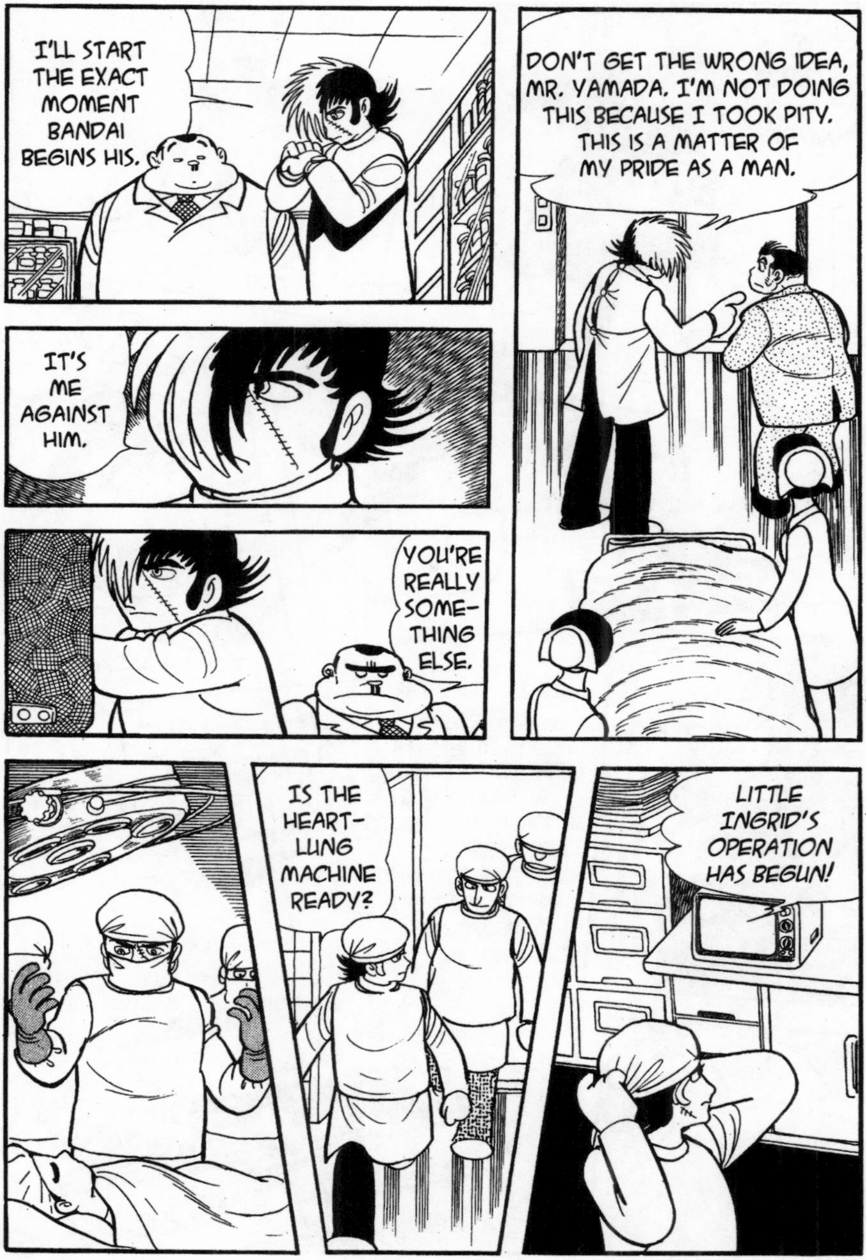
DON'T GET THE WRONG IDEA, MR. YAMADA. I'M NOT DOING THIS BECAUSE I TOOK PITY. THIS IS A MATTER OF MY PRIDE AS A MAN.
I'LL START THE EXACT MOMENT BANDAI BEGINS HIS.
IT'S ME AGAINST HIM.
YOU'RE REALLY SOMETHING ELSE.
LITTLE INGRID'S OPERATION HAS BEGUN!
IS THE HEART-LUNG MACHINE READY?

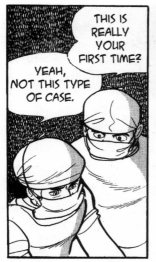

THIS IS REALLY YOUR FIRST TIME?
YEAH, NOT THIS TYPE OF CASE.
I WOULD NEVER HAVE GUESSED.
KOCHER...
NO, PÉAN FORCEPS!
THE HEART'S BEEN EXPOSED ...
READY THE HEART-LUNG MACHINE.

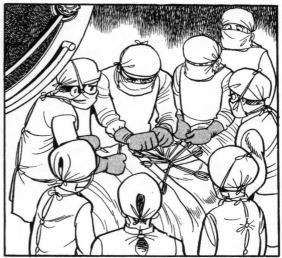

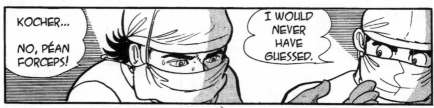

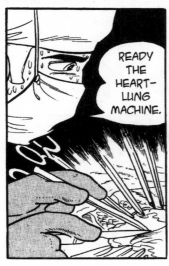

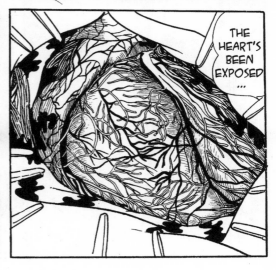

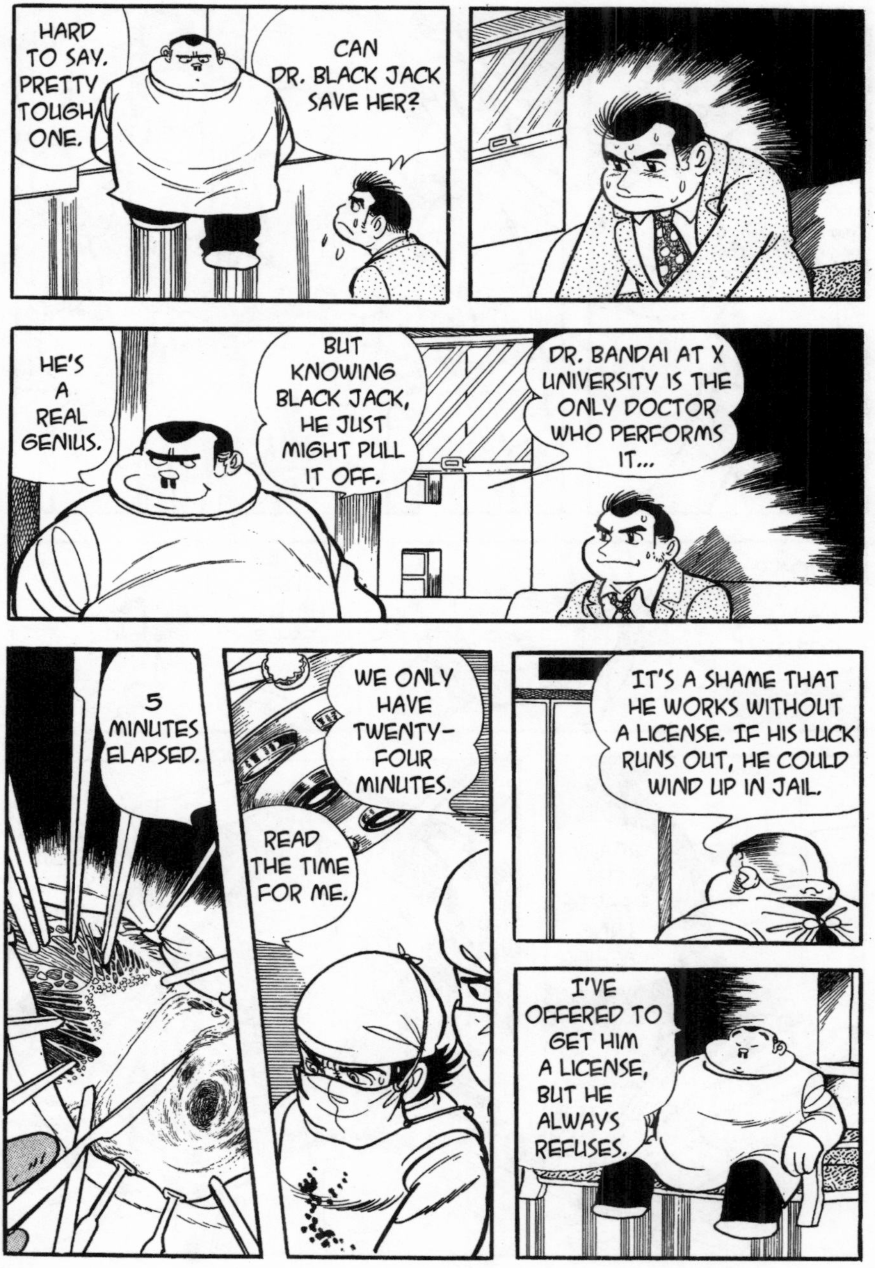
CAN DR. BLACK JACK SAVE HER?
HARD TO SAY. PRETTY TOUGH ONE.
DR. BANDAI AT X UNIVERSITY IS THE ONLY DOCTOR WHO PERFORMS IT...
BUT KNOWING BLACK JACK, HE JUST MIGHT PULL IT OFF.
HE'S A REAL GENIUS.
IT'S A SHAME THAT HE WORKS WITHOUT A LICENSE. IF HIS LUCK RUNS OUT, HE COULD WIND UP IN JAIL.
I'VE OFFERED TO GET HIM A LICENSE, BUT HE ALWAYS REFUSES.
WE ONLY HAVE TWENTY-FOUR MINUTES.
READ THE TIME FOR ME.
5 MINUTES ELAPSED.

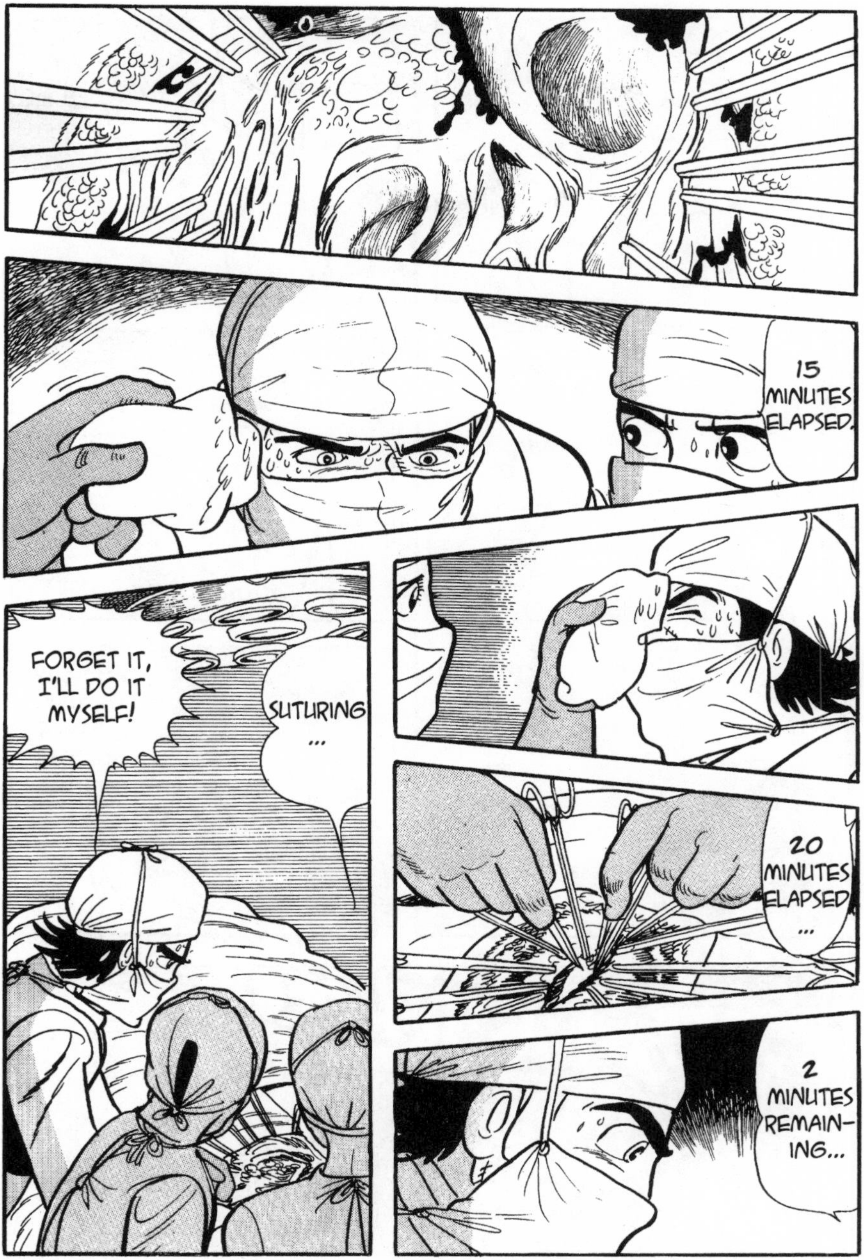
15 MINUTES ELAPSED.
20 MINUTES ELAPSED ...
2 MINUTES REMAINING...
SUTURING ...
FORGET IT, I'LL DO IT MYSELF!

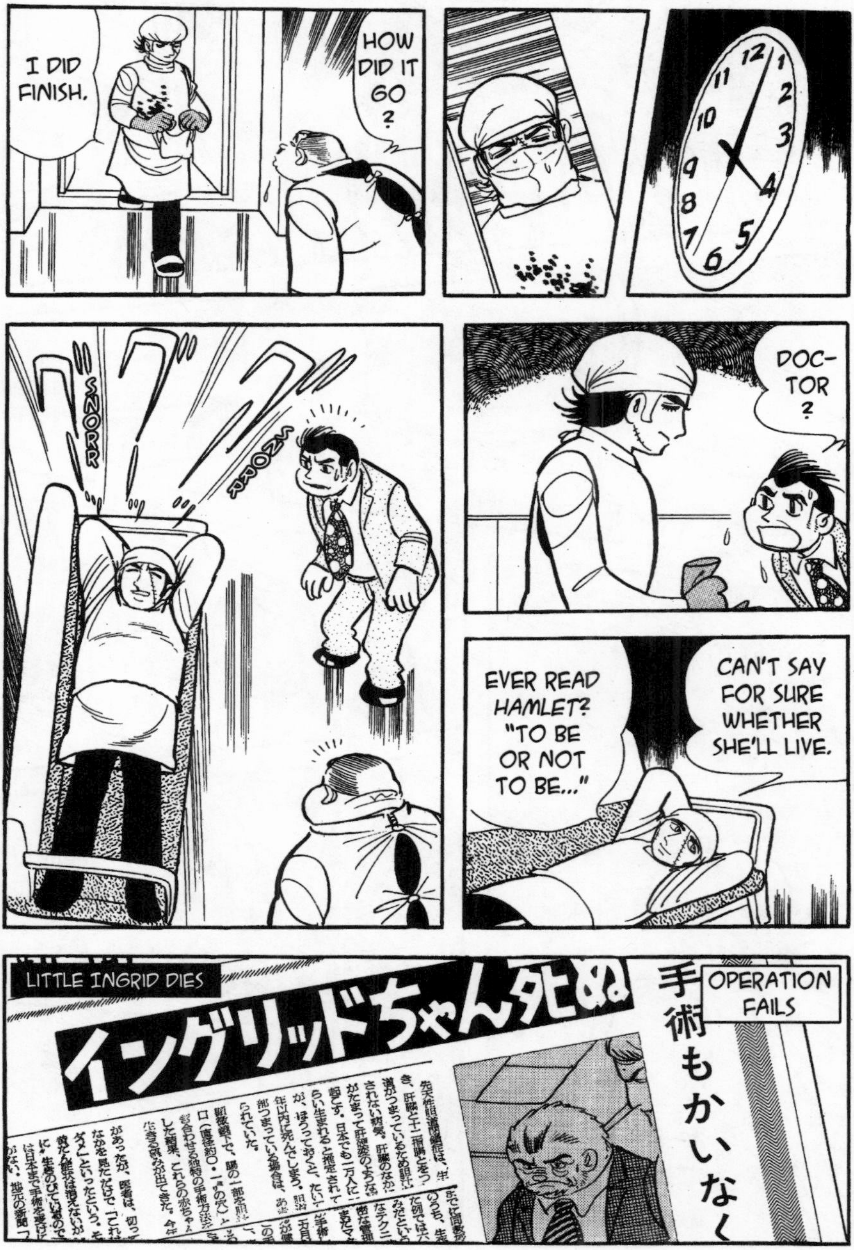
HOW DID IT GO?
I DID FINISH.
DOC-TOR?
CAN'T SAY FOR SURE WHETHER SHE'LL LIVE.
EVER READ HAMLET? "TO BE OR NOT TO BE..."
SNORRR
SNORRR
手術もかいなく
OPERATION FAILS
イングリッドちゃん死ぬ
LITTLE INGRID DIES

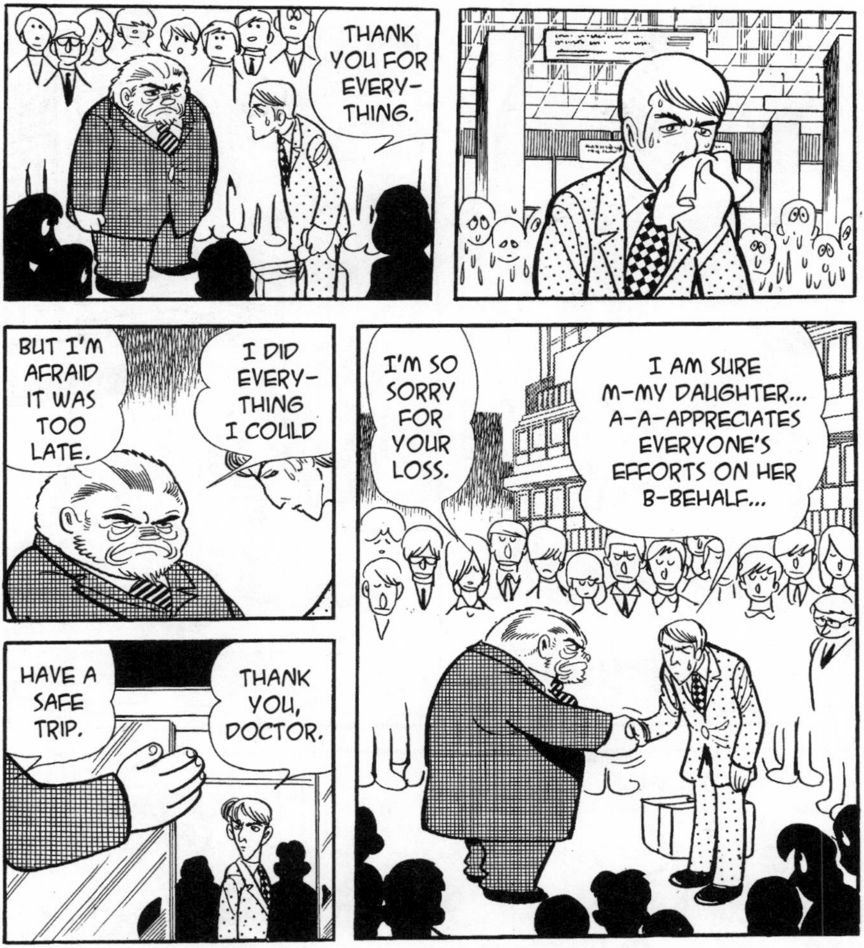
THANK YOU FOR EVERY-THING.
I AM SURE M-MY DAUGHTER... A-A-APPRECIATES EVERYONE'S EFFORTS ON HER B-BEHALF...
I'M SO SORRY FOR YOUR LOSS.
I DID EVERY-THING I COULD
BUT I'M AFRAID IT WAS TOO LATE.
THANK YOU, DOCTOR.
HAVE A SAFE TRIP.
AH, WELL. THESE THINGS HAPPEN.

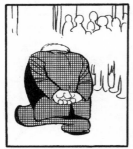

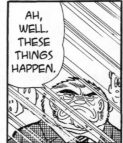

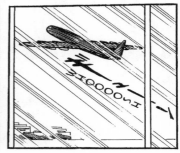

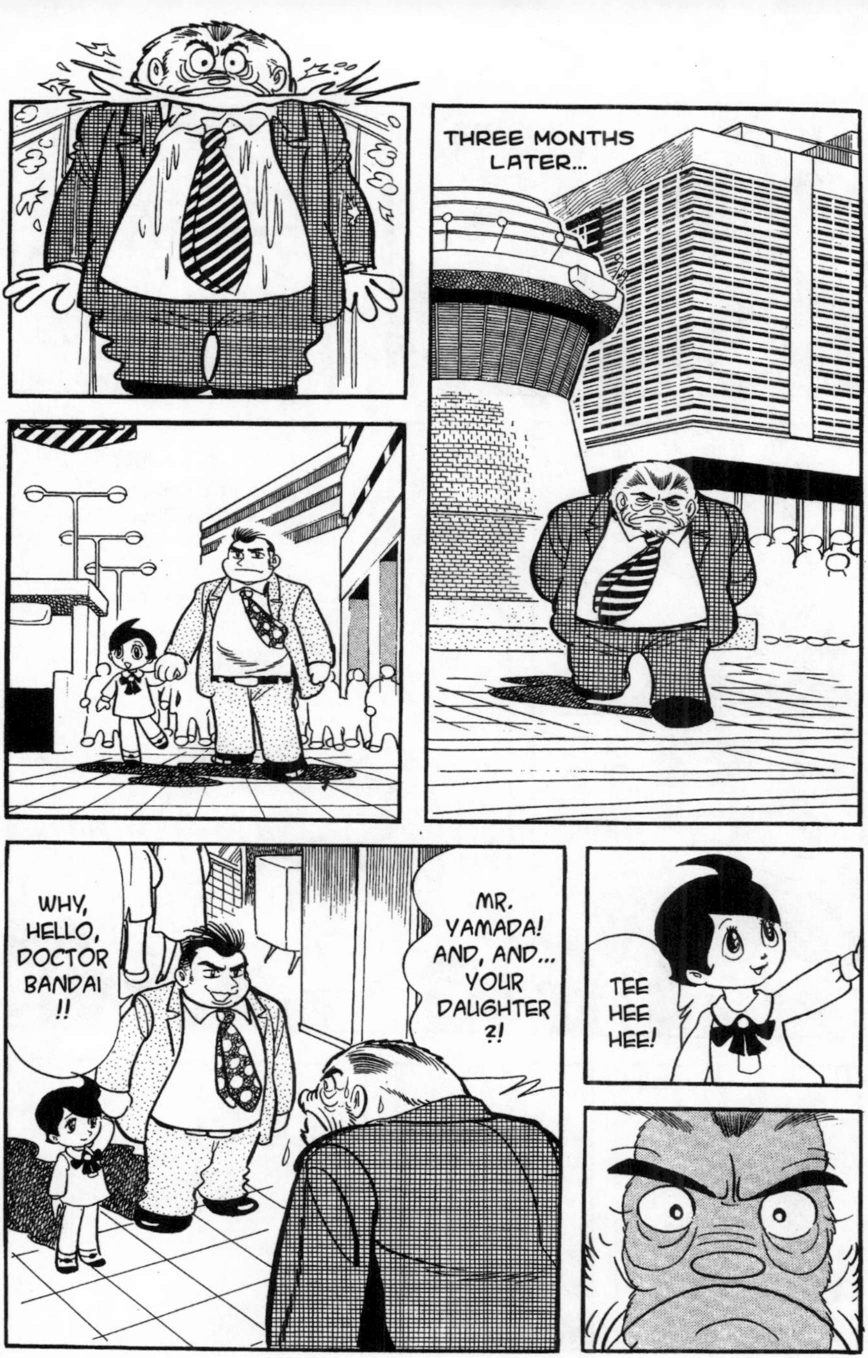
THREE MONTHS LATER...
TEE HEE HEE!
MR. YAMADA! AND, AND... YOUR DAUGHTER ?!
WHY, HELLO, DOCTOR BANDAI !!

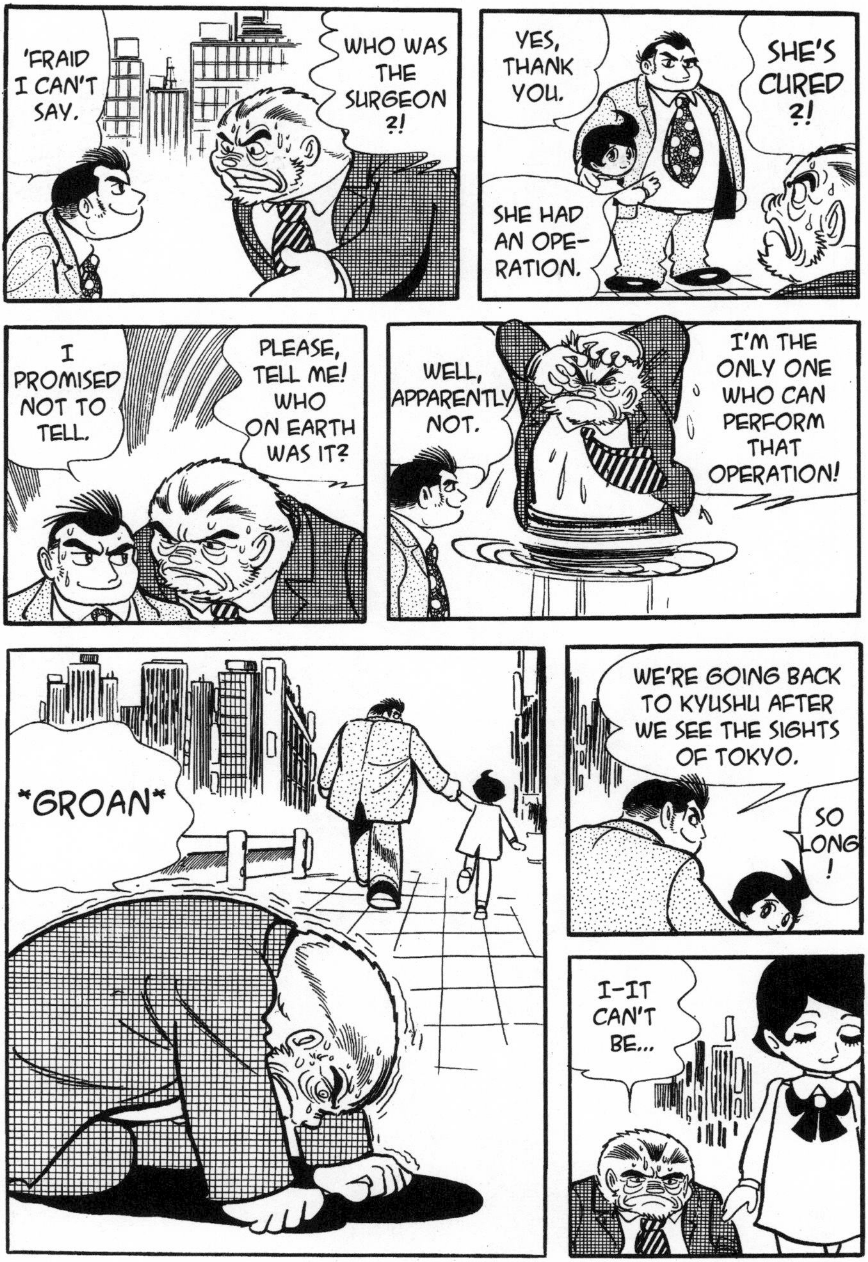
SHE'S CURED ?!
YES, THANK YOU.
SHE HAD AN OPERATION.
WHO WAS THE SURGEON ?!
'FRAID I CAN'T SAY.
I'M THE ONLY ONE WHO CAN PERFORM THAT OPERATION!
WELL, APPARENTLY NOT.
PLEASE, TELL ME! WHO ON EARTH WAS IT?
I PROMISED NOT TO TELL.
WE'RE GOING BACK TO KYUSHU AFTER WE SEE THE SIGHTS OF TOKYO.
SO LONG!
I-IT CAN'T BE...
GROAN

THIEVING DOG

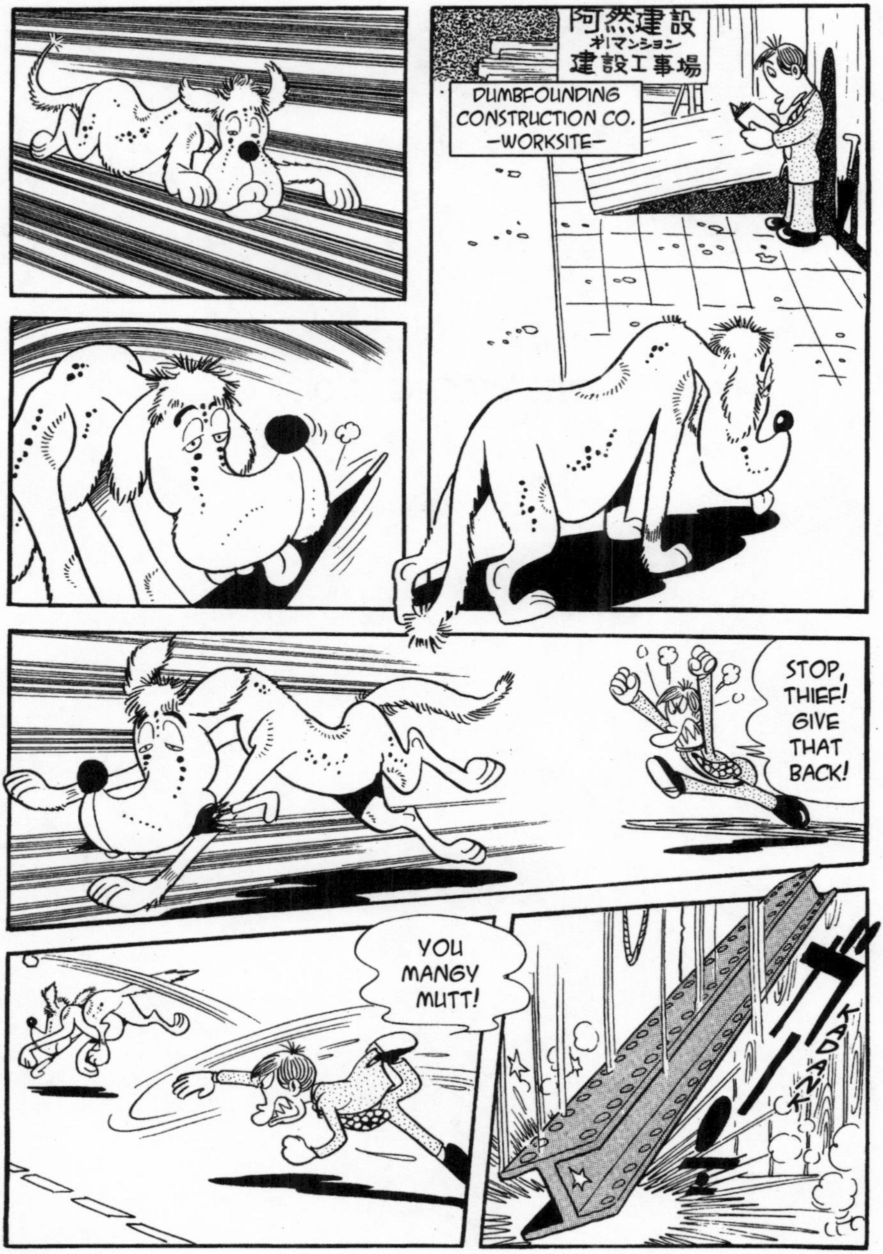
阿然建設
建設工事場
DUMBFOUNDING CONSTRUCTION CO. —WORKSITE—
STOP, THIEF! GIVE THAT BACK!
KADANK
YOU MANGY MUTT!

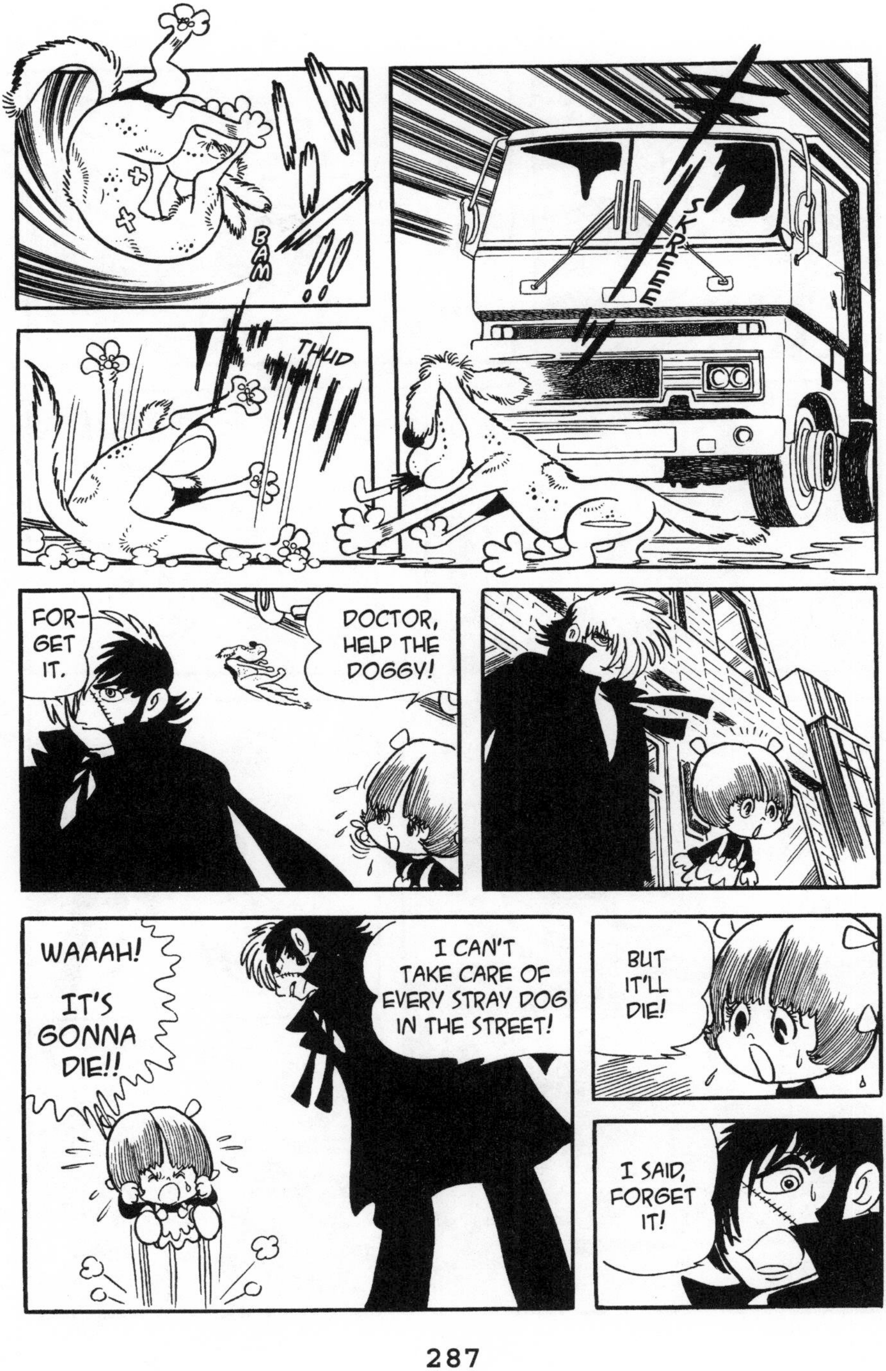
SKREEEE
BAM
THUD
DOCTOR, HELP THE DOGGY!
FOR-GET IT.
BUT IT'LL DIE!
I SAID, FORGET IT!
I CAN'T TAKE CARE OF EVERY STRAY DOG IN THE STREET!
WAAAH!
IT'S GONNA DIE!!

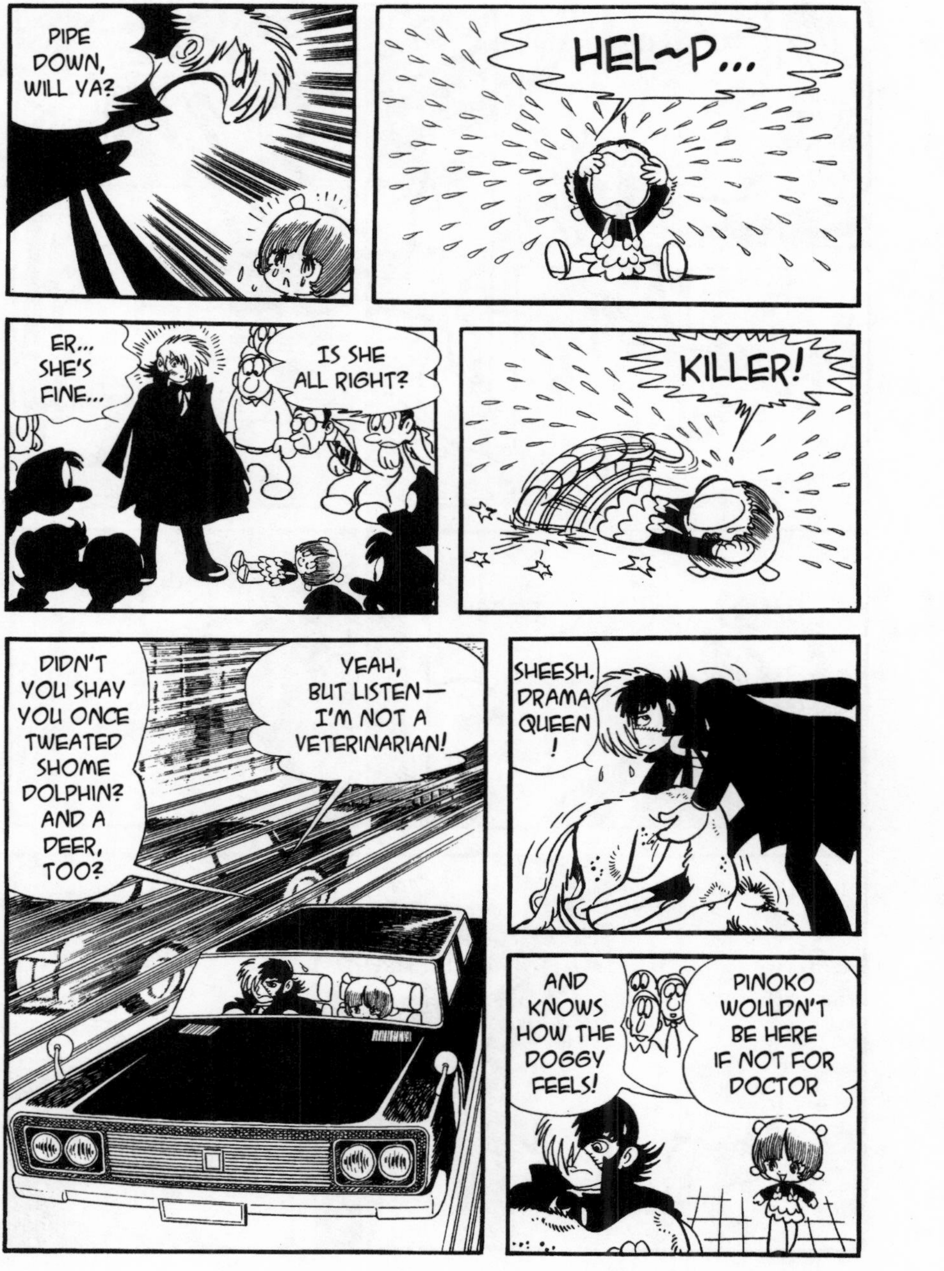
HEL~P...
PIPE DOWN, WILL YA?
KILLER!
IS SHE ALL RIGHT?
ER... SHE'S FINE...
SHEESH. DRAMA QUEEN!
PINOKO WOULDN'T BE HERE IF NOT FOR DOCTOR
AND KNOWS HOW THE DOGGY FEELS!
DIDN'T YOU SHAY YOU ONCE TWEATED SHOME DOLPHIN? AND A DEER, TOO?
YEAH, BUT LISTEN— I'M NOT A VETERINARIAN!

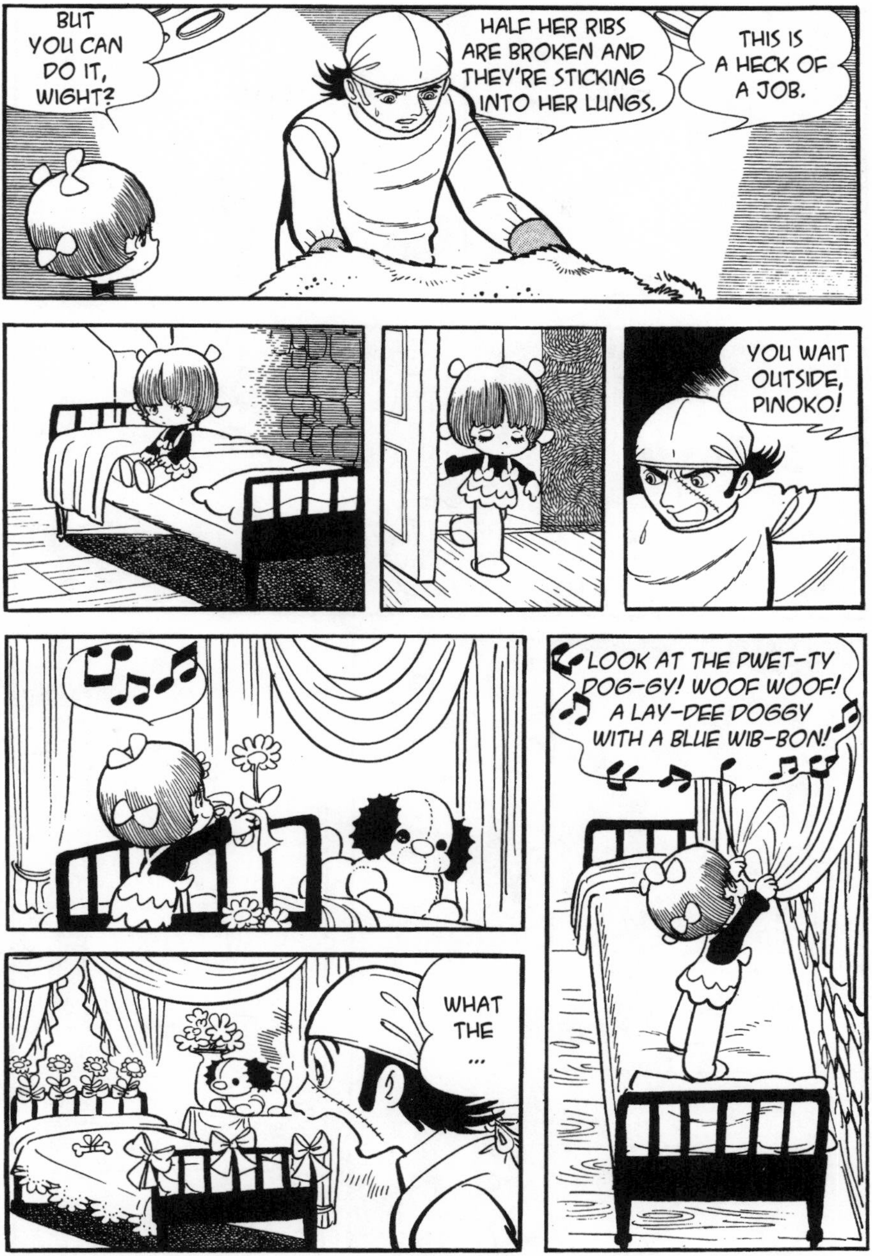
THIS IS A HECK OF A JOB.
HALF HER RIBS ARE BROKEN AND THEY'RE STICKING INTO HER LUNGS.
BUT YOU CAN DO IT, WIGHT?
YOU WAIT OUTSIDE, PINOKO!
LOOK AT THE PWET-TY DOG-GY! WOOF WOOF! A LAY-DEE DOGGY WITH A BLUE WIB-BON!
WHAT THE ...

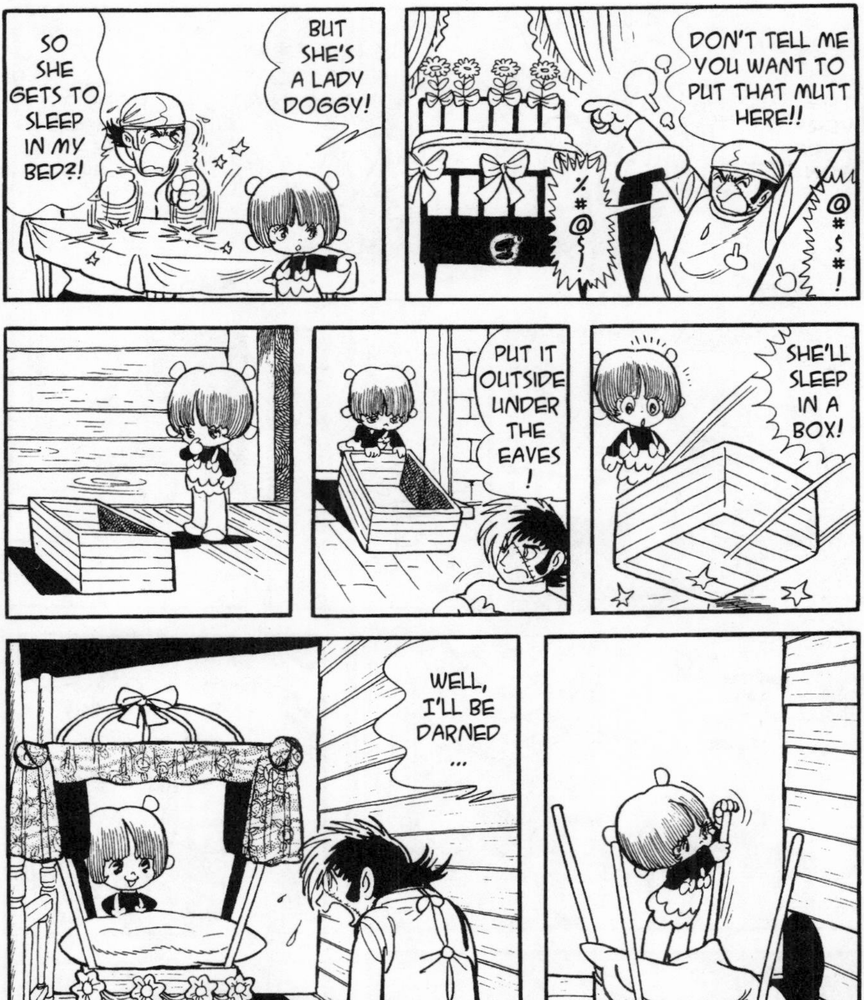
DON'T TELL ME YOU WANT TO PUT THAT MUTT HERE!!
@#$#!
%#@~!
BUT SHE'S A LADY DOGGY!
SO SHE GETS TO SLEEP IN MY BED?!
SHE'LL SLEEP IN A BOX!
PUT IT OUTSIDE UNDER THE EAVES!
WELL, I'LL BE DARNED...

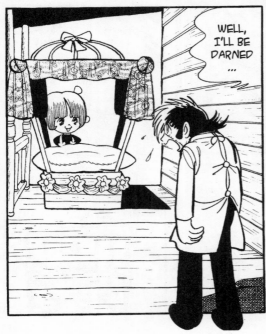

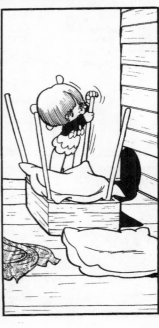

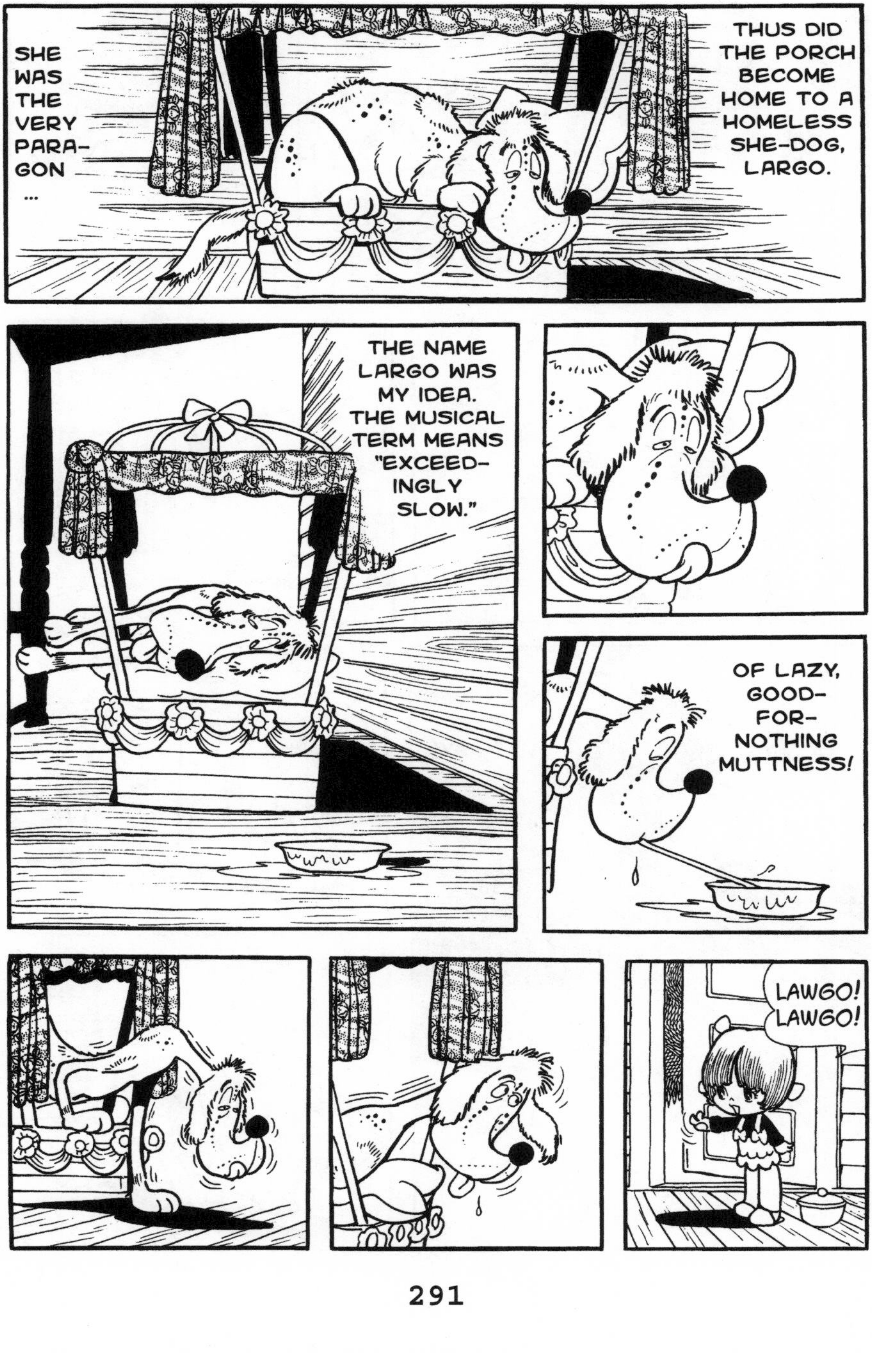
THUS DID THE PORCH BECOME HOME TO A HOMELESS SHE-DOG, LARGO.
SHE WAS THE VERY PARA-GON ...
OF LAZY, GOOD-FOR-NOTHING MUTTNESS!
THE NAME LARGO WAS MY IDEA. THE MUSICAL TERM MEANS "EXCEED-INGLY SLOW."
LAWGO! LAWGO!

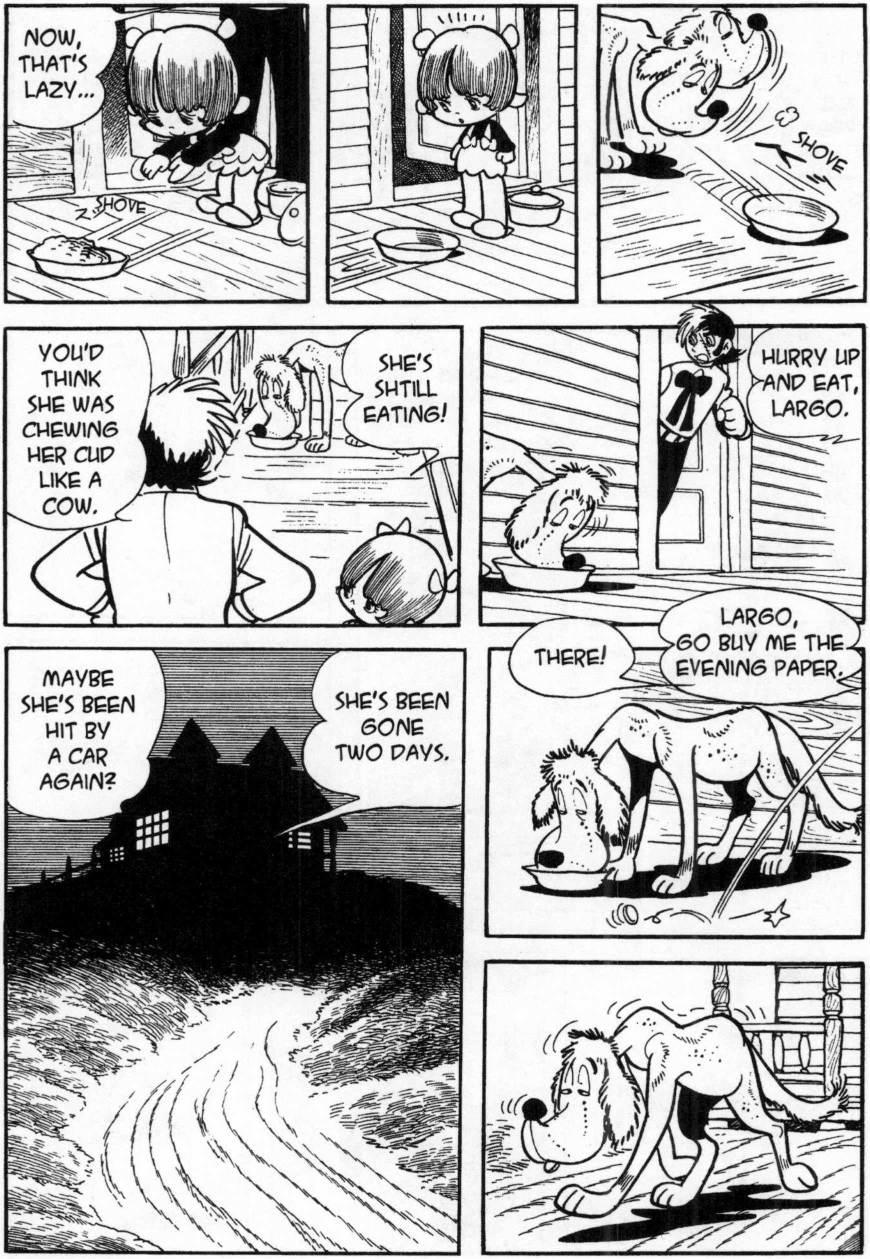
SHOVE
NOW, THAT'S LAZY...
SHOVE
HURRY UP AND EAT, LARGO.
SHE'S SHTILL EATING!
YOU'D THINK SHE WAS CHEWING HER CUD LIKE A COW.
LARGO, GO BUY ME THE EVENING PAPER.
THERE!
SHE'S BEEN GONE TWO DAYS.
MAYBE SHE'S BEEN HIT BY A CAR AGAIN?

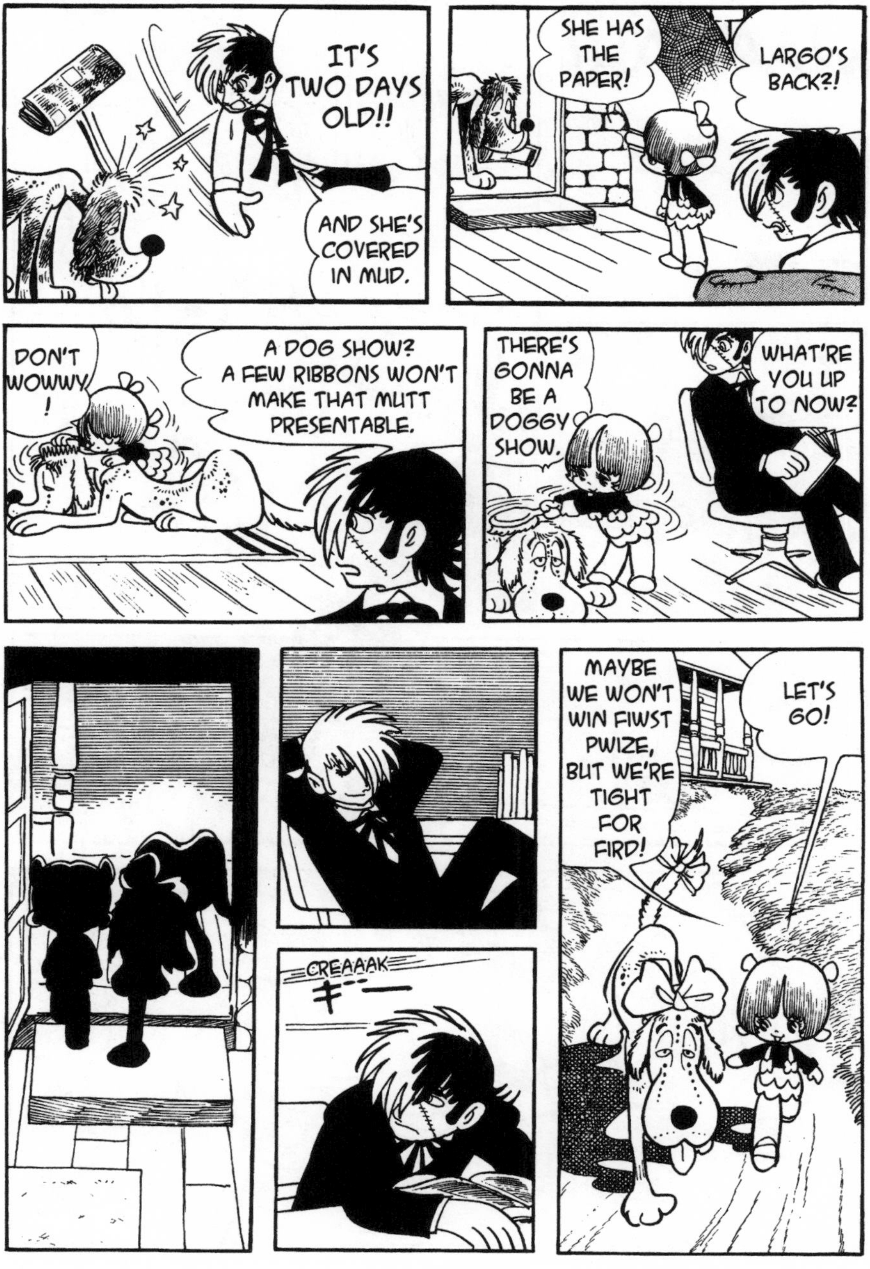
LARGO'S BACK?!
SHE HAS THE PAPER!
IT'S TWO DAYS OLD!!
AND SHE'S COVERED IN MUD.
WHAT'RE YOU UP TO NOW?
THERE'S GONNA BE A DOGGY SHOW.
A DOG SHOW? A FEW RIBBONS WON'T MAKE THAT MUTT PRESENTABLE.
DON'T WOWWY!
LET'S GO!
MAYBE WE WON'T WIN FIWST PWIZE, BUT WE'RE TIGHT FOR FIRD!
CREAAAK
キー

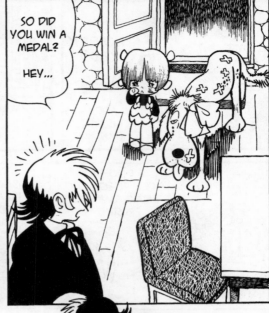

SO DID YOU WIN A MEDAL?
HEY...
WAAAAH!
STOP CRYING AND TELL ME WHAT HAPPENED.
WHAT? LARGO STOLE A JEWEL AT THE CONTEST?
SHE GWABBED A NECKLESH FWOM A LADY JUDGE...

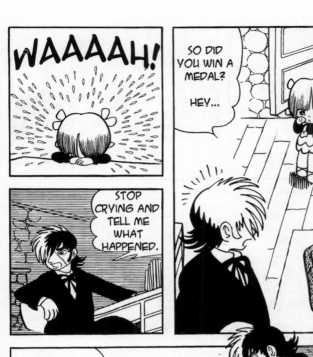

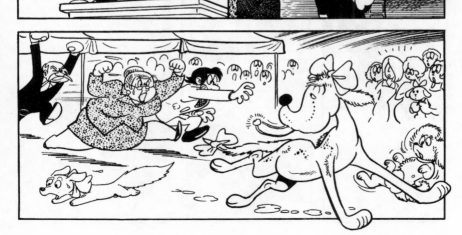

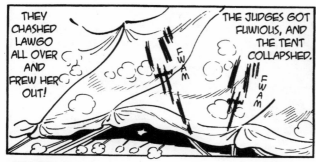

THEN WHAT?
THE JUDGES GOT FUWIOUS, AND THE TENT COLLAPSHED.
FWAM
FWAM
THEY CHASHED LAWGO ALL OVER AND FREW HER OUT!
YOU MISERABLE, ROTTEN MONGREL!
BUT WE'D HAVE WON, WIGHT?
OH YEAH, SURE!
THEN GIVE US A PWIZE INSHTEAD.
FIRD PWIZE IS OKAY!
WHY DO I HAVE TO GIVE OUT A PRIZE?
POOR LAWGO! IT ISN'T FAAAIR!
AWARDING LARGO THIRD PRIZE!
GIMME A BREAK ...
GOOD JOB, LAWGO!

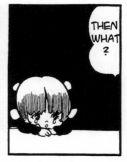

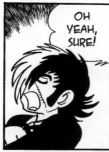

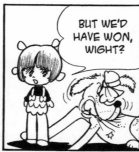

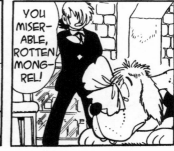

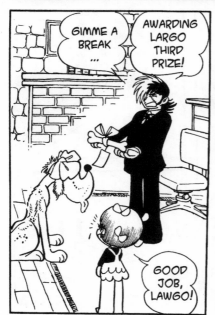

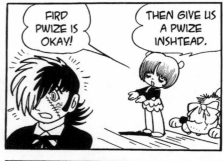

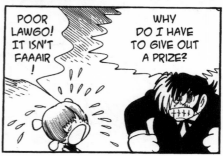

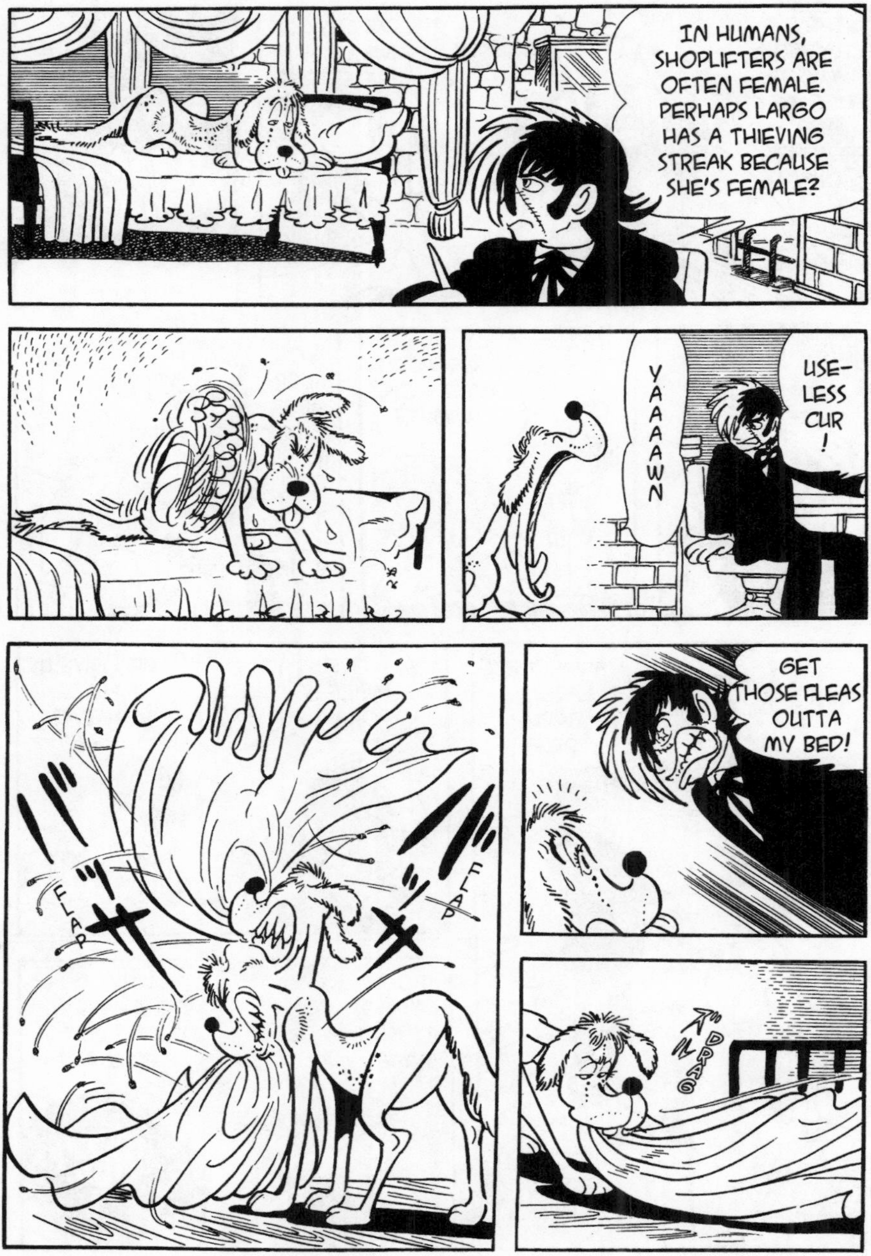
IN HUMANS, SHOPLIFTERS ARE OFTEN FEMALE. PERHAPS LARGO HAS A THIEVING STREAK BECAUSE SHE'S FEMALE?
USE-LESS CUR!
YAAAAAWN
GET THOSE FLEAS OUTTA MY BED!
DRAG
FLAP
FLAP

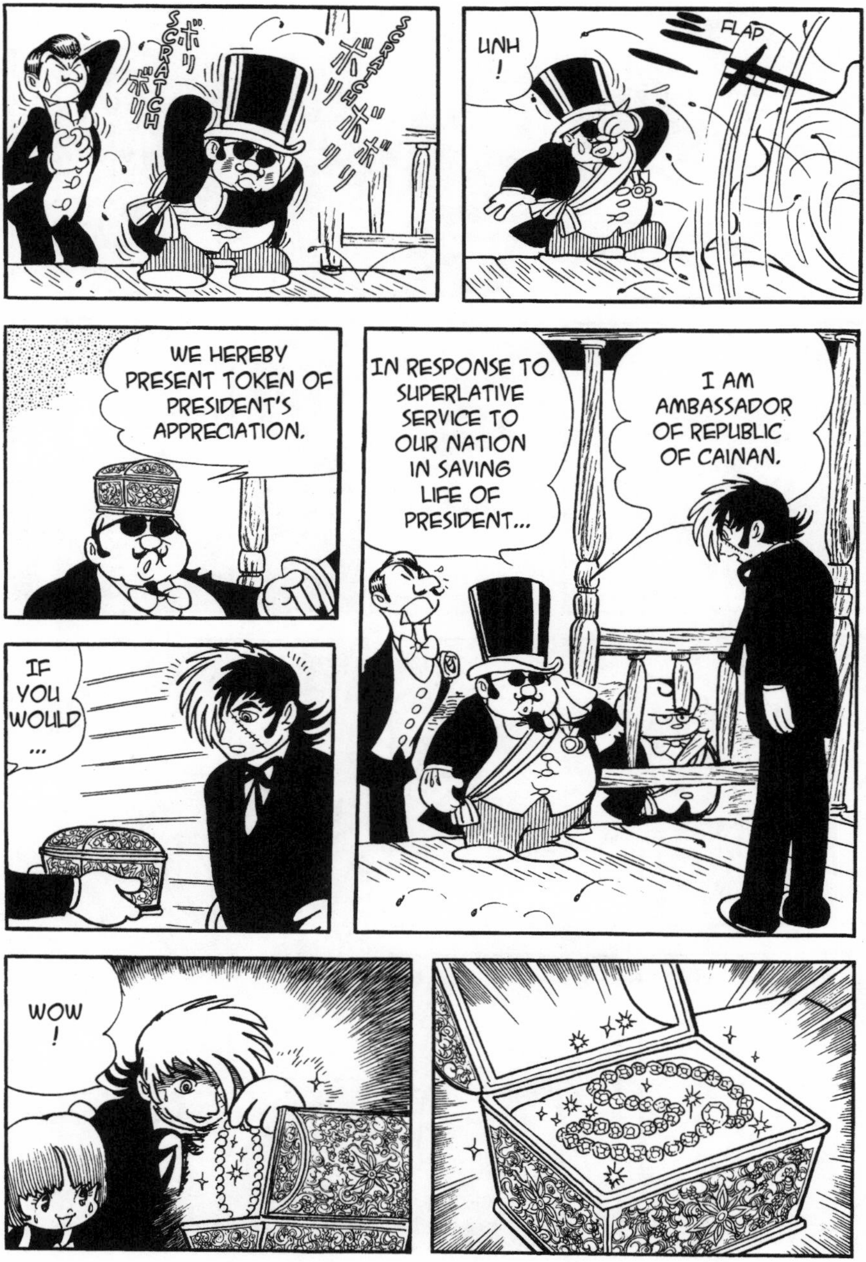
UNH!
FLAP
SCRATCH
ボリボリボリ
SCRATCH
ボリボリ
I AM AMBASSADOR OF REPUBLIC OF CAINAN.
IN RESPONSE TO SUPERLATIVE SERVICE TO OUR NATION IN SAVING LIFE OF PRESIDENT...
WE HEREBY PRESENT TOKEN OF PRESIDENT'S APPRECIATION.
IF YOU WOULD ...
WOW!

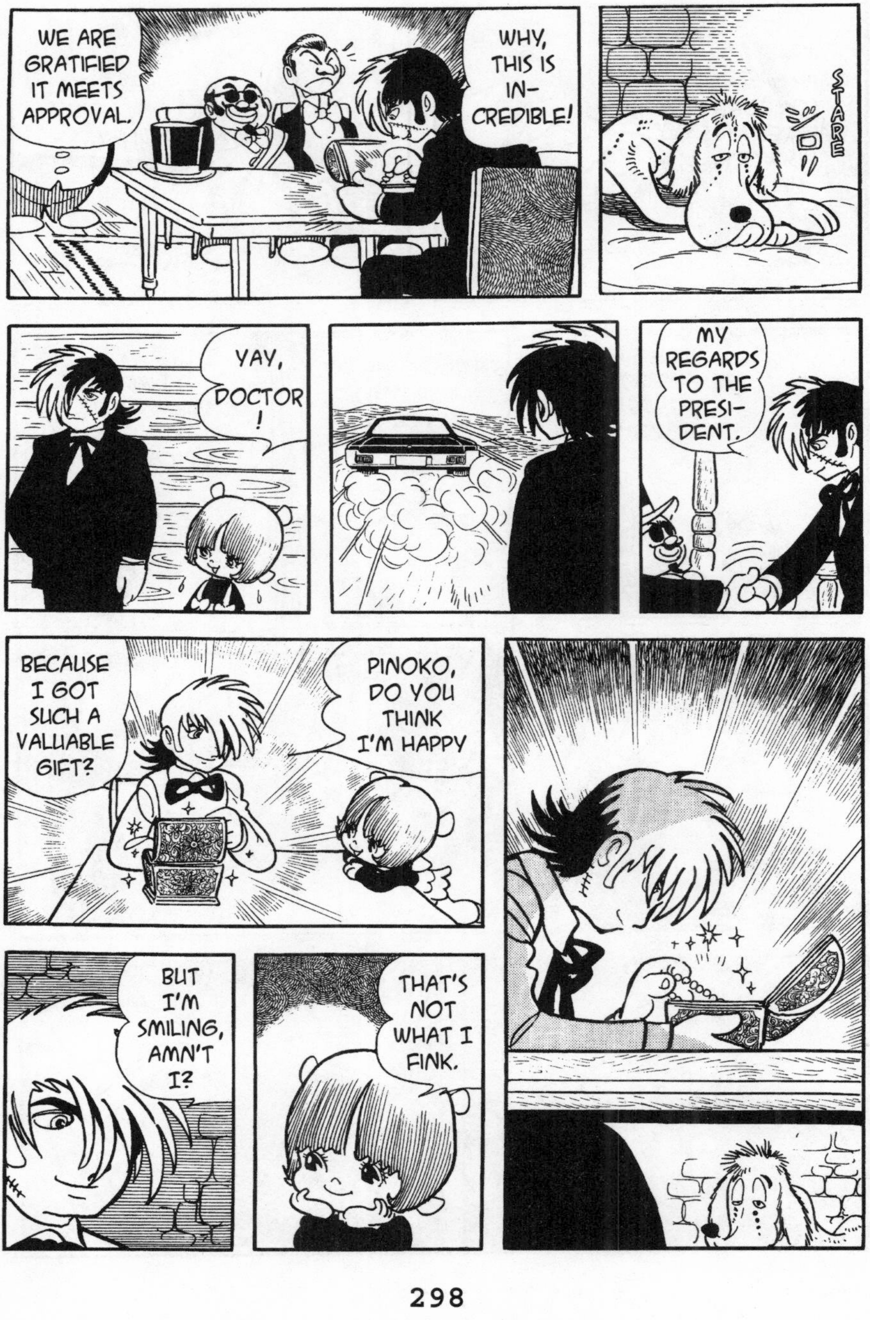
STARE
WHY, THIS IS IN-CREDIBLE!
WE ARE GRATIFIED IT MEETS APPROVAL.
MY REGARDS TO THE PRESI-DENT.
YAY, DOCTOR!
PINOKO, DO YOU THINK I'M HAPPY
BECAUSE I GOT SUCH A VALUABLE GIFT?
THAT'S NOT WHAT I FINK.
BUT I'M SMILING, AMN'T I?

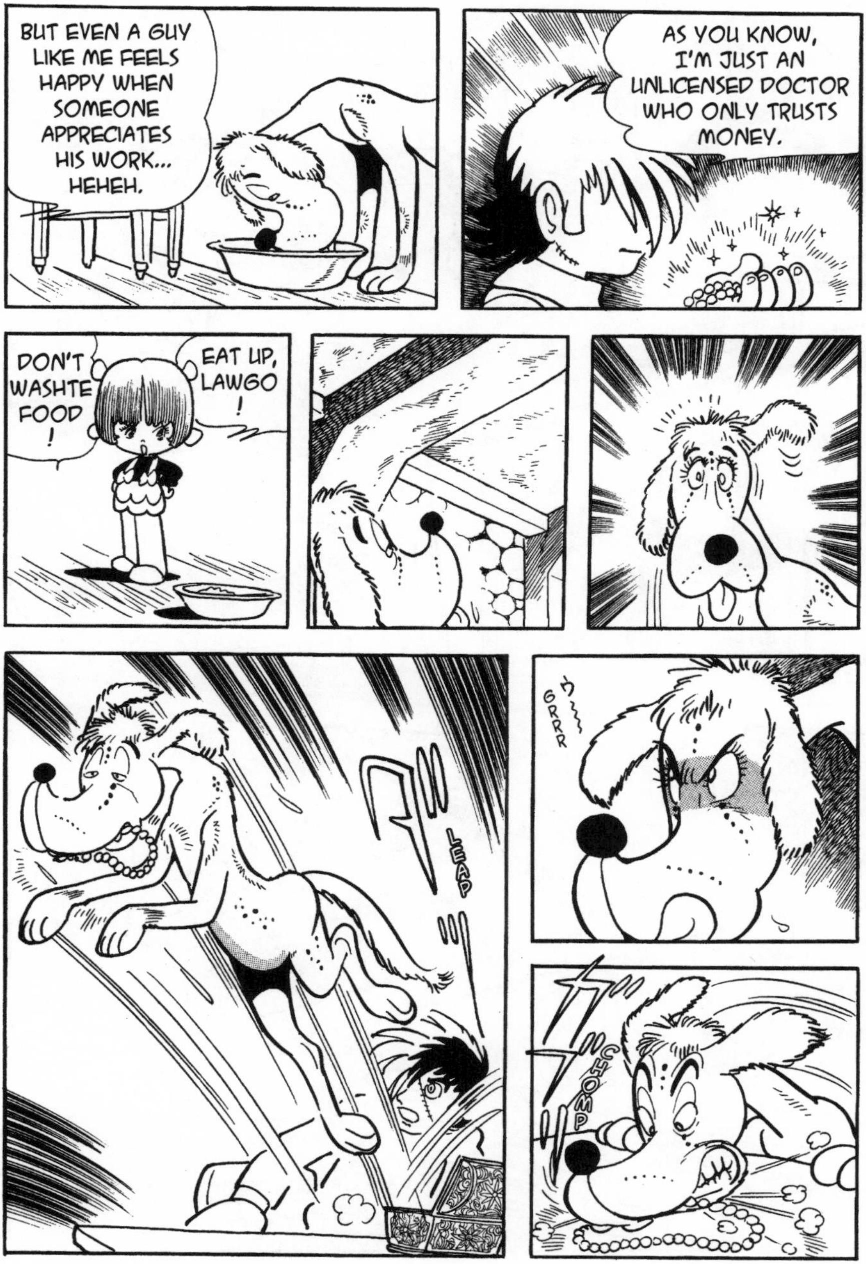
AS YOU KNOW, I'M JUST AN UNLICENSED DOCTOR WHO ONLY TRUSTS MONEY.
BUT EVEN A GUY LIKE ME FEELS HAPPY WHEN SOMEONE APPRECIATES HIS WORK... HEHEH.
EAT UP, LAWGO!
DON'T WASHTE FOOD!
GRRR
CHOMP
LEAP

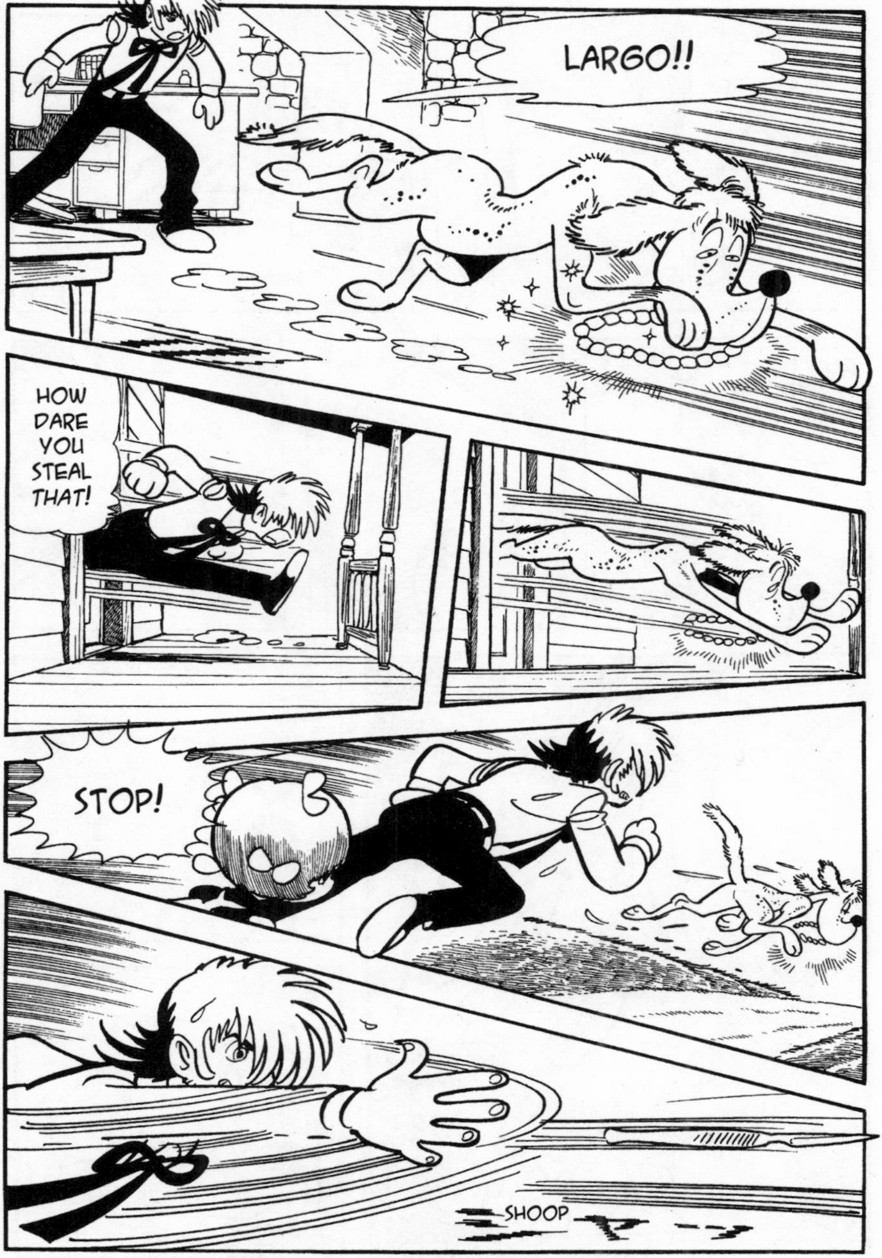
LARGO!!
HOW DARE YOU STEAL THAT!
STOP!
SHOOP

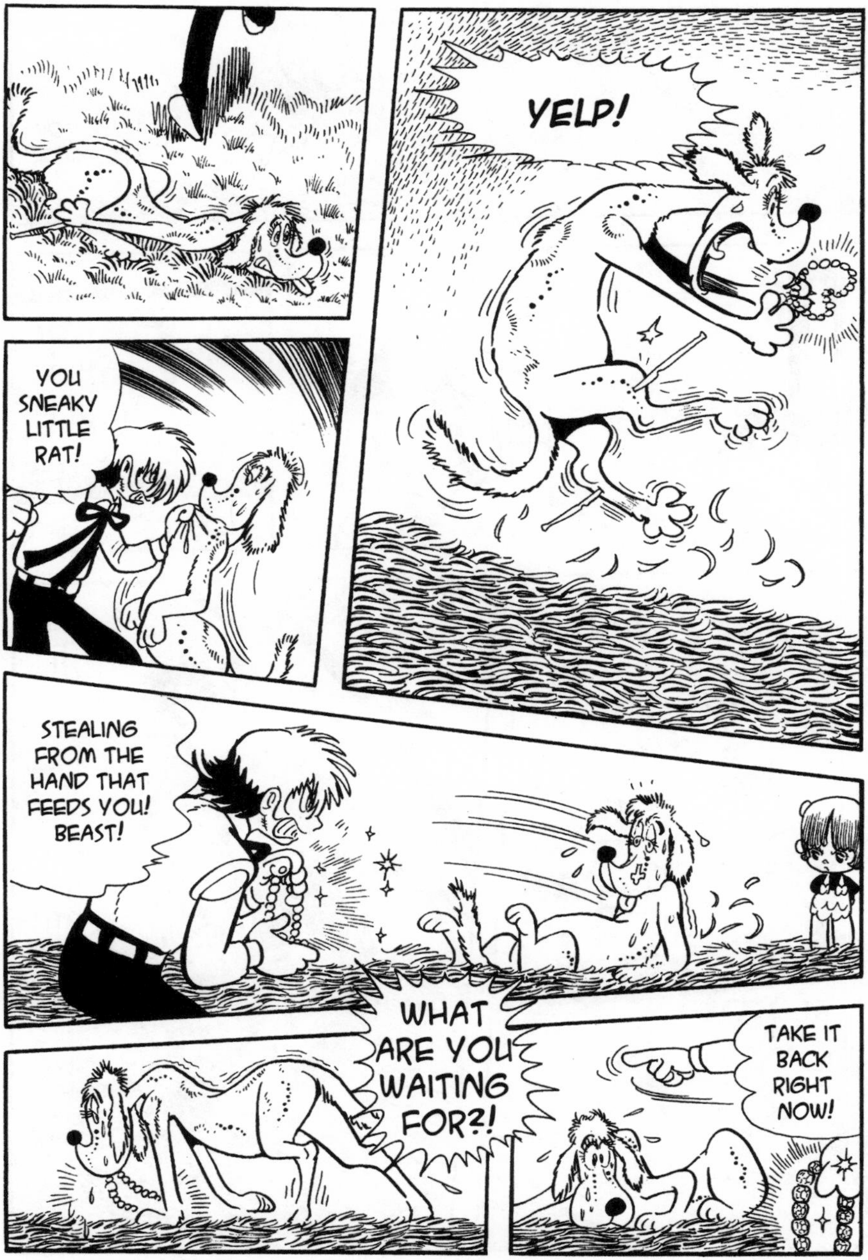
YELP!
YOU SNEAKY LITTLE RAT!
STEALING FROM THE HAND THAT FEEDS YOU! BEAST!
TAKE IT BACK RIGHT NOW!
WHAT ARE YOU WAITING FOR?!

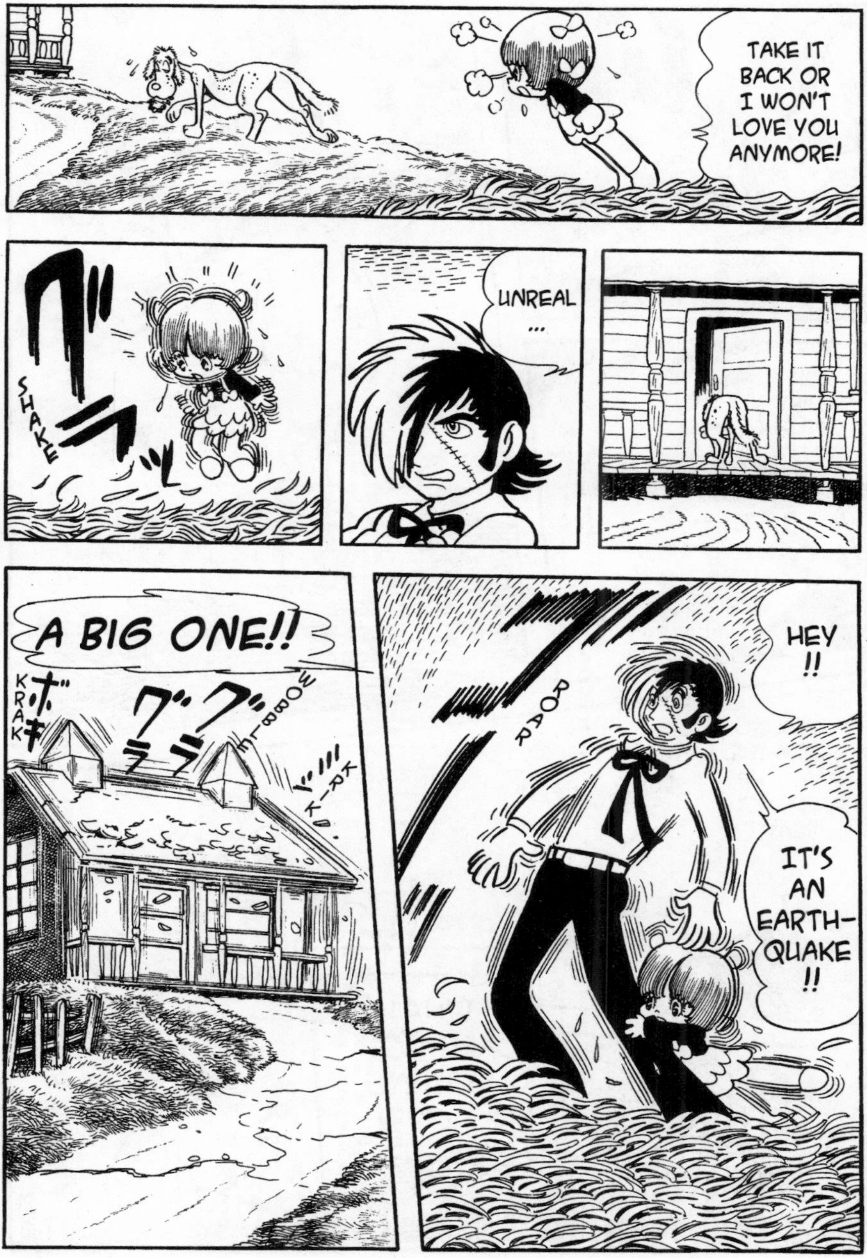
TAKE IT BACK OR I WON'T LOVE YOU ANYMORE!
UNREAL ...
SHAKE
HEY !!
ROAR
IT'S AN EARTH-QUAKE !!
A BIG ONE!!
KRAK
ボキ
グラグラ
WOBBLE
K-RRK

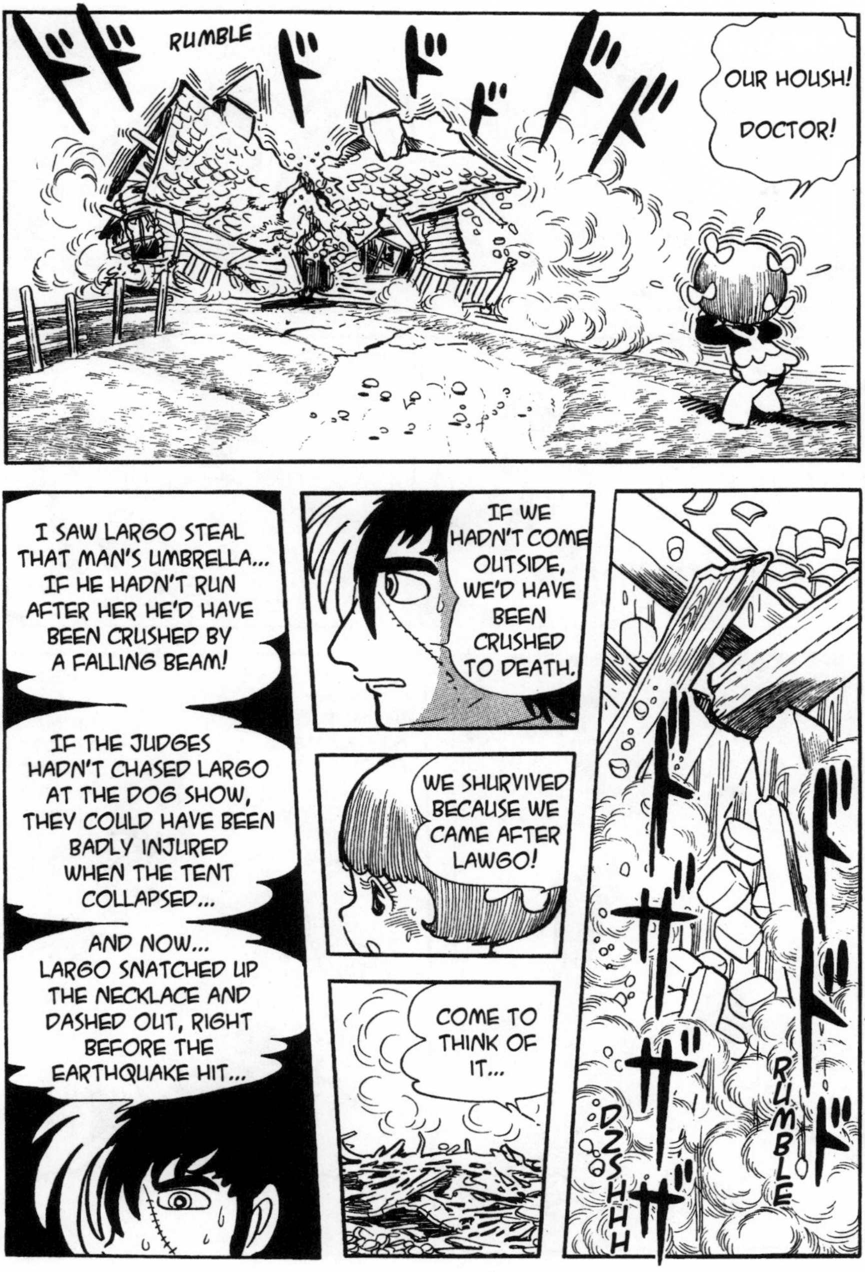
RUMBLE
OUR HOUSH! DOCTOR!
RUMBLE
DZSHHH
IF WE HADN'T COME OUTSIDE, WE'D HAVE BEEN CRUSHED TO DEATH.
WE SHURVIVED BECAUSE WE CAME AFTER LAWGO!
COME TO THINK OF IT...
I SAW LARGO STEAL THAT MAN'S UMBRELLA... IF HE HADN'T RUN AFTER HER HE'D HAVE BEEN CRUSHED BY A FALLING BEAM!
IF THE JUDGES HADN'T CHASED LARGO AT THE DOG SHOW, THEY COULD HAVE BEEN BADLY INJURED WHEN THE TENT COLLAPSED...
AND NOW... LARGO SNATCHED UP THE NECKLACE AND DASHED OUT, RIGHT BEFORE THE EARTHQUAKE HIT...

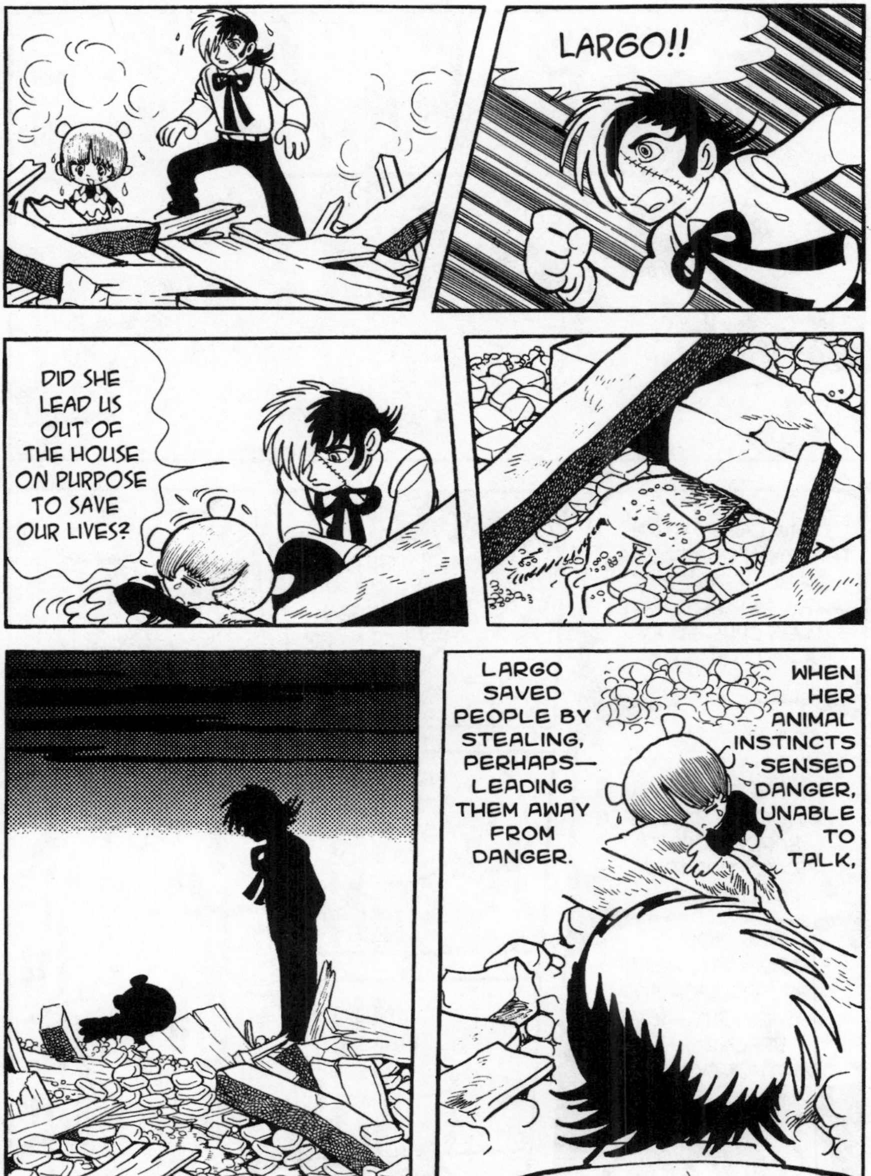
LARGO!!
DID SHE LEAD US OUT OF THE HOUSE ON PURPOSE TO SAVE OUR LIVES?
WHEN HER ANIMAL INSTINCTS SENSED DANGER, UNABLE TO TALK,
LARGO SAVED PEOPLE BY STEALING, PERHAPS— LEADING THEM AWAY FROM DANGER.